FREE Study Skills Videos/DVD Offer

Dear Customer,

Thank you for your purchase from Mometrix! We consider it an honor and a privilege that you have purchased our product and we want to ensure your satisfaction.

As a way of showing our appreciation and to help us better serve you, we have developed Study Skills Videos that we would like to give you for FREE. These videos cover our *best practices* for getting ready for your exam, from how to use our study materials to how to best prepare for the day of the test.

All that we ask is that you email us with feedback that would describe your experience so far with our product. Good, bad, or indifferent, we want to know what you think!

To get your FREE Study Skills Videos, you can use the **QR code** below, or send us an **email** at studyvideos@mometrix.com with *FREE VIDEOS* in the subject line and the following information in the body of the email:

- The name of the product you purchased.
- Your product rating on a scale of 1-5, with 5 being the highest rating.
- Your feedback. It can be long, short, or anything in between. We just want to know your impressions and experience so far with our product. (Good feedback might include how our study material met your needs and ways we might be able to make it even better. You could highlight features that you found helpful or features that you think we should add.)

If you have any questions or concerns, please don't hesitate to contact me directly.

Thanks again!

Sincerely,

Jay Willis
Vice President
jay.willis@mometrix.com
1-800-673-8175

SCAN HERE

Mometrix
TEST PREPARATION

NCLEX PN 2021 and 2022 Exam Secrets Study Guide

LPN NCLEX Review Book

3 Full-Length Practice Tests

Step-by-Step Prep

Video Tutorials

Includes Detailed Answer Explanations

Written and edited by Mometrix Test Prep

Printed in the United States of America

This paper meets the requirements of ANSI/NISO Z39.48-1992 (Permanence of Paper).

Paperback
ISBN 13: 978-1-5167-1840-5
ISBN 10: 1-5167-1840-2

Dear Future Exam Success Story

First of all, **THANK YOU** for purchasing Mometrix study materials!

Second, congratulations! You are one of the few determined test-takers who are committed to doing whatever it takes to excel on your exam. **You have come to the right place.** We developed these study materials with one goal in mind: to deliver you the information you need in a format that's concise and easy to use.

In addition to optimizing your guide for the content of the test, we've outlined our recommended steps for breaking down the preparation process into small, attainable goals so you can make sure you stay on track.

We've also analyzed the entire test-taking process, identifying the most common pitfalls and showing how you can overcome them and be ready for any curveball the test throws you.

Standardized testing is one of the biggest obstacles on your road to success, which only increases the importance of doing well in the high-pressure, high-stakes environment of test day. Your results on this test could have a significant impact on your future, and this guide provides the information and practical advice to help you achieve your full potential on test day.

Your success is our success

We would love to hear from you! If you would like to share the story of your exam success or if you have any questions or comments in regard to our products, please contact us at **800-673-8175** or **support@mometrix.com**.

Thanks again for your business and we wish you continued success!

Sincerely,
The Mometrix Test Preparation Team

TABLE OF CONTENTS

Introduction

Thank you for purchasing this resource! You have made the choice to prepare yourself for a test that could have a huge impact on your future, and this guide is designed to help you be fully ready for test day. Obviously, it's important to have a solid understanding of the test material, but you also need to be prepared for the unique environment and stressors of the test, so that you can perform to the best of your abilities.

For this purpose, the first section that appears in this guide is the **Secret Keys**. We've devoted countless hours to meticulously researching what works and what doesn't, and we've boiled down our findings to the five most impactful steps you can take to improve your performance on the test. We start at the beginning with study planning and move through the preparation process, all the way to the testing strategies that will help you get the most out of what you know when you're finally sitting in front of the test.

We recommend that you start preparing for your test as far in advance as possible. However, if you've bought this guide as a last-minute study resource and only have a few days before your test, we recommend that you skip over the first two Secret Keys since they address a long-term study plan.

If you struggle with **test anxiety**, we strongly encourage you to check out our recommendations for how you can overcome it. Test anxiety is a formidable foe, but it can be beaten, and we want to make sure you have the tools you need to defeat it.

Secret Key #1 – Plan Big, Study Small

There's a lot riding on your performance. If you want to ace this test, you're going to need to keep your skills sharp and the material fresh in your mind. You need a plan that lets you review everything you need to know while still fitting in your schedule. We'll break this strategy down into three categories.

Information Organization

Start with the information you already have: the official test outline. From this, you can make a complete list of all the concepts you need to cover before the test. Organize these concepts into groups that can be studied together, and create a list of any related vocabulary you need to learn so you can brush up on any difficult terms. You'll want to keep this vocabulary list handy once you actually start studying since you may need to add to it along the way.

Time Management

Once you have your set of study concepts, decide how to spread them out over the time you have left before the test. Break your study plan into small, clear goals so you have a manageable task for each day and know exactly what you're doing. Then just focus on one small step at a time. When you manage your time this way, you don't need to spend hours at a time studying. Studying a small block of content for a short period each day helps you retain information better and avoid stressing over how much you have left to do. You can relax knowing that you have a plan to cover everything in time. In order for this strategy to be effective though, you have to start studying early and stick to your schedule. Avoid the exhaustion and futility that comes from last-minute cramming!

Study Environment

The environment you study in has a big impact on your learning. Studying in a coffee shop, while probably more enjoyable, is not likely to be as fruitful as studying in a quiet room. It's important to keep distractions to a minimum. You're only planning to study for a short block of time, so make the most of it. Don't pause to check your phone or get up to find a snack. It's also important to **avoid multitasking**. Research has consistently shown that multitasking will make your studying dramatically less effective. Your study area should also be comfortable and well-lit so you don't have the distraction of straining your eyes or sitting on an uncomfortable chair.

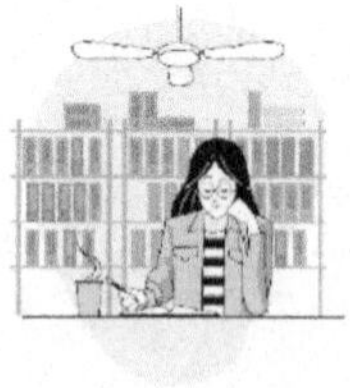

The time of day you study is also important. You want to be rested and alert. Don't wait until just before bedtime. Study when you'll be most likely to comprehend and remember. Even better, if you know what time of day your test will be, set that time aside for study. That way your brain will be used to working on that subject at that specific time and you'll have a better chance of recalling information.

Finally, it can be helpful to team up with others who are studying for the same test. Your actual studying should be done in as isolated an environment as possible, but the work of organizing the information and setting up the study plan can be divided up. In between study sessions, you can discuss with your teammates the concepts that you're all studying and quiz each other on the details. Just be sure that your teammates are as serious about the test as you are. If you find that your study time is being replaced with social time, you might need to find a new team.

Secret Key #2 – Make Your Studying Count

You're devoting a lot of time and effort to preparing for this test, so you want to be absolutely certain it will pay off. This means doing more than just reading the content and hoping you can remember it on test day. It's important to make every minute of study count. There are two main areas you can focus on to make your studying count.

Retention

It doesn't matter how much time you study if you can't remember the material. You need to make sure you are retaining the concepts. To check your retention of the information you're learning, try recalling it at later times with minimal prompting. Try carrying around flashcards and glance at one or two from time to time or ask a friend who's also studying for the test to quiz you.

To enhance your retention, look for ways to put the information into practice so that you can apply it rather than simply recalling it. If you're using the information in practical ways, it will be much easier to remember. Similarly, it helps to solidify a concept in your mind if you're not only reading it to yourself but also explaining it to someone else. Ask a friend to let you teach them about a concept you're a little shaky on (or speak aloud to an imaginary audience if necessary). As you try to summarize, define, give examples, and answer your friend's questions, you'll understand the concepts better and they will stay with you longer. Finally, step back for a big picture view and ask yourself how each piece of information fits with the whole subject. When you link the different concepts together and see them working together as a whole, it's easier to remember the individual components.

Finally, practice showing your work on any multi-step problems, even if you're just studying. Writing out each step you take to solve a problem will help solidify the process in your mind, and you'll be more likely to remember it during the test.

Modality

Modality simply refers to the means or method by which you study. Choosing a study modality that fits your own individual learning style is crucial. No two people learn best in exactly the same way, so it's important to know your strengths and use them to your advantage.

For example, if you learn best by visualization, focus on visualizing a concept in your mind and draw an image or a diagram. Try color-coding your notes, illustrating them, or creating symbols that will trigger your mind to recall a learned concept. If you learn best by hearing or discussing information, find a study partner who learns the same way or read aloud to yourself. Think about how to put the information in your own words. Imagine that you are giving a lecture on the topic and record yourself so you can listen to it later.

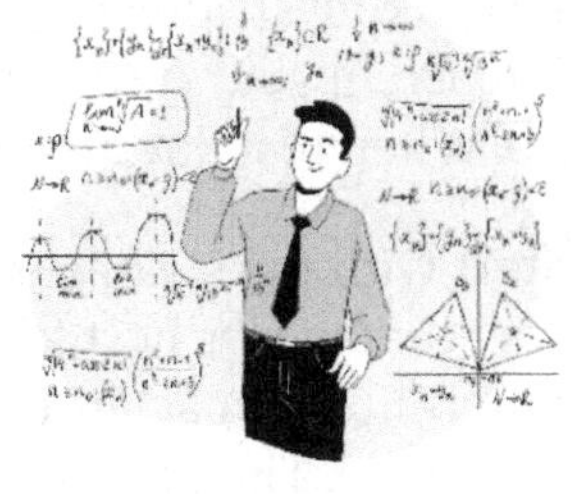

For any learning style, flashcards can be helpful. Organize the information so you can take advantage of spare moments to review. Underline key words or phrases. Use different colors for different categories. Mnemonic devices (such as creating a short list in which every item starts with the same letter) can also help with retention. Find what works best for you and use it to store the information in your mind most effectively and easily.

Secret Key #3 – Practice the Right Way

Your success on test day depends not only on how many hours you put into preparing, but also on whether you prepared the right way. It's good to check along the way to see if your studying is paying off. One of the most effective ways to do this is by taking practice tests to evaluate your progress. Practice tests are useful because they show exactly where you need to improve. Every time you take a practice test, pay special attention to these three groups of questions:

- The questions you got wrong
- The questions you had to guess on, even if you guessed right
- The questions you found difficult or slow to work through

This will show you exactly what your weak areas are, and where you need to devote more study time. Ask yourself why each of these questions gave you trouble. Was it because you didn't understand the material? Was it because you didn't remember the vocabulary? Do you need more repetitions on this type of question to build speed and confidence? Dig into those questions and figure out how you can strengthen your weak areas as you go back to review the material.

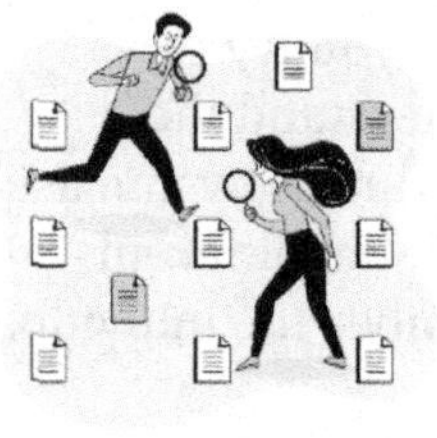

Additionally, many practice tests have a section explaining the answer choices. It can be tempting to read the explanation and think that you now have a good understanding of the concept. However, an explanation likely only covers part of the question's broader context. Even if the explanation makes perfect sense, **go back and investigate** every concept related to the question until you're positive you have a thorough understanding.

As you go along, keep in mind that the practice test is just that: practice. Memorizing these questions and answers will not be very helpful on the actual test because it is unlikely to have any of the same exact questions. If you only know the right answers to the sample questions, you won't be prepared for the real thing. **Study the concepts** until you understand them fully, and then you'll be able to answer any question that shows up on the test.

It's important to wait on the practice tests until you're ready. If you take a test on your first day of study, you may be overwhelmed by the amount of material covered and how much you need to learn. Work up to it gradually.

On test day, you'll need to be prepared for answering questions, managing your time, and using the test-taking strategies you've learned. It's a lot to balance, like a mental marathon that will have a big impact on your future. Like training for a marathon, you'll need to start slowly and work your way up. When test day arrives, you'll be ready.

Start with the strategies you've read in the first two Secret Keys—plan your course and study in the way that works best for you. If you have time, consider using multiple study resources to get different approaches to the same concepts. It can be helpful to see difficult concepts from more than one angle. Then find a good source for practice tests. Many times, the test website will suggest potential study resources or provide sample tests.

Practice Test Strategy

If you're able to find at least three practice tests, we recommend this strategy:

Untimed and Open-Book Practice

Take the first test with no time constraints and with your notes and study guide handy. Take your time and focus on applying the strategies you've learned.

Timed and Open-Book Practice

Take the second practice test open-book as well, but set a timer and practice pacing yourself to finish in time.

Timed and Closed-Book Practice

Take any other practice tests as if it were test day. Set a timer and put away your study materials. Sit at a table or desk in a quiet room, imagine yourself at the testing center, and answer questions as quickly and accurately as possible.

Keep repeating timed and closed-book tests on a regular basis until you run out of practice tests or it's time for the actual test. Your mind will be ready for the schedule and stress of test day, and you'll be able to focus on recalling the material you've learned.

Secret Key #4 – Pace Yourself

Once you're fully prepared for the material on the test, your biggest challenge on test day will be managing your time. Just knowing that the clock is ticking can make you panic even if you have plenty of time left. Work on pacing yourself so you can build confidence against the time constraints of the exam. Pacing is a difficult skill to master, especially in a high-pressure environment, so **practice is vital**.

Set time expectations for your pace based on how much time is available. For example, if a section has 60 questions and the time limit is 30 minutes, you know you have to average 30 seconds or less per question in order to answer them all. Although 30 seconds is the hard limit, set 25 seconds per question as your goal, so you reserve extra time to spend on harder questions. When you budget extra time for the harder questions, you no longer have any reason to stress when those questions take longer to answer.

Don't let this time expectation distract you from working through the test at a calm, steady pace, but keep it in mind so you don't spend too much time on any one question. Recognize that taking extra time on one question you don't understand may keep you from answering two that you do understand later in the test. If your time limit for a question is up and you're still not sure of the answer, mark it and move on, and come back to it later if the time and the test format allow. If the testing format doesn't allow you to return to earlier questions, just make an educated guess; then put it out of your mind and move on.

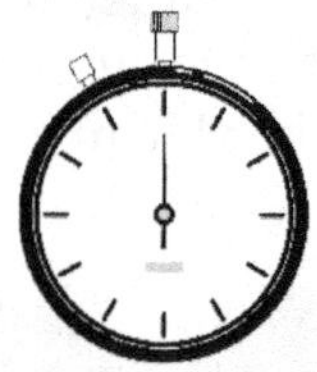

On the easier questions, be careful not to rush. It may seem wise to hurry through them so you have more time for the challenging ones, but it's not worth missing one if you know the concept and just didn't take the time to read the question fully. Work efficiently but make sure you understand the question and have looked at all of the answer choices, since more than one may seem right at first.

Even if you're paying attention to the time, you may find yourself a little behind at some point. You should speed up to get back on track, but do so wisely. Don't panic; just take a few seconds less on each question until you're caught up. Don't guess without thinking, but do look through the answer choices and eliminate any you know are wrong. If you can get down to two choices, it is often worthwhile to guess from those. Once you've chosen an answer, move on and don't dwell on any that you skipped or had to hurry through. If a question was taking too long, chances are it was one of the harder ones, so you weren't as likely to get it right anyway.

On the other hand, if you find yourself getting ahead of schedule, it may be beneficial to slow down a little. The more quickly you work, the more likely you are to make a careless mistake that will affect your score. You've budgeted time for each question, so don't be afraid to spend that time. Practice an efficient but careful pace to get the most out of the time you have.

Secret Key #5 – Have a Plan for Guessing

When you're taking the test, you may find yourself stuck on a question. Some of the answer choices seem better than others, but you don't see the one answer choice that is obviously correct. What do you do?

The scenario described above is very common, yet most test takers have not effectively prepared for it. Developing and practicing a plan for guessing may be one of the single most effective uses of your time as you get ready for the exam.

In developing your plan for guessing, there are three questions to address:

- When should you start the guessing process?
- How should you narrow down the choices?
- Which answer should you choose?

When to Start the Guessing Process

Unless your plan for guessing is to select C every time (which, despite its merits, is not what we recommend), you need to leave yourself enough time to apply your answer elimination strategies. Since you have a limited amount of time for each question, that means that if you're going to give yourself the best shot at guessing correctly, you have to decide quickly whether or not you will guess.

Of course, the best-case scenario is that you don't have to guess at all, so first, see if you can answer the question based on your knowledge of the subject and basic reasoning skills. Focus on the key words in the question and try to jog your memory of related topics. Give yourself a chance to bring the knowledge to mind, but once you realize that you don't have (or you can't access) the knowledge you need to answer the question, it's time to start the guessing process.

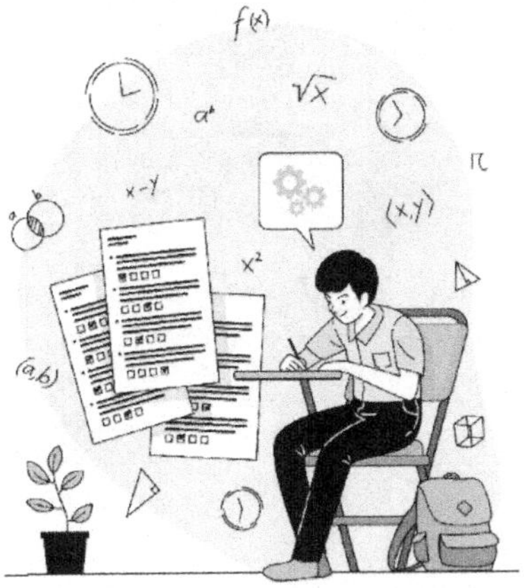

It's almost always better to start the guessing process too early than too late. It only takes a few seconds to remember something and answer the question from knowledge. Carefully eliminating wrong answer choices takes longer. Plus, going through the process of eliminating answer choices can actually help jog your memory.

Summary: Start the guessing process as soon as you decide that you can't answer the question based on your knowledge.

How to Narrow Down the Choices

The next chapter in this book (**Test-Taking Strategies**) includes a wide range of strategies for how to approach questions and how to look for answer choices to eliminate. You will definitely want to read those carefully, practice them, and figure out which ones work best for you. Here though, we're going to address a mindset rather than a particular strategy.

Your odds of guessing an answer correctly depend on how many options you are choosing from.

Number of options left	5	4	3	2	1
Odds of guessing correctly	20%	25%	33%	50%	100%

You can see from this chart just how valuable it is to be able to eliminate incorrect answers and make an educated guess, but there are two things that many test takers do that cause them to miss out on the benefits of guessing:

- Accidentally eliminating the correct answer
- Selecting an answer based on an impression

We'll look at the first one here, and the second one in the next section.

To avoid accidentally eliminating the correct answer, we recommend a thought exercise called **the $5 challenge**. In this challenge, you only eliminate an answer choice from contention if you are willing to bet $5 on it being wrong. Why $5? Five dollars is a small but not insignificant amount of money. It's an amount you could afford to lose but wouldn't want to throw away. And while losing $5 once might not hurt too much, doing it twenty times will set you back $100. In the same way, each small decision you make—eliminating a choice here, guessing on a question there—won't by itself impact your score very much, but when you put them all together, they can make a big difference. By holding each answer choice elimination decision to a higher standard, you can reduce the risk of accidentally eliminating the correct answer.

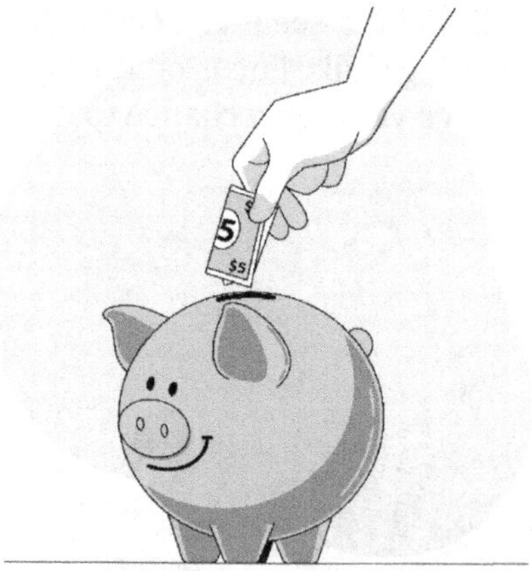

The $5 challenge can also be applied in a positive sense: If you are willing to bet $5 that an answer choice *is* correct, go ahead and mark it as correct.

Summary: Only eliminate an answer choice if you are willing to bet $5 that it is wrong.

Which Answer to Choose

You're taking the test. You've run into a hard question and decided you'll have to guess. You've eliminated all the answer choices you're willing to bet $5 on. Now you have to pick an answer. Why do we even need to talk about this? Why can't you just pick whichever one you feel like when the time comes?

The answer to these questions is that if you don't come into the test with a plan, you'll rely on your impression to select an answer choice, and if you do that, you risk falling into a trap. The test writers know that everyone who takes their test will be guessing on some of the questions, so they intentionally write wrong answer choices to seem plausible. You still have to pick an answer though, and if the wrong answer choices are designed to look right, how can you ever be sure that you're not falling for their trap? The best solution we've found to this dilemma is to take the decision out of your hands entirely. Here is the process we recommend:

Once you've eliminated any choices that you are confident (willing to bet $5) are wrong, select the first remaining choice as your answer.

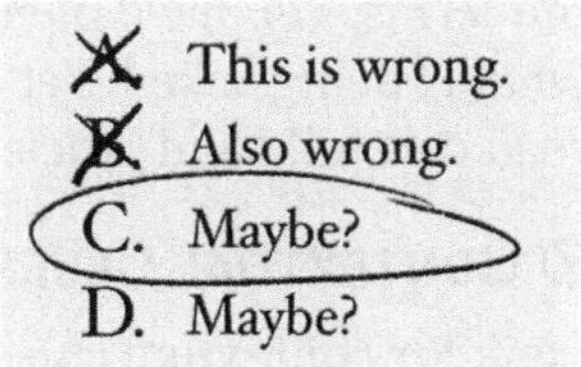

Whether you choose to select the first remaining choice, the second, or the last, the important thing is that you use some preselected standard. Using this approach guarantees that you will not be enticed into selecting an answer choice that looks right, because you are not basing your decision on how the answer choices look.

This is not meant to make you question your knowledge. Instead, it is to help you recognize the difference between your knowledge and your impressions. There's a huge difference between thinking an answer is right because of what you know, and thinking an answer is right because it looks or sounds like it should be right.

Summary: To ensure that your selection is appropriately random, make a predetermined selection from among all answer choices you have not eliminated.

Test-Taking Strategies

This section contains a list of test-taking strategies that you may find helpful as you work through the test. By taking what you know and applying logical thought, you can maximize your chances of answering any question correctly!

It is very important to realize that every question is different and every person is different: no single strategy will work on every question, and no single strategy will work for every person. That's why we've included all of them here, so you can try them out and determine which ones work best for different types of questions and which ones work best for you.

Question Strategies

✓ Read Carefully

Read the question and the answer choices carefully. Don't miss the question because you misread the terms. You have plenty of time to read each question thoroughly and make sure you understand what is being asked. Yet a happy medium must be attained, so don't waste too much time. You must read carefully and efficiently.

✓ Contextual Clues

Look for contextual clues. If the question includes a word you are not familiar with, look at the immediate context for some indication of what the word might mean. Contextual clues can often give you all the information you need to decipher the meaning of an unfamiliar word. Even if you can't determine the meaning, you may be able to narrow down the possibilities enough to make a solid guess at the answer to the question.

✓ Prefixes

If you're having trouble with a word in the question or answer choices, try dissecting it. Take advantage of every clue that the word might include. Prefixes and suffixes can be a huge help. Usually, they allow you to determine a basic meaning. *Pre-* means before, *post-* means after, *pro-* is positive, *de-* is negative. From prefixes and suffixes, you can get an idea of the general meaning of the word and try to put it into context.

✓ Hedge Words

Watch out for critical hedge words, such as *likely, may, can, sometimes, often, almost, mostly, usually, generally, rarely*, and *sometimes*. Question writers insert these hedge phrases to cover every possibility. Often an answer choice will be wrong simply because it leaves no room for exception. Be on guard for answer choices that have definitive words such as *exactly* and *always*.

✓ Switchback Words

Stay alert for *switchbacks*. These are the words and phrases frequently used to alert you to shifts in thought. The most common switchback words are *but, although*, and *however*. Others include *nevertheless, on the other hand, even though, while, in spite of, despite*, and *regardless of*. Switchback words are important to catch because they can change the direction of the question or an answer choice.

☑ FACE VALUE

When in doubt, use common sense. Accept the situation in the problem at face value. Don't read too much into it. These problems will not require you to make wild assumptions. If you have to go beyond creativity and warp time or space in order to have an answer choice fit the question, then you should move on and consider the other answer choices. These are normal problems rooted in reality. The applicable relationship or explanation may not be readily apparent, but it is there for you to figure out. Use your common sense to interpret anything that isn't clear.

Answer Choice Strategies

☑ ANSWER SELECTION

The most thorough way to pick an answer choice is to identify and eliminate wrong answers until only one is left, then confirm it is the correct answer. Sometimes an answer choice may immediately seem right, but be careful. The test writers will usually put more than one reasonable answer choice on each question, so take a second to read all of them and make sure that the other choices are not equally obvious. As long as you have time left, it is better to read every answer choice than to pick the first one that looks right without checking the others.

☑ ANSWER CHOICE FAMILIES

An answer choice family consists of two (in rare cases, three) answer choices that are very similar in construction and cannot all be true at the same time. If you see two answer choices that are direct opposites or parallels, one of them is usually the correct answer. For instance, if one answer choice says that quantity *x* increases and another either says that quantity *x* decreases (opposite) or says that quantity *y* increases (parallel), then those answer choices would fall into the same family. An answer choice that doesn't match the construction of the answer choice family is more likely to be incorrect. Most questions will not have answer choice families, but when they do appear, you should be prepared to recognize them.

☑ ELIMINATE ANSWERS

Eliminate answer choices as soon as you realize they are wrong, but make sure you consider all possibilities. If you are eliminating answer choices and realize that the last one you are left with is also wrong, don't panic. Start over and consider each choice again. There may be something you missed the first time that you will realize on the second pass.

☑ AVOID FACT TRAPS

Don't be distracted by an answer choice that is factually true but doesn't answer the question. You are looking for the choice that answers the question. Stay focused on what the question is asking for so you don't accidentally pick an answer that is true but incorrect. Always go back to the question and make sure the answer choice you've selected actually answers the question and is not merely a true statement.

☑ EXTREME STATEMENTS

In general, you should avoid answers that put forth extreme actions as standard practice or proclaim controversial ideas as established fact. An answer choice that states the "process should be used in certain situations, if..." is much more likely to be correct than one that states the "process should be discontinued completely." The first is a calm rational statement and doesn't even make a definitive, uncompromising stance, using a hedge word *if* to provide wiggle room, whereas the second choice is far more extreme.

✓ Benchmark

As you read through the answer choices and you come across one that seems to answer the question well, mentally select that answer choice. This is not your final answer, but it's the one that will help you evaluate the other answer choices. The one that you selected is your benchmark or standard for judging each of the other answer choices. Every other answer choice must be compared to your benchmark. That choice is correct until proven otherwise by another answer choice beating it. If you find a better answer, then that one becomes your new benchmark. Once you've decided that no other choice answers the question as well as your benchmark, you have your final answer.

✓ Predict the Answer

Before you even start looking at the answer choices, it is often best to try to predict the answer. When you come up with the answer on your own, it is easier to avoid distractions and traps because you will know exactly what to look for. The right answer choice is unlikely to be word-for-word what you came up with, but it should be a close match. Even if you are confident that you have the right answer, you should still take the time to read each option before moving on.

General Strategies

✓ Tough Questions

If you are stumped on a problem or it appears too hard or too difficult, don't waste time. Move on! Remember though, if you can quickly check for obviously incorrect answer choices, your chances of guessing correctly are greatly improved. Before you completely give up, at least try to knock out a couple of possible answers. Eliminate what you can and then guess at the remaining answer choices before moving on.

✓ Check Your Work

Since you will probably not know every term listed and the answer to every question, it is important that you get credit for the ones that you do know. Don't miss any questions through careless mistakes. If at all possible, try to take a second to look back over your answer selection and make sure you've selected the correct answer choice and haven't made a costly careless mistake (such as marking an answer choice that you didn't mean to mark). This quick double check should more than pay for itself in caught mistakes for the time it costs.

✓ Pace Yourself

It's easy to be overwhelmed when you're looking at a page full of questions; your mind is confused and full of random thoughts, and the clock is ticking down faster than you would like. Calm down and maintain the pace that you have set for yourself. Especially as you get down to the last few minutes of the test, don't let the small numbers on the clock make you panic. As long as you are on track by monitoring your pace, you are guaranteed to have time for each question.

✓ Don't Rush

It is very easy to make errors when you are in a hurry. Maintaining a fast pace in answering questions is pointless if it makes you miss questions that you would have gotten right otherwise. Test writers like to include distracting information and wrong answers that seem right. Taking a little extra time to avoid careless mistakes can make all the difference in your test score. Find a pace that allows you to be confident in the answers that you select.

✓ Keep Moving

Panicking will not help you pass the test, so do your best to stay calm and keep moving. Taking deep breaths and going through the answer elimination steps you practiced can help to break through a stress barrier and keep your pace.

Final Notes

The combination of a solid foundation of content knowledge and the confidence that comes from practicing your plan for applying that knowledge is the key to maximizing your performance on test day. As your foundation of content knowledge is built up and strengthened, you'll find that the strategies included in this chapter become more and more effective in helping you quickly sift through the distractions and traps of the test to isolate the correct answer.

Now that you're preparing to move forward into the test content chapters of this book, be sure to keep your goal in mind. As you read, think about how you will be able to apply this information on the test. If you've already seen sample questions for the test and you have an idea of the question format and style, try to come up with questions of your own that you can answer based on what you're reading. This will give you valuable practice applying your knowledge in the same ways you can expect to on test day.

Good luck and good studying!

Coordinated Care

Client Rights, Client Advocacy, and Delegation of Care

Advance Directive

An **advance directive** is a legal list of the wishes a patient may have regarding the level and type of health care they want provided in a specific situation. Typical advance directives include code status, (limited treatment measures and Do-Not-Resuscitate [DNR] orders), most often stating the client's wishes regarding end-of-life issues, including feeding decisions and life support. In order to be legally binding, the document is witnessed, and clearly states the wishes of the client regarding health care–related situations. The directive must be drawn up when the patient is of sound mind and mentally and emotionally capable of making these types of decisions. It is encouraged for every patient to have some sort of advance directive, regardless of age or health. On admission to an acute care facility, every patient should be asked and offered the opportunity to execute advance directives, and a copy placed on the patient's record. The nurse has some responsibilities when it comes to helping patients with advance directives. First, the nurse helps the patient obtain copies of advance directives, ensuring the forms are filled out correctly. The nurse educates the patient and their family about keeping papers in a safe place and submitting copies to the physician, attorney, and others who may need them. The nurse ensures that copies of all documents are in the chart, and that they are copied and sent if the patient is transferred.

End-of-Life Care Decisions

In accordance to Federal and state laws, individuals have the right to self-determination in health care, including decisions about end of life care through advanced directives such as living wills and the right to assign a surrogate person (healthcare proxy) to make decisions through a **durable power of attorney (POA)**. A durable power of attorney allows the designated person to make all legal decisions for a client, including decisions about health care, even if the client remains competent. A **living will** provide instructions to medical staff regarding end-of-life care and may include provisions regarding organ donation. An advance directive may include a living will, and DNR, and designation of a healthcare proxy. A **healthcare proxy** designates a person to make decisions about healthcare and DNR if the client becomes incapable of making the decisions. Clients should routinely be questioned about advanced directives as they may present at a healthcare organization without the document. Clients who have indicated they desire a **do-not-resuscitate** (DNR) order should not receive resuscitative treatments for terminal illness or conditions in which meaningful recovery cannot occur. More specifically, a **do-not-intubate** (DNI) order may also be requested by clients who, in the case of respiratory failure, do not want to be intubated.

Advocacy

Advocacy is an ethical concept that means the act or incidence of beseeching for, supporting, urging public argument, recommending publicity, and espousing actively things that promote the health and well-being of individuals and communities. In simpler terms, advocacy is speaking for those who cannot speak for themselves. Nurses are responsible for recognizing situations that might compromise patients' rights, and advocating for their patients. Nurse advocates accept responsibility to safeguard patient rights, and ensure quality of care for the patients they care for. The role of nurse advocate involves informing the patient of their own rights, providing information needed to make informed decisions, and supporting patient decisions and autonomy.

Resources to Use for Client Advocacy

The following can be utilized for **client advocacy**:

- **Social worker**: Can assess the needs of the client and determine if the client is eligible for assistance, such as through Medicaid or SSI, food stamps, or other government or community programs. Social workers also respond to complaints of abuse and carry out observations and investigations.
- **Chain of command**: Leadership comprises the governing body, chief executive officer, nurse executive, and senior managers, department leaders, leaders (both elected and appointed) of staff or departments, and other nurse leaders as well as team members and support staff. The chain of command provides a system by which a client or nurse can appeal for assistance or advice.
- **Interpreter**: Ensures that the client/family are accurately informed and able to communicate needs and wants.

Patient Rights

Patients have certain **rights** when it comes to their medical treatment. A patient's bill of rights is a document that clearly states what rights a patient should be entitled to. Typical rights include:

- **Right to health services** provided with dignity and respect for personal and medical needs; this includes effective pain management and cultural consideration.
- **Right to privacy**: HIPAA, protection of PHI.
- **Right to self-determination**: Patients have the right to make health care decisions, and to receive information regarding their care; this includes informed consent and education on procedures, prognosis, and course of treatment.
- **Right to information**: Patients should know the cost of health care services being provided and receive notification of discharge or if services are to be terminated.
- **Right to refuse treatment**: refuse certain medications, withdraw from a case management program, file a grievance if they feel they have been treated unfairly, and choose a community service agency of their choice.
- **Right to non-discrimination**: All patients should receive appropriate care regardless of race, religion, ethnicity, or economic status. Patients cannot be denied care based on age, sexual orientation, marital status, disability, or ability to pay.

Informed Consent

Informed consent is the patient's voluntary, autonomous authorization to undergo a medical or surgical procedure. Informed consent is intended to facilitate appropriate, knowledgeable decision making among clients who are hospitalized, receiving specialty services, and/or making any type of decision regarding health care. Informed consent must contain the following elements:

- Detailed information on the prognosis.
- Potential benefits and risks of the treatment.
- Information related to alternative treatments.
- Risks of refusing treatment.
- Must be directed toward the education and cognitive level of the client; it is the physician's duty to ensure proper understanding of procedure (may require interpreter for language barrier).
- Signed and acknowledged by both the physician and patient; also includes signature of witness.

**Nursing role in informed consent is NOT to obtain informed consent.* The physician is responsible for obtaining consent. The nurses' duty is to validate the patient's understanding/ that the patient did indeed give informed consent. The nurse usually witnesses informed consent and may educate the client on informed consent.

Exceptions and Barriers

There are several prominent situations **when obtaining informed consent may not be required.** These include:

- **Emergent situations to save life or limb***:* often occurs in trauma patients, when the client is unconscious, and there is no legal representative of the client available to give consent.
- **Disclosures of therapeutic privilege***:* where these privileges would have adverse effects on the client/patient (seen in psychiatric patients mostly).
- **Lack of decision-making capacity***:* patient does not have the capacity to make decisions; this includes patients with dementia, delirium, or other cognitive impairments. Informed consent should be obtained from HCPOA/closest family member.
- **Waived Right***:* Patient may waive his/her right to informed consent.
- **Court Order***:* Physician does not believe the decisions being made are in the best interest of the individual; this will involve a court order to treat against patient/client will.

Client's Right to Refuse Care and Leave AMA

The **Patient Self Determination Act** (1991) provides clients the right to make decisions about end-of-life care through advance directives, to refuse care, and to make informed consent. Autonomy is the ethical principle that the individual has the right to make decisions about his/her own care. Some clients want to be discharged before treatment is complete or simply refuse treatments **against medical advice** (AMA). Before asking the client to sign an AMA form (which should be witnessed), the healthcare provider should ensure that the client has the ability to make decisions and should remain supportive while explaining the need for care and the risks associated with refusing care or leaving the hospital. The client's refusal of care should be carefully documented as well as details about the encounter and the risks associated with the refusal. Any efforts, such as explanations, made to convince the client and encourage followup should be documented as well. The client should be urged to have followup or to return if the client's condition worsens or does not improve.

Delegation

Tasks Delegated to Members of the Healthcare Team

The delegating nurse must be aware of the state laws and regulations regarding ***delegation*** and must understand the responsibility and the risks and benefits of delegation. Generally, an RN cannot delegate tasks to LPNs/LVNs that require the person to teach, assess, plan, or evaluate because these tasks are in the scope of practice of the RN. LPNs/LVNs can delegate duties to other LPNs within their scope responsibilities to which they have adequate knowledge and training. Members of the healthcare team to whom tasks can be delegated include:

- **Other LPNs/LVNs**: May delegate specific tasks and procedures, report observations, gather data (vital signs, wound condition), implement interventions outlined in the care plan (in accordance with scope of practice). State laws vary, so some may be able to give medications, administer IV, and delegate to UAPs but others may not.
- **Assistive personnel (PCTs, CNAs)**: May carry out routine care, such as bathing, linen changes, toileting, and vital signs (for stable clients). May not give medications or carry out invasive procedures. State laws may vary in relation to allowed practice.

5 Rights of Delegation

Practical Nurses (PNs) have the right to ***delegate*** certain tasks to appropriate personnel. Delegation involves handing over the responsibility to complete a task, while maintaining the responsibility for how the task is completed, including the final outcome. It is crucial for the nurse to follow the Five Rights of Delegation to prevent liability if the delegate does not perform the task in an acceptable manner.

- **Right task** – "Is this a task that can be delegated to another person/does it require a higher level of skill?"
- **Right circumstances** – "Is there a circumstance that makes this task require more critical thinking/assessment than normal?"
- **Right person** – "Is this person trained and licensed to complete this task and do I have confidence in them personally to complete it correctly?"
- **Right directions/communication** – "Did I thoroughly explain what was expected and how to perform this task?"
- **Right supervision/evaluation** – "Did I adequately supervise this task/ did I personally follow up to ensure the task was done correctly?"

Case Management

Managed Care and Case Management

Managed care is a broad term referring to an organized delivery of care or services. It involves a select panel of care providers who give out their services based on a prepayment arrangement between the provider and the managed care organization. For instance, a hospital may be the managed care organization, and the physicians who are part of the hospital staff are prepaid for the services they render to patients who seek care from that institution. HMOs and PPOs are examples of those types of managed care services.

Case management is an individual patient care delivery system specific to the patient, their diagnosis, and their individual needs. The main difference is that managed care is the function of the health care reimbursement system, while case management is the structure used to provide individual patient care to affect expected treatments and outcomes.

Well-Organized Case Management Plan

A good **case management plan** must include all of the disciplines that are relevant to the patient's care, and it must be clinically specific to the patient and their condition. The plan must be outcome based, with the best possible outcome for the patient as the goal. The plan must be flexible so that it can be adapted to each individual patient. It must also, however, be standardized for each disease process so that a health care team from any institution could easily implement the plan for a patient with the same condition. An example of this would be a case management plan with community-acquired pneumonia as the disease process. The standard treatments and expected outcomes would be listed in the plan, but the entire plan would be individualized for each patient with pneumonia based on factors such as age, response, health history, and compliance. The plan must also have a financial component emphasizing the most cost-effective way to care for the individual patient.

Increasing Patient Involvement in the Plan of Care

When developing a plan of care, the nurse should keep the patient's individual needs in mind. By specializing the care to the particular patient, the nurse will increase compliance and involvement by the patient. Ways to **involve the patient with the plan of care** include:

- Interviewing the patient personally, along with the family, allows the patient to have input and to verbalize what issues they feel are priority.
- Asking the patient what goals they have and what they expect the outcomes of their care to be can help the nurse to be realistic about the plan of care.
- Including the family and all members of the health care team to ensure that information is complete and accurate.
- Setting goals that the patient feels are achievable will help avoid discouragement.
- Ensuring that all education provided within the plan of care is easily understood/appropriate to the educational level and cultural needs of the patient.

Providing Cost Effective Care

Principles and strategies of providing **cost effective care** include:

- Providing evidence-based client care in order to improve outcomes.
- Assessing and modifying procedures if indicated to increase efficiency.
- Avoiding waste through just-in-time ordering of supplies and dispensing supplies only as needed.
- Educating clients about self-care and self-management.
- Avoiding duplicative care procedures and testing.
- Administering generic drugs rather than brand name.
- Following protocols for administration of antibiotics to reduce resistance.
- Utilizing careful handwashing and infection control procedures to avoid the spread of infection.
- Providing follow up for discharge clients.
- Coordinating care.
- Purchasing in bulk and from fewer vendors.
- Continually reviewing data and using the data to make decisions.
- Focusing programs on those with the greatest need, such as clients with multiple health conditions and multiple hospitalizations.
- Providing preventive programs, such as screenings, family planning, and immunizations.
- Utilizing telehealth and other interventions to provide health services.
- Reducing absenteeism.

Discharge Planning

Discharge planning begins as soon as a patient is admitted to hospital. With hospital stays becoming increasingly shorter, the practical nurse needs to help the patient prepare for discharge as soon as possible to ensure a safe transition into the community. This could include medication management, home safety evaluations, and scheduling/transport to follow-up appointments. It is critical for the nurse to work closely with the case management team, as many different disciplines often need to be consulted, such as physical therapy, social services, etc. The nurse will need to act as a liaison between the patient and different members of the health care team, to ensure a safe and timely discharge. The practical nurse may be directly involved in patient transfer or discharge by assisting in the gathering of belongings and the appropriate method of transport (wheelchair, bed, standby assist). They may also be involved in following up after discharge and communicating any questions or concerns to the appropriate health care team member.

Discharge planning must also include assessment of the client's needs for materials, supplies and equipment. The registered nurse should review those that the client required during hospitalization and determine ongoing needs, such as for oxygen, wound care supplies, or catheters. The practical nurse can assist the registered nurse in this process. Some clients, such as those with tracheostomies, may need suction equipment. Additionally, clients may need supportive equipment, such as elevated toilet seats, canes, and/or walkers, which are not directly related to medical care but reflect the clients' general conditions and needs for safety. The nurse is often in a better position to assess equipment needs than physicians, who are not involved in direct care of the client. The nurse should ask the client what equipment the client will need (such as a walker) and ask what types of tasks they will need to do when they return home because this can help to determine equipment they may need.

Collaborative Care Management

Roles of Health Care Team Members

Health and human service professions that collaborate with the RN through co-treatment, consultation, and referral include:

- **Speech therapist**: Evaluate and treat communication and swallowing disorders.
- **Occupational therapist**: Evaluate abilities and assist clients to manage activities of daily living, such as cooking, bathing, and other personal care and usual activities.
- **Physical therapist**: Evaluates and provides exercise regiments in order to improve or restore function, reduce discomfort, and prevent complications.
- **Social worker**: Evaluates, serves as case manager, makes referrals, identifies resources available to the client, educates, and assists with financial and housing needs.
- **Charge nurse**: Supervises and manages other nursing staff, monitors client care, and serves as a resource.
- **Physician**: Prescribes treatments as appropriate for client needs.
- **Respiratory therapist**: Evaluates, tests, and treats clients with respiratory and cardiopulmonary disorders.
- **Case manager**: Evaluates clients' needs and determines the types of care they require, monitors their progress, and links them to services, such as community resources and rehabilitation programs.

Reporting Critical Information

The nurse must report significant client information to various **disciplines**:

- **Primary physician**: Information should include the client's current condition and any changes or problems noted. The physician should be alerted to laboratory reports and results of diagnostic tests as well as any client concerns or reports and response to treatments.
- **Pharmacist**: Information should include the client's name, age, and diagnoses, a list of current medications (including supplements and herbal preparations), and allergies as well as any medication errors that may occur (such as missed or wrong medication or dosage) and reports of adverse reactions.

- **Social worker**: Information should include that needed by the social worker to assist the client, such as demographic information and information about living situation or abuse, although most information will come directly from the client or family.
- **Respiratory therapist**: Information should include the client's name, age, diagnoses, medications, mobility status, cognitive status, and respiratory status (short of breath, coughing, cyanotic). If on a ventilator, the ventilator settings should be reviewed and any oxygen delivery outlined.

Concepts of Management

Management is the process by which a person leads and directs the employees under them in order to achieve institutional and financial goals to improve patient care and outcomes. The nurse manager is usually the first level of authority after the charge nurse, and often has to balance clinical skills and expertise with the business aspects of management, such as creation of a budget and conflict resolution between employees. A good manager will set clear expectations for their employees and create attainable long and short-term goals for their floor. They will also focus on building an environment and culture of teamwork with their employees; often this may be accomplished using *shared governance* (when employees have a say in the policies and procedures of the floor/unit) or creating committees to help identify and improve different areas.

Types of Power

One concept of management is **types of power**. They include

- **Authority***:* Power granted by position.
- **Reward***:* Power inspired by the promise of retribution (bonuses, time-off, food, etc.).
- **Expertise***:* Power granted to an individual based on the belief that they are the expert in an area/ more skilled than most.
- **Coercion***:* Power gained by threatening physical/physiological/financial pain if expectations are not met.

Conflict Management

Conflict is an almost inevitable product of teamwork, and the leader must assume responsibility for conflict resolution. While conflicts can be disruptive, they can produce positive outcomes by forcing team members to listen to different perspectives and opening dialogue. The team should make a plan for dealing with conflict resolution. The best time for conflict resolution is when differences emerge but before open conflict and hardening of positions occur. The leader must pay close attention to the people and problems involved, listen carefully, and reassure those involved that their points of view are understood. Steps to conflict resolution include:

- Allow both sides to present their side of conflict without bias, maintaining a focus on opinions rather than individuals.
- Encourage cooperation through negotiation and compromise.
- Maintain the focus, providing guidance to keep the discussions on track and avoid arguments.
- Evaluate the need for renegotiation, formal resolution process, or third party.
- Utilize humor and empathy to diffuse escalating tensions.
- Summarize the issues, outlining key arguments.
- Avoid forcing resolution if possible.

Continuity of Care

Continuity of care refers to the idea that every patient should receive the same quality of care throughout their healthcare experience, and that care should be congruous within itself. The nurse plays an integral part of maintaining continuity of care in several areas:

- **Report:** Nurses should use SBAR or some other standardized method for giving/receiving report. This prevents errors/omissions in the report, and ensures that the patient gets the same care throughout the different changes of shift.
- **Terminology:** The use of abbreviations should be limited, and only used if they are nationally-approved. Medical jargon should be avoided when speaking with patients to avoid miscommunication.
- **Safe Procedures**: There should **ALWAYS** be a "time-out" before surgical or invasive procedures to ensure consent is signed, and that it is the right patient/procedure/body-part, etc. It should also be determined before major or life-altering procedures that the patient will have the resources at home needed for a safe and full recovery; this may mean that the nurse will assist in setting up home-healthcare services or a short-term stay in a rehabilitation center.
- **Follow-up:** Continuity of care continues after hospitalization as the patient transfers into the community. Every patient should have a follow-up visit scheduled before leaving the facility, and the nurse should ensure they have the time and transport necessary to get there. The patient should also have access to the contact information of the physicians on their care team, and leave with written post-discharge instructions.

Verbal Orders

Telephone and direct **verbal orders** both pose a risk of misinterpretation and error because they rely on the nurse correctly understanding and remembering the orders, especially if there are multiple orders. According to the National Patient Safety Goals, telephone and verbal orders should be written in their entirety and read back and confirmed before the orders are carried out. If the ordering physician is present, the physician should write the orders rather than giving verbal orders.

SBAR Technique

The **SBAR technique** is used to hand-off a patient from one caregiver to another to provide a systematic method so that important information is conveyed:

- **(S) Situation**: Overview of current situation and important issues.
- **(B) Background**: Important history and issues leading to current situation.
- **(A) Assessment**: Summary of important facts and condition.
- **(R) Recommendation**: Actions needed.

Recording and Communicating Client Information

Documents used to record and **communicate client information** include:

- **Medical records**: Include demographic information, history and physical, progress notes, lists of allergies, treatment plan, physician's orders, and various reports as well as the discharge planning form. Medical records may be in paper form or electronic.
- **Referral forms**: Include client's name, birthdate, contact information, address, and insurance information. The reason for the consultation, the diagnosis and ICD-10-CM code, and information about the referring physician/therapist are included.

- **Transfer forms**: May vary but include the client's name, date of birth, gender, contact person, physicians name and telephone number, any code status (such as DNR), the date and time of transfer and the reason for transfer as well as vital signs, report of pain, client diagnosis, use of restraints, respiratory needs, allergies, sensory status, skin condition, diet, list of personal items, risk alert, mobility/weight-bearing status, mental status, functional ability, immunization record, bowel and bladder status, and list of medication as well as any attached documents, such as operative reports, advance directives, and medication reconciliation.
- **Various report forms**: May include laboratory and imaging reports, consultation reports, and therapy reports.

Common Nursing Abbreviations

The following **abbreviations** are important for the nurse to know when communicating with health care team members regarding the health status of the client:

Abbreviation	Meaning
ADL	activities of daily living
BMP	basic metabolic panel
CBC	complete blood count
CNS	central nervous system
DOE	dyspnea on exertion
ESRD	End-stage Renal Disease
GI	gastrointestinal
h	hours
HA	headache
MI	myocardial infarction (heart attack)
MOA	mechanism of action
N/V/D	nausea, vomiting, and diarrhea.
ORIF	open reduction internal fixation
RBC	red blood cell
ROM	Range of Motion
S&S	signs and symptoms
SOB	shortness of breath
URI	upper respiratory infection
US	ultrasound
UTI	urinary tract infection
WBC	white blood cells

HIPAA

HIPAA stands for the **Health Insurance Portability and Accountability Act.** It protects a patient's privacy and prevents that patient from being denied insurance because of a preexisting condition. It creates a standard for privacy protection among health care providers and institutions, and protects the patient's health record. It is based on the principle of "Need to Know," stating that those not directly involved in the patient's care do not have the right to access his/her health records or other PHI (private health information). It also allows the patient to know how and with whom their information will be shared. Employers are required by law to train employees to practice confidentiality and ensure they understand the consequences of a HIPAA breach.

CONFIDENTIALITY

Confidentiality is the principle of maintaining the privacy of client information by not giving out any information about the client without the express permission of the client or his/her health care power of attorney (HCPOA). This includes the client's medical status, location, treatments, and condition. Confidentiality respects the patient's autonomy and privacy, supports a trusting relationship between the nurse and the client, and assists in preventing harm to the client. It is also of legal concern, as the Health Insurance Portability and Accountability Act (HIPAA) has made the sharing of private health information (PHI) a prosecutable offense. However, there are some notable exceptions to patient confidentiality. These include:

- Information essential to patient's care to other health care providers (Principle of "Need-to-Know").
- Testifying in court.
- Reporting communicable diseases.
- Reporting child abuse, spouse abuse, and/or elder abuse.
- Reporting suspicious or gunshot wounds.
- Information relating to workers' compensation issues.

BREACHES OF CONFIDENTIALITY

HIPAA Breach Notification Rule requires covered entities to report any breaches in confidentiality/protected health information:

- **Individuals**: Notification by standard mail or email (if the individual has agreed) as soon as possible but no later than 60 days after the breach. If lacking contact information for 10 or more individuals, notice must be placed on the organization's website for 90 days with a tollfree telephone number or notice provided in print or broadcast media. For fewer than 10 individuals, alternate notification, such as by telephone, is permitted. Individual breaches are reported to the HHS Secretary annually.
- **500 or more individuals**: In addition to individual notification, notice must be given in prominent media outlet serving the affected states no later than 60 days after the breach. The HHS Secretary must be notified electronically within 60 days after the breach. If the breach affected fewer than 500 individuals, the HHS Secretary must be notified within 60 days of the end of the calendar year in which the breaches occurred.

MASLOW'S HIERARCHY OF NEEDS

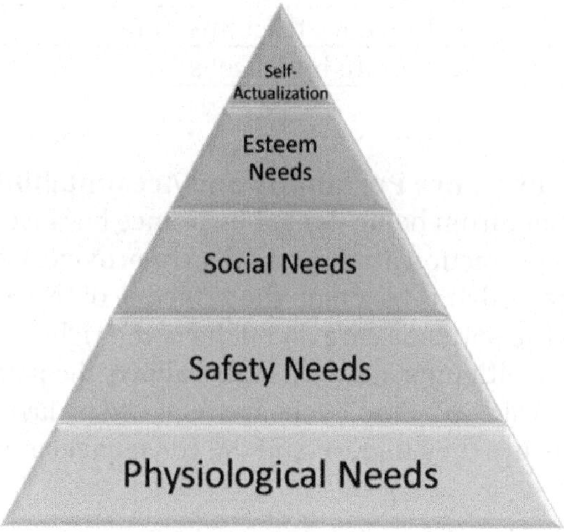

Maslow's Hierarchy of Needs was created by Abraham Maslow as a way to discuss the prioritization of human needs. It is generally represented as a pyramid, with the most basic human needs at the bottom. The principle is that the needs must be met in order, working from bottom to top. Maslow is also used extensively in nursing as a way to prioritize patient needs. It is also a tenet that is basic to the NCLEX exam.

- Physiological Needs
  - Physiological needs are basic life needs, including air, water, food, sex, sleep, etc. Failure to satisfy these needs can lead to sickness, irritation, pain, etc.
- Safety Needs
  - Safety needs entail establishing stability and consistency in life for psychological health.
- Social Needs
  - Social needs of love and belongingness come next on the priority ladder. Humans have a desire for connection and belong to groups like clubs, work groups, families, religious groups, etc.
- Esteem Needs
  - Esteem needs can be one of two types. Self-esteem results from task competence or mastery. Another type of esteem comes from the attention and recognition from others.
- Self-Actualization Needs
  - Self-actualization is one's desire to become everything that he or she is capable of becoming.

Prioritizing Interventions

CPR Approaches

ABC	CAB
Airway, breathing, circulation	Circulation, airway, breathing
Utilized by those trained for: * Adults with **respiratory arrest**, such as those with drug overdose or drowning. * Newborns.	Utilized by those trained for: * Adults with sudden **cardiac arrest**. * Infants and children.
Administer the following for respiratory arrest (with a pulse): A. Maintain **airway** (consider advanced airway if necessary). B. Provide rescue **breaths**, 1 every 5 to 6 seconds. *Rescue breaths provided to newborns and infants should cover both the nose and mouth. C. Check pulse (**circulation**) every 2 minutes. If no pulse is present, move to cardiac arrest algorithm.	Administer the following for adults, infants and children with cardiac arrest: 1. Call 9-1-1 or ask for someone else to/Shout for help. 2. 30 compressions at rate of 100/min (120/min for infants/newborns). 3. Two rescue breaths. 4. Shock with defibrillator if available. 5. Continue compressions/ventilation at 30:2 rate for adults. 6. For infants and children with one rescuer, continue at rate of 30:2 or 15:2 if two rescuers. 7. Repeat shock with defibrillator every 2 minutes.

Ethical Practice

Standards of Care and the ANA's Code of Ethics

Standards of care are the current practice standards used to ensure capable and skillful health care delivery. They are used as a measurement tool for providing quality care; an established norm as a mechanism of providing safe and appropriate care to the public. Nursing standards discuss what would be done in and under the same circumstance by any other nurse with the same level of expertise and knowledge. By following the established standards of care or practice standards, the nurse reduces his/her chances of being found negligent in a court of law.

Additionally, nurses must abide by the **Nurses' Code of Ethics.** Since nursing involves providing for the care and well-being of the sick, injured, and those at risk, nurses must have a code of ethics to govern their behavior and practices. The ANA has developed a Code of Ethics to serve several purposes. First, the code discusses the essential obligations to be upheld by every person who works as a nurse. These obligations set *standards of care* that are universal to those throughout the nursing profession and include such concepts as patient autonomy and respect for human dignity. The ethics involved in the code are obligatory and are not optional practice. Finally, the code of ethics reflects the nurse's understanding of his/her role as a professional and the requirements of respect and compassion that he/she must give to patients.

ANA's Ethical Principles for Nurses

The **American Nurses Association** lists **six ethical principles** that a nurse must maintain to be excellent in his/her practice. These include:

1. **Autonomy**: Autonomy is the individual's self-determination. Autonomy involves personal respect for others. Nurses have an obligation to respect the rights of patients to make unforced, voluntary decisions.
2. **Beneficence**: Beneficence involves doing well and acting in the patient's best interest.
3. **Nonmaleficence**: Nonmaleficence is the principle of doing no harm.
4. **Justice**: The principle of justice involves fair treatment and equal care for all.
5. **Veracity**: Veracity involves telling the truth. Health care providers are required and responsible to be truthful when providing care to patients.
6. **Fidelity**: Fidelity is the health care provider's obligation to keep the promises they make to their patients, maintain patient confidentiality, and keep patient information private.

Theories of Bioethics

Bioethics is a type of philosophy used to guide ethical decisions in health care and nursing. There are several different theories followed by different practices that are used to establish their ethics. The more popular theories of bioethics include:

1. **Utilitarianism**: Utilitarianism believes that ethical conflicts can be resolved by considering the individuals affected by the decision being made. Utilitarianism works under the premise of doing the most good for the greatest number of people. The theory of utilitarianism believes that maximization of good consequences automatically minimizes bad consequences.
2. **Deontology**: Deontology functions on the premise of duty or obligation. The deontological theory states that nurses are bound to always do what is right for their patients.

3. **Virtue**: Virtue is a theory that involves making ethical decisions or taking ethical stands related to health care. The intent is the driving force behind virtue. With virtue, functioning under good intentions makes actions ethical.
4. **Egoist**: The egoist theory cites objectivism as the main focus. Egoist thought is centered on self-interest of the individual.

ETHICAL DECISION MAKING

ETHICAL DECISION MAKING

Nurses are required to follow the ethical guidelines set by the American Nurses Association (ANA) to make ethical decisions*. To decide the most ethical decision, the nurse must use the following steps:

1. Identify or determine the health problem.
2. Determine the ethical issue.
3. Obtain additional information.
4. Identify the decision maker.
5. Assess ethical and moral principles.
6. Research and consider alternative options.
7. Implement decisions as needed.
8. Assess and modify actions.

NEGLIGENCE AND MALPRACTICE

Nurses use ethical decision making to avoid negligence and malpractice:

Negligence	An unintentional tort that causes patient harm from either a breach of duty or an omission or failure to meet the accepted standard of care.
Malpractice	A liability on negligence in which a health care professional is held accountable for a breach of a duty of care involving special knowledge and skill.

**The nurse should realize that the legality and ethicality of the decision are not the same thing; sometimes, ethics and legality will conflict.*

CASE AND STATUTORY LAW FOR NURSES

The practical nurse should know the **ten ethical principles** that are used to govern court decisions regarding nursing and medical malpractice:

1. Nurses have a legal duty to always act in the best interest of the individuals they care for.
2. Informed consent is required for testing, procedures, and treatment.
3. All patients should be informed of the consequences of refusing treatment. This should be documented in the permanent patient record.
4. All mentally sound adult patients have the right to refuse treatment, including life-saving treatment.
5. Patients have the right of advance directives to direct care when they are incapacitated.
6. The state may require documented evidence related to refusal of care.
7. Decisions that involve children should be made with the child's best interest in mind.
8. Adolescents are capable of making health care decisions.
9. Health care providers are legally bound to abide by privacy laws.
10. Privacy laws are only breached when the patient is endangering others with his or her decisions.

Information Technology

Correct Nursing Documentation

Documentation is an essential component of nursing to support communication between caregivers, prevent errors and adverse outcomes, and maintain a record of work should nursing care or judgment come into question. The following are components of correct nursing documentation:

- **Detailed and Factual***:* avoiding opinion or blame; only observations, not diagnosis. Example "Patient speaking with raised voice, asking to speak to manager," not "Patient is angry at staff, being belligerent; probably due to negligence by night shift staff."
- **Thorough***:* Should include all actions that were performed for the patient's plan of care, communication/instructions from physicians, educational information given to the patient and family: "If it's not documented, it's not done!"
- **Mistakes***:* correct mistakes with a single line through the error and mark with initials; NEVER use Wite-Out or scribble out the mistake.
- **Timely***:* Chart in real time whenever possible. Charting that is performed late should be noted within documentation that it is a late entry, to avoid questions about time lapses.

Use of Data Management to Plan Care

Data management is a crucial tool to help improve patient outcomes. To effectively use this tool, the interdisciplinary team would meet on a regular basis and utilize the following steps:

1. Discuss the goals/expectations for new plan of care.
2. Determine method and criteria for data collection.
3. Collect the data.
4. Analyze the data and begin evaluating the information.
5. Report all of the data, the analysis, and the evaluation.
6. Begin documenting the care plan for any patient with the disease.
7. Develop expected outcomes and needed interventions.
8. Develop the treatment plan.
9. Implement the new treatment plan.
10. Evaluate effectiveness of new treatment plan; revise as needed.

The ultimate purpose of data management would be to put together a new clinical pathway, to improve outcomes for those patients with that disease. The entire process of developing a pathway for each disease entity takes several months, and requires evaluation after the initial application in the clinical setting.

Legal Issues and Performance Improvement

Legal Issues Related to Nursing Care

Negligence

The four necessary **elements of negligence** (failure to follow standards of care) are:

- **Duty of care**: The defendant (healthcare provider) had a duty to provide adequate care and/or protect the plaintiff's (client's) safety.
- **Breach of duty**: The defendant failed to carry out the duty to care, resulting in danger, injury, or harm to the plaintiff.
- **Damages**: The plaintiff experienced illness or injury as a result of the breach of duty.
- **Causation**: The plaintiff's illness or injury is directly caused by the defendant's negligent breach of duty.

Types of negligence include:

- **Negligent conduct**: An individual failed to provide reasonable care or to protect/assist another, based on standards and expertise.
- **Gross negligence**: Willfully providing inadequate care while disregarding the safety and security of another.
- **Contributory negligence**: injured party contributing to his/her own harm.
- **Comparative negligence**: The percentage amount of negligence attributed to each individual involved.

FACT System of Documentation

The medical record is a legal document, and the nurse must meet legal responsibilities in documentation. The **FACT (Bergerson) system of documentation** helps to ensure legal requirements are met:

- **Factual**: The nurse should record objective factual information. Subjective information, such as statements of the client, must be clearly identified and not presented as facts ("The client states she has pain in the abdomen.")
- **Accurate**: The correct date, time, treatments, and observations must be recorded, using approved abbreviations only so that the information cannot be misinterpreted.
- **Complete**: The information should be complete and contain all relevant details. All aspects of the nursing process should be addressed.
- **Timely**: Documentation should be done as soon as possible after interventions and/or interactions with the client to ensure that information is not forgotten or excluded and to prevent errors, such as double medicating a client.

Every entry must be signed, late entries properly documented, and errors in documentation crossed out with a single line. No blank lines should be left between documentation and signature.

Managing Client Valuables

Clients should be advised to leave all **valuables** at home when planning for admission or to send all valuables home. However, if client's bring valuable items (such as jewelry, watches, cash, credit cards, electronic readers, and computers), the nurse and client or family member (if client unable) should together fill out a valuable receipt form, place the items in an envelope or container, and immediately place them in the safe until discharge. When the items are requested, they should be obtained by security and the contents reviewed by the client and nurse together to ensure the contents match the receipt. If the client insists on keeping valuable items at bedside, the client should be advised that clients are responsible for their own belongings in the event they are lost and this information should be documented. If clients have dentures or partial plates, a denture cup should be provided and labeled. Hearing and vision aids (glasses) should be kept in their original case or a container provided and labeled. Any assistive devices should be labeled with the client's name, ID number, and room number.

Serving as an Interpreter

Each healthcare institution should have guidelines in place for nurses serving as **interpreters.** Ideally, the nurse should have training in healthcare interpretation. The nurse should begin an interpreting session by advising those involved that the nurse will respect confidentiality and will interpret all comments so the client should not say anything ("Don't tell the doctor!") the client does not want interpreted. The nurse interpreter should avoid giving any advice or stating personal opinions or expressing opinions through body language and should attempt to replicate the speaker's tone and expressions. Interpreting involves several elements:

- Converting the message from one language to another with as much accuracy as possible.
- Paying attention to words or concepts that may be misinterpreted and seeking clarification when necessary.
- Clarifying cultural ideas or manners of expression that may lack an exact equivalence.
- Remembering always to be an advocate for the client, especially if aware of discriminatory actions or comments.

Mandatory Reporting

While laws about **mandatory reporting** vary from state to state, healthcare providers are considered mandatory reporters in all states and must report suspected cases of child, disabled, and elder abuse and neglect. The nurse must follow state guidelines for reporting as simply notifying the receiving facility of suspected child abuse is not adequate. The nurse should be familiar with the signs of abuse and neglect (certain types of fractures, unexplained or multiple bruises, suspicious bruise patterns, burns, hair loss, and inadequate food, clothing, shelter). Additionally, in most states, certain types of injuries or assaults must be reported to law enforcement, including stab wounds, gunshot wounds, and sexual assaults. Each state has lists of specific communicable diseases (such as TB and measles) that must be reported—some required by the CDC but others specific to the state or local area. Those classified as urgent (such as Ebola) must be reported immediately while others may be reported within one to seven working days. Reporting procedures vary.

Nurse's Scope of Practice and Regulatory Bodies

Each state has its own Nurse Practice Act, which is administered by the state Board of Nursing. The Nurse Practice Act outlines requirements for licensure and certification and delineates the **scope of practice** of registered nurses, practical nurses, and advanced practice nurses, including duties and delegation. Typically, licensure is granted to those who complete an accredited LVN/LPN or RN program and pass the nursing exam (NCLEX) or receive endorsement because of licensure in another state. The nurse must function legally under the nurse practice act of the state in which the nurse resides. In some cases, a license/certification in one state is automatically recognized in other states through the Compact agreement, but advance practice nurses are often excluded from these agreements. The American Nurses Association does not itself have regulatory authority but works closely with federal and state agencies to provide guidance regarding the roles of nurses and to monitor regulations. The ANA has issued many position statements and leads lobbying efforts on the behalf of the nursing profession.

Nurses' Rights and Responsibilities

Responsibility of Nurses

The primary responsibility of the nurse is to provide safety in health care for all individuals. Nurses are responsible for knowing their scope of practice, the patient's rights, hospital policies and procedures, and standards of care and community norms.

Rights of Nurses

Because their primary objective is safety, nurses have the right to refuse assignments that jeopardize the client or the nurse, or place the client in immediate or serious danger. Nurses have the right to refuse to treat patients who are beyond their scope of practice. Nurses have the right to not be abused by clients, coworkers, or employers. Nurses have the right to ask for clarity with assignments, assess his or her personal abilities as they relate to clients and client situations, and assist in identifying options that will fulfill the assignment.

Performance Improvement

Performance improvement, a focus on assessing outcomes, gathering data, and using that data to improve performance, should begin at the top level of management with a commitment to effecting change at all levels and to providing the financial resources that make these changes possible. This entails beginning with a clear definition of quality as it applies to clients and relating this to mission and vision statements, goals and objectives. Nurses and all members of an organization should share equally in the goal of working toward performance improvement. The act of setting goals alone often leads to improved performance. The nurse should be alert to possible methods of improving practice in all nursing activities. An organization-wide model for performance improvement should include:

- Assessment: Identifying processes that can be improved.
- Planning: Brainstorming different possible actions.
- Implementation: Pilot or organizational.
- Evaluation of continuous improvement.

A number of different models may be utilized for performance improvement, including Plan-Do-Check-Act (PDCA) and Find-Organize-Clarify-Uncover-Start (FOCUS).

Continuous Quality Improvement

Continuous Quality Improvement (CQI) emphasizes the organization and systems and processes within that organization rather than individuals. It recognizes internal customers (staff) and external customers (clients) and utilizes data to improve processes. CQI represents the concept that most processes can be improved. CQI uses the scientific method of experimentation to meet needs and improve services and utilizes various tools, such as brainstorming, multivoting, various charts and diagrams, storyboarding, and meetings. Core concepts include:

- Quality and success are meeting or exceeding internal and external customer's needs and expectations.
- Problems relate to processes, and variations in process lead to variations in results.
- Change can be in small steps.

Steps to CQI include:

1. Forming a knowledgeable team.
2. Identifying and defining measures used to determine success.

3. Brainstorming strategies for change.
4. Planning, collecting, and utilizing data as part of making decisions.
5. Testing changes and revising or refining as needed.

Strategies for Reducing Infections

Intravascular Devices

Strategies for reducing infection risks associated with intravascular devices include:

- **Site selection** away from the internal jugular or femoral veins, using PICC if possible.
- **Tunneled catheter or ports** used if possible, because of lower infection rates than non-tunneled catheters.
- **TPN catheters** used only for TPN and not other procedures.
- **Experienced trained staff** to insert intravascular devices.
- **Dressings** should be transparent, and the site examined frequently by palpation. Change dressings at least weekly.
- Using maximum aseptic technique for insertion.
- **Rotation of catheter sites** every 72-96 hours (for adults) for short peripheral venous catheters but only as needed for others.
- **Avoid antibiotic ointments** at insertion site because of danger of fungal infections or resistance.

Urinary Catheters

Strategies for reducing infection risks associated with urinary catheters include:

- **Using aseptic technique** for both straight and indwelling catheter insertion.
- **Limiting catheter use** by establishing protocols for use, duration, and removal, training staff, issuing reminders to physicians, using straight catheterizations rather than indwelling, using ultrasound to scan the bladder, and using condom catheters.
- Utilizing closed-drainage systems for indwelling catheters.
- **Avoiding irrigation** unless required for diagnosis or treatment.
- **Using sampling port** for specimens rather than disconnecting catheter and tubing.
- **Maintaining proper urinary flow** by proper positioning, securing of tubing and drainage bag, and keeping drainage bag below the level of the bladder.
- **Changing catheters** only when medically needed.
- **Cleansing external meatal** area gently each day, manipulating the catheter as little as possible.
- **Avoid** placing catheterized patients adjacent to those infected or colonized with antibiotic-resistant bacteria to reduce cross-contamination.

Referrals

Referrals occur when a physician consults another physician or specialty group to help care for the patient. Referrals are made in both the inpatient and outpatient settings, and may be from physician to physician (such as the attending physician consulting a pulmonologist for a COPD patient) or physician to a group (social services, dietary, etc.) Physicians should call their own referrals, but it is part of the nurses' responsibilities to ensure all referrals are properly called and charted, and that the patient is aware of them. It is the physician's responsibility to ensure all critical referrals are made, especially if the patient's problem is outside the area of their own expertise. However, the nurse should advocate for the patient if a problem arises, and respect the patient's wishes if the patient requests for a certain referral to be made. It is important that when referrals are made, that the entire care team is aware and communicates together to ensure optimal care for the patient.

Assessing the Need for Referrals to Specialties

Clients may need **referrals** to the following services:

- **Physical therapists**: Clients with musculoskeletal injuries, disease, or problems (such as paralysis) may be referred for therapy to improve or maintain mobility and to increase strength. Patients in long term care units, such as intensive care, who have been immobile and/or seriously ill may also require an in-hospital physical therapy consult to approve progress in mobility orders (from bed rest to using the bedside commode, for instance) prior to transfer to a step-down unit.
- **Speech therapists**: Clients with speech impediments, such as those resulting from a stroke, may be referred for therapy to improve communication ability or to teach compensatory methods. Speech therapists also assess the ability to chew and swallow and assist clients with methods of improving swallowing and preventing choking and aspiration. Speech therapists may be responsible for progressing a client's diet order from NPO to full liquids to regular on critical care and intermediate care units.
- **Respite care**: Clients under Hospice care may receive respite care for 4 to 5 days when caregivers are exhausted or unable to care for them.
- **Social services**: Social services can aid clients in applying for assistance, such as Medicaid, and accessing community resources, and can investigate possible cases of abuse.
- **Shelters**: Homeless clients who are in need of ongoing treatment or followup are especially at risk if living on the streets, so efforts should be made to find housing in shelters before a homeless client is discharged from hospital or other care.

Referral Form

Clients are often given referrals to other healthcare providers, such as a specialist (ophthalmologist, neurologist, orthopedist), therapist (physical therapist, occupational therapist, speech therapist, recreational therapist, psychologist), or community resource (home health agency, meals-on-wheels). Necessary information that must be included on the **referral form** includes the client's name, telephone number, date of birth, admission diagnosis, and insurance information as well as the name of the referring healthcare provider and the reason for the consultation/referral. Additional reports may be attached to the referral form if necessary. For example, a referral for speech therapy may include a neurological report about the nerves affected by a stroke. The referral includes the number of anticipated visits (such as PT three times a week for a month). Preauthorization may be required for consultations/referrals. One copy of the referral form is stored in the client's medical record and another given to the client or sent directly to the consultant/therapist/community resource. The client may be instructed to make an appointment independently or the healthcare provider may make the initial appointment after discussing time eligibility with the client.

Safety and Infection Control

Accident, Error, and Injury Prevention

Assessing Clients for Allergies

When assessing clients for **allergies** it's important to determine the type of symptoms they have, when the initial reaction occurred, and what type of treatment they have used (including antihistamines). Allergies of particular interest include:

- **Food**: Ask clients about any specific foods that cause an adverse reaction as some foods may have cross-reactivity to latex (such as kiwi, papaya, avocado, and bananas), so clients may be at risk of developing latex allergy and should avoid contact with latex. Some medications may contain substances derived from food, such as eggs, fish, gelatin, lactose, and soy.
- **Latex**: Sensitivity to latex can result in mild reactions, such as itching and rash, to severe anaphylactic reactions and is common among those with repeated contact with healthcare, such as those with spina bifida or multiple surgeries, so it should be suspected with these clients. While non-latex options are more readily available in most hospitals (non-latex gloves and Foley catheters, for instance), latex continues to be used in hospital materials, therefore this allergy must be assessed immediately upon arrival so that appropriate materials can be substituted if necessary.
- **Environmental**: The most common environmental allergies include pollens, dust mites, animals, cigarette smoke, cockroaches, and mold/mildew, so the nurse should be sure to ask about these as well as any other environmental allergies. Some clients are sensitive to strong colognes and perfumes, so the use of these are often regulated by hospital dress codes on units with immunocompromised patients.

Deficits That Can Impede Client Safety

Deficits that can impede client safety include:

- **Visual impairment**: Clients are at risk of trips, slips, falls, burn injuries, poisoning (mistaken containers, ingredients), and medication errors because of taking the wrong medication or wrong dosage.
- **Hearing impairment**: Clients are at increased risk of falls and may not hear danger signals, such as fire alarms, smoke detectors, police/fire sirens, and tornado warning sirens, and may, therefore, not be aware that they are in danger. Most smoke detectors emit a high-frequency alarm that cannot always be detected by those with high-frequency hearing loss.
- **Sensory/Perceptual impairment**: Clients (such as those with stroke or brain injury) may exhibit a wide variety of impairments so safety concerns may vary. For example, those with one-sided neglect may have injuries to the neglected side, such as from running into doors or other things. Those with face blindness may easily get lost if away from familiar places or people.

Non-Pharmacologic Prescription Precautions

Some **non-pharmacologic prescriptions** may contribute to accident or injury, including the following:

- **Oxygen supplies**: Oxygen may be administered at the wrong liters (too much or too little), and the oxygen supply may be inadvertently obstructed or disconnected. Oxygen concentrators may not have backup batteries and may fail to function if electricity goes off. If people smoke around oxygen, this increases the risk of fires. Nasal cannulas and face masks that delivery oxygen, when used over prolonged periods of time, can cause pressure injuries, therefore appropriate assessment and skin care is also necessary.
- **Assistive devices**: If equipment, such as canes and walkers, are improperly fitted, they may increase risk of falls.
- **Dialysis equipment**: Contamination of equipment is always a concern and can result in peritonitis (peritoneal dialysis) and sepsis (hemodialysis). If the lines become separated, the client may exsanguinate.
- **Hot/Cold compresses**: If cold compresses are placed directly on the skin, they may damage the tissue, especially if left in place for too long. Hot compresses may cause burns if temperature is too high and may damage wounds if placed directly over them.

Correct Use of Car Seats

All infants, regardless of age, must be placed properly in an **infant car seat** during transit. Holding an infant while the car is in motion is not safe. Car seats should be new or in very good condition and fastened according to manufacturer's guidelines to ensure safety:

- Place the car seat in the back seat and away from any side airbags.
- Always securely buckle the child into the seat.
- Face the infant seat toward the rear of the car.
- Recline the seat so that the infant's head does not fall forward.
- Place padding around (not under) the infant if the infant slouches to one side.
- Place blankets OVER the straps and buckles, not under.

The infant/toddler should be placed in the rear-facing seat to the maximum weight and height allowed by the seat (some accommodate up to 65 pounds). Once transitioned to front-facing seats, children should be placed in belt-positioning booster seats until the vehicle's seat/shoulder belts fit properly (usually until 4' 9" and 8-12 years old). Until age 13, children should sit secured in the back seat and not the front.

Aspects of Client Safety in the Hospital

Aspects of **client safety** include:

- **Signaling staff**: The client must be educated about the use of the call light, and the call light placed within easy reach. If the client is unable to use the call light, then an alternative means of calling for help, such as a handheld bell, should be available for the client. If the client is unable to manage any type of signaling system, then the nurse should check on the client at least every hour.

- **Protecting from falls and electrical hazards**: All clutter should be removed from floors and cords secured away from walkways. All electrical appliances should be checked to ensure they are working properly and have no frayed cords. Clients should be provided assistive devices, such as walkers, if necessary, to improve stability.
- **Making appropriate room assignments**: Clients with the greatest need for supervision should be placed closest to the nursing desk and within the line of sight whenever possible.

Seizure Disorders and Safety

Seizure disorders are broadly categorized as partial seizures (which begin locally) or generalized seizures (which are bilateral and symmetrical and may be convulsive or non-convulsive):

- **Partial seizures** include *simple partial* (with motor, sensory, and/or autonomic symptoms but without impaired consciousness), *complex partial* (with cognitive, affective, psychosensory, and/or psychomotor symptoms, as well as impaired consciousness), or *partial secondarily generalized.*
- **Generalized seizures** include seizures that are bilateral and symmetric without local onset and may be convulsive or non-convulsive. These seizures include *tonic-clonic, tonic, clonic, absence* (petit mal), *atonic*, and *myoclonic seizures*, as well as *unclassified seizures.*

First aid for a seizure includes ensuring privacy and providing supportive care, such as easing the patient to the floor and providing padding to protect the head. Side rails should be raised and pillow removed if the patient is in bed. The patient should be placed on one side with the head flexed so the tongue does not block the airway. The patient should **not** be restrained or a padded tongue-blade inserted between the teeth.

R.A.C.E. Acronym for Fire Safety

RACE for Fire Safety is explained below:

- Rescue – remove all patients from area of danger
- Activate alarm - pull fire alarm/call 9-1-1
- Confine the fire - close doors to unit/place
- Evacuate/Extinguish (NFPA/OSHA fire safety) - Use **PASS** for fire extinguisher
    - Pull
    - Aim at the base of the flames
    - Squeeze the trigger
    - Sweep – use a sweeping motion across the flames

Emergency Response

Emergency Response Plans

Emergency response plans must include plans for communication, resources and assets available, safety and security measures, responsibilities of staff, utilities, and measure to support clinical activities.

Bomb Threats

The response depends on the type of bomb threat and the information gleaned from the threat. The first response is to notify the police and designated staff by landlines (avoiding cell phones, which can trigger some devices) or overhead paging. An initial search may be carried out by staff in each area to try to locate possible bombs. Administration should make the decision about evacuation, and plans for evacuation should be in place. With terrorist bombing and improvised explosive devices (IEDs), situational awareness is critical because multiple explosive devices (some undetonated) may be at the scene. IEDs may be inside backpacks, suitcases, and packages left unattended. Additionally, people wearing suicide vests or belts may mix in with other victims or people escaping the blast area.

Natural Disasters

Plans vary according to type of natural disaster. If anticipated, extra food, clothing, and supplies should be stockpiled for both clients and staff (who may be required to stay at the facility for extended periods). A command structure should be in place. With a hurricane or tornado, clients may need to be moved away from windows and to more secure areas, such as interior hallways, during the storm. The hospital must prepare plans to evacuate clients if necessary (such as with flooding, earthquakes, or storm damage) and transfer them to other facilities and must also be prepared for an influx of clients.

Community Planning

Healthcare providers, such as hospitals, should work closely with the community to identify community resources that are available for emergency response and the needs that may arise in response to disasters, including the number of people who may depend on the hospital for care.

Identifying Clients to Discharge in Disaster Situations

In the event of a **disaster situation**, the surge capacity of a hospital may need to increase markedly with a large influx of clients in need of emergency care and hospitalization, so appropriate clients must be quickly identified for possible discharge. All elective admissions and procedures should be cancelled and non-critical clients, such as those with non-life-threatening conditions or those near discharge, should be discharged or transferred to other facilities if possible. Generally, hospitalists, charge nurses, or team leaders may be in the best position to identify clients for discharge as well as the person tasked with monitoring length of stay. If an acuity-based model of client care is utilized, then those already categorized as the least acute should be quickly assessed for discharge. Ideally, each unit should have plans in place for rapid discharge so that assessment and discharge can be carried out quickly and safely.

Organizational Plan for Bioterrorism

The ICP and the infection control team should develop specific plans for dealing with different **bioterrorism** agents, and training should be provided to staff. An organized approach should include the following:

- Be on the alert for possible bioterrorism-related infections, based on clusters of patients or symptoms.
- Use personal protection equipment, including respirators when indicated.
- Complete thorough assessment of patient, including medical history, physical examination, immunization record, and travel history.
- Provide a probable diagnosis based on symptoms and lab findings, including cultures.
- Provide treatment, including prophylaxis, while waiting for laboratory findings.
- Use transmission precautions as well as isolation for suspected biologic agents.
- Notify local, state, and federal authorities per established protocol.
- Conduct surveillance and epidemiological studies to identify at-risk populations.

- Develop plans to accommodate large numbers of patients:
  - Restricting elective admissions.
  - Transferring patients to other facilities.

Principles of Triage During Mass Casualty Events

Primary triage is a rapid method (30 to 60 seconds) of prioritizing clients based on severity of condition and carried out at the scene of multiple casualty incidents. All clients are triaged and tagged according to international color-coding priority (P) guidelines on foot or wrist (not clothing):

- P1—Red: Immediate care needed for urgent systemic life-threatening conditions, such as airway/breathing problems, severe bleeding, severe burns (especially with breathing problems), decreased mental status, shock, and severe medical problems, Glasgow Coma Score ≤13.
- P2—Yellow: Delayed care and able to wait 45-60 minutes for treatment. Conditions include burns (without breathing problems), multiple bone/joint injuries, back and/or spinal cord injuries (unless in respiratory distress).
- P3—Green: Hold, able to wait hours for treatment of minor injuries.
- P4—Black: Deceased or with injuries so extensive that they are not survivable.

Resource management involves identifying a triage officer, who remains at the scene during the event, and identifying the need for additional personnel and equipment and providing those to the clients with the highest priority.

Infections with Biological Weapons

Anthrax

A number of different infections could be part of a bioterrorism attack. The type of barrier/isolation needed is dependent upon the symptoms and the mode of transmission. Knowledge of typical presenting symptoms and prompt precautions are essential to prevent spread of disease. **Anthrax (Bacillus anthracis)** usually occurs from contact with animals, but as a bioterrorism weapon, anthrax would most likely be aerosolized and inhaled. It is not transferred from person to person. There are 3 types:

- **Inhalation**: Fever, cough, shortness of breath, and general debility.
- **Cutaneous**: Small non-painful sores that blister and ulcerate with necrosis at the center.
- **Gastrointestinal**: Nausea, vomiting, diarrhea, and abdominal pain.

The inhaled form of anthrax is the most severe with about a 50% mortality rate. The vaccine for anthrax is not yet available to the public.

Precautions are as follows:

- Prophylaxis with antibiotics after exposure.
- Standard precautions.
- Contact precautions for wounds if there are cutaneous lesions.

Pneumonic Plague

Yersinia pestis causes **pneumonic plague**, which is normally carried by fleas from infected rats but can be aerosolized to use as a biologic weapon. There are 3 forms of plague, but they sometimes occur together and bubonic and septicemic plague can develop into pneumonic, which is the primary concern related to bioterrorism:

- **Bubonic** occurs when a person is bitten by an infected flea.
- **Pneumonic** occurs with inhalation and results in pneumonia with fever, headache, cough, and progressive respiratory failure.
- **Septicemic** occurs when *Y. pestis* invades the bloodstream, often after initial bubonic or pneumonic plague.

Pneumonic plague can spread easily from person to person. There is no vaccine available. Precautions include the following:

- Immediate antibiotics within first 24 hours are necessary, so early diagnosis is critical.
- Prophylaxis with antibiotics may protect those exposed.
- Droplet precautions should be used with appropriate barriers, such as surgical mask.

Botulism

Clostridium botulinum produces an extremely poisonous toxin that causes botulism. The organism can be aerosolized or used to infect food. There are 3 primary forms of botulisms:

- **Foodborne botulism** results from contamination of food. This type poses the greatest threat from bioterrorism. Symptoms usually appear 12-36 hours after ingestion but may be delayed for 2 weeks, and include nausea, vomiting, dyspnea, dysphagia, slurred speech, progressive weakness, and paralysis.
- **Infant botulism** results from *C. botulinum* ingested into the intestinal tract. Constipation, poor feeding, and progressive weakness are presenting symptoms.
- **Wound botulism** results from contamination of open skin, but symptoms are similar to foodborne botulism.

Botulism is not transmitted from person to person, but contaminated food has the potential to infect many people, especially if the contaminated food is manufactured and widely distributed.

Precautions include the following:

- Antitoxin after exposure and as early in disease as possible.
- Standard precautions.
- Do not feed honey to infants, as there is a risk of spore ingestion.

Tularemia

Francisella tularensis causes tularemia, which is usually transmitted from small mammals to humans through insect bites, ingestion of contaminated food or water, inhalation, or handling of infected animals. Although there is no evidence of person-to-person transmission, *F. tularensis* has the potential to be aerosolized for use in bioterrorism because it is highly infective and requires only about 10 organisms to infect. Flu-like symptoms appear in 3-5 days after exposure and progress to severe respiratory infection and pneumonia. A vaccine for laboratory workers was available until recently, but the FDA is currently reviewing it, and it is unavailable in the United States.

- Prophylaxis with antibiotics within 24 hours may prevent disease.
- Standard precautions are sufficient.

- Biologic safety measures should be used for laboratory specimens.
- Autopsy procedures that may cause tissue to be aerosolized should be avoided.

Smallpox

The variola virus causes **smallpox**, which has been eradicated worldwide since 1980, but has the potential for use as a biological weapon because people are no longer vaccinated. Smallpox is extremely contagious and has a high mortality rate (about 30%). Flu-like symptoms appear about 7-17 days after exposure with fever, weakness, vomiting, and rash that begins on the face and arms and spreads. The rash becomes pustular, crusts, scabs over, and then sloughs off, leaving scars. People remain infective from the first rash until all scabs are gone. The disease can spread through contact with infective fluid from lesions or from contact with clothes or bedding. Aerosol spread is theoretically possible. Precautions are as follows:

- Vaccination must be done before symptoms appear and as soon as possible after exposure as vaccination after rash appears will not affect the severity of the disease; vaccination is done by scratching the skin with a small needle on the upper arm, leaving a characteristic pox scar.
- Contact precautions should be used, which includes the use of gowns and gloves to enter the room and keeping the patient in a private or cohorted room.

Viral Hemorrhagic Fevers

Viral hemorrhagic fevers are zoonoses (spread from animals to humans) and comprise a number of different diseases: Ebola, Lassa, Marburg, yellow, Argentine and Crimean-Congo. Some hemorrhagic fevers can spread person to person, notably Ebola, Marburg, and Lassa, through close contact with body fluids or contaminated items. Hemorrhagic fevers are extremely contagious multi-system diseases, and those in contact with infected patients are at risk of infection. Symptoms vary somewhat according to the disease but present with flu-like symptoms that progress to bleeding under the skin and internally, and some people develop kidney failure and central nervous system symptoms, such as coma and seizures. Treatment is supportive and mortality rates are high. Only yellow fever and Argentine have vaccines.

Precautions are as follows:

- **Maximum precautions** must be used with full barrier precautions, with care used in any handling of blood and body fluids or wastes.
- **Screening**: ask patient if they have been out of the country in the last 3-6 months.

Security Plan

A **security plan** is a plan that is set in place to help guide the actions of employees in case of a breach in security at a healthcare facility. All employees must be educated and comfortable with their facilities plan, in order to facilitate the safety of staff and patients alike. The security plan usually has several components:

- **Security workers**: Most facilities have securities guards who patrol the campus and help maintain patient and visitor safety. If a patient/visitor threatens violence or becomes combative, security should be called immediately.
- **Silent Alarms:** Most units have "silent alarms", which are usually buttons or switches underneath the secretary's desk or in some other discreet location. These are pushed in the case of a threat to security in which a call cannot safely be made.

- **Locked units**: Certain units in the hospital (such as Mother/Baby, critical care units, psychiatric floors, etc.) are locked and require an access code to enter.
- **"Do Not Acknowledge":** Certain patients may be deemed as "do not acknowledge", meaning that the nurse cannot give out any information regarding these patients, including acknowledging the patients' presence in the facility. Examples include psychiatric patients, victims of crime, celebrities, and others. If someone calls asking about the patient, it is appropriate and ethical for the nurse to state "I do not have any information regarding a patient with that name."
- **Over-head Announcements**: Many facilities have different codes that they may call overhead to alert staff of emergences/safety threats.
- **Newborn nursery security**: Measure include matching ID bands for infant and parents/caregivers, footprinting and photographing the infant after birth, transporting infants in bassinets rather than carrying them, utilizing a tracking and security alarm system that can trigger automatic lockdown, limiting access to obstetrics and nursery areas, having staff wear easily-identifiable ID badges, and utilizing video surveillance.
- **Violence prevention**: Measures include educating staff about de-escalation techniques, having an alarm system in place, providing adequate security, utilizing video surveillance, limiting access, identifying clients who may be at risk for behaving violently, and requiring visitors' badges.
- **Controlled access**: Measures include locked areas that require a password, biologic ID (fingerprint, eye scan), or access card for entry, turnstiles at entry and/or metal detectors, security personal stationed at entry points, and video surveillance of entries, exits, stairwells, hallways, elevators, and storage areas.

Principles of Evacuation in a Security Plan

Principles of evacuation in a security plan, according to OSHA, should include:

- Conditions that would trigger an evacuation.
- Chain of command for decision making.
- Procedures for evacuation, including methods of evacuation and preferred routes. Exits should be clearly identified.
- Procedures for assisting clients who are disabled and those who do not speak English.
- Procedures for determining who are responsible for terminating critical operations.
- Procedures for tracking personnel and clients.
- Transportation plans for transferal of clients to other facilities.

The path of least resistance is an important concept to understand for evacuation, especially if they involve fire and any products of combustion (smoke, heat, gas). Fire's path of least resistance is usually vertical and upward although fire also spreads horizontally, especially if a vertical path is not available. Water, on the other hand, also flows vertically, but downward and then horizontally if the downward flow is blocked. Clients should be evacuated according to the path of least resistance; that is, the route that is the easiest and safest.

Handling Hazardous Materials

Hazardous Materials

Hazardous materials, those that are ignitable, corrosive, reactive, or toxic, are any that are harmful to humans or the environment and may be solids, liquids, solid gases, or sludges. Each facility should have a plan in place for appropriate handling of hazardous materials:

- Staff must be trained in safe handling of hazardous materials with training repeated at least annually.
- Appropriate personal protective equipment (PPE) should be available for staff members handling hazardous materials.
- Hazardous materials should be clearly labeled for easy identification.
- All hazardous materials must be safely and securely stored in appropriate environmental temperatures and conditions.
- Materials Safety Data Sheets (SDS) must be readily available for all hazardous materials.
- Decontamination procedures must be reviewed and appropriate decontamination facilities (such as eyewash stations and showers) must be available.
- Records must be maintained for any accidental exposures (with or without injury) and reported to the appropriate authorities.

Internal Radiation Therapy

Internal radiation therapy (brachytherapy) may be utilized to treat a variety of cancers, including prostate, breast, and cervical cancer. Radiation implants may be permanent or temporary. Temporary implants may have high-dose radiation (HDR) or low-dose radiation (LDR). Systemic brachytherapy may be administered per IV with radioactive isotopes; intraluminal and intracavity, per catheters or tubes; and interstitial, per seeds, needles, small implants, or wires. Symptoms relate to the area being irradiated, but the skin and GI tract are usually the most sensitive. Bone marrow suppression may occur if the source of radiation is near bone marrow, and clients may experience fatigue and weakness. Because clients emit radiation during therapy, safeguards include:

- Specific limitations and safeguards posted at room by X-ray department outlining requirements, such as time limits for contact time.
- Visitors limited to non-pregnant adults who must be 6 feet from the client and remain in room no longer than 30 minutes each day.
- Staff, limited to those who are non-pregnant, must wear dosimeters for contact with client.
- Client placed in private room.
- Staff limit time in room to only that necessary to carry out care (in accordance with posted guidelines).

Infectious Diseases and Infection Control

Norwalk Family of Virus Infections

Viral gastroenteritis, more commonly known as food poisoning, has at its root a member of the Norwalk family of viruses. It is a preeminent cause of illness in the United States, occurring mostly during winter months. It is estimated that Norwalk viruses are behind about a third of all viral gastroenteritis cases, and the only viral illness reported to a greater extent is the common cold. Though not permanent (people can become reinfected), half the population over 18 develops immunity because it gradually increases with age.

Norwalk gastroenteritis is transmitted through drinking water or foods that have been contaminated with human feces, water being the most common source of outbreaks. Eating raw or insufficiently steamed clams and oysters that come from polluted beds makes for a high risk of Norwalk virus infection. But other foods, not just shellfish, may be contaminated by food handlers. Illness usually comes on about 24 to 48 hours after eating or drinking. The disease is self-limiting, lasting between 24 and 60 hours, and is mild. It is characterized by diarrhea, nausea, vomiting, and abdominal pain.

Treatment includes:

- Supportive treatment

Prevention includes the following:

- Eat thoroughly cooked foods
- Wash hands, disinfect common areas

Entamoeba Histolytica Infections

Amebiasis (or *amoebiasis*), the infection caused by *E. histolytica*, can last for up to 4 years with no symptoms, some gastrointestinal distress, or dysentery, complete with blood and mucus. Potential complications include pain from ulcers or abscesses, and, rarely, intestinal blockage.

The amoeba's cysts survive, especially under moist conditions, in water, soils, and on foods. They result in infections when they are swallowed; they excyst to the trophozoite stage in the digestive tract, with the possibility of other tissues being invaded. Ingestion of one viable cyst, it is thought, is enough to cause an infection.

Amebiasis is transmitted primarily by fecal contamination of drinking water and foods, and also through direct contact with dirty hands or objects. Because sexual contact may also transmit the disease, AIDS/AIDS-related complex (ARC) patients are very vulnerable. Fatalities are infrequent.

Treatment includes:

- Supportive care: rehydration

Prevention is as follows:

- Wash hands, drink clean drinking water, wash fruits/vegetables.
- Close mouth when swimming/avoid swallowing pond water.

Clostridium Botulinum Infections

The heat-resistant spores of **Clostridium botulinum** can produce a deadly neurotoxin in poorly processed foods, with most of the outbreaks reported annually in the United States (from 10 to 30) associated with home-canned foods. Occasionally, though, commercially produced foods are at fault—canned meat products, canned vegetables, and canned seafood products are the most frequent sources.

The organism and its spores occur widely in soils as well as stream, lake, and ocean sediments, intestinal tracts of fish and mammals, and in the gills and viscera of crabs and other shellfish. It also appears in honey, which is definitively linked to infant botulism but not in any cases involving adults. Foods are not involved in the botulism sometimes found in wounds; it results when *C.*

botulinum infects a wound, producing toxins that travel via the bloodstream to infect other parts of the body.

Treatment includes:

- Supportive Care
- Antitoxin

Prevention is as follows:

- Heat canned foods to 80 °C for 10 minutes or longer to destroy spores
- Never feed infants younger than 12 months raw honey
- Difficulty breathing/muscle rigidity—report immediately!

Gram-Negative Campylobacter Jejuni Infections

While seldom deadly, **Campylobacter** is the most common cause of diarrhea in the United States. Of some 100,000 who contract it yearly in the United States, only about 100 die. It can sometimes occur in outbreaks, and there may be long-term consequences of infection. Some people may develop arthritis following campylobacteriosis. Others may develop Guillain-Barré syndrome, which is a rare autoimmune disease that affects nerves throughout the body, beginning several weeks after the diarrheal illness. Paralysis may last several weeks and usually requires intensive care. As many as 40% of Guillain-Barré syndrome cases in this country may be triggered by campylobacteriosis, usually as a result of eating or handling raw or undercooked poultry meat. An outbreak in 1988 was caused by milk that had been improperly pasteurized.

Treatment is as follows:

- IV fluids/electrolytes, supportive care
- Should resolve in a week; may prescribe antibiotics

Prevention is as follows:

- Cook meat thoroughly, use separate cutting boards for meat/vegetables, wash hands before and after handling raw meat
- Wash hands after petting animals/before eating

Escherichia Coli (E. Coli)

Escherichia coli, the coliform bacteria most abundant in the colon and normally innocuous, can upon acquiring a virulence factor, cause enteric infections such as traveler's diarrhea. This can lead to osmotic diarrhea by inhibiting uptake of salt. It can also cause hemolytic uremic syndrome (HUS), making possible acute renal failure as well as urinary tract infections such as cystitis and pyelonephritis, neonatal meningitis, respiratory infection, and bacteremia. Particularly bad strains can produce hemorrhagic colitis with severe cramping and bloody diarrhea. The illness, usually self-limited, lasts for an average of 8 days.

Treatment is as follows:

- Fluid Resuscitation – IV fluids and electrolytes
- Antibiotics are discouraged, due to the germ's resistance; urinary tract infections can be treated with trimethoprim/sulfamethoxazole or ampicillin, and meningitis with third-generation cephalosporin (ceftriaxone)

Prevention is as follows:

- Cook meat thoroughly and wash all vegetables before eating.
- Wash hands after petting animals/before eating.

Cryptosporidium Parvum

Severe watery diarrhea marks intestinal **cryptosporidiosis**, while tracheal cryptosporidiosis causes coughing and mild fever, and sometimes severe intestinal distress. They are both caused by a single-celled obligate intracellular parasite. Herd animals (cows, goats, sheep) and humans may be infected with the *Cryptosporidium parvum* sporocysts, which are resistant to most chemical disinfectants. Drying and the ultraviolet portion of sunlight are deadly to them.

Presumably, one organism in infected food touched by a contaminated food handler can initiate an infection. Incidence is high in child day care centers where food is served. Another possible source of human infection is raw manure that has been spread over garden vegetables, but large outbreaks invariably have contaminated water supplies as their source. Up to 80% of the population has been infected with cryptosporidiosis. There is no effective treatment, and the severe watery diarrhea is often a contributor in the death of AIDS victims; invasion of the pulmonary system may also be fatal.

Treatment includes:

- Supportive care: rehydration.

Prevention is as follows:

- Wash hands, clean drinking water, wash fruits/vegetables.

Giardia Lamblia Infections

Giardia lamblia is a parasite and the causative agent of giardiasis, the most frequent source of non-bacterial diarrhea in North America. Ingestion of 1 or more protozoan cysts may bring on diarrhea within a week; however, for most bacterial illnesses, at least thousands of organisms may have to be consumed to produce illness. Illness normally lasts for 7-14 days, but there are cases of chronic infections lasting months to years. Chronic cases, both those with defined immune deficiencies and those without, are difficult to treat.

Giardiasis most frequently results from drinking contaminated water, though outbreaks have been traced to food contamination, and it is impossible to rule out contaminated vegetables eaten raw as sources of infection. It is more prevalent in children, possibly because many adults seem to have a lasting immunity after infection. It can also spread through anal sex.

Treatment includes the following:

- Supportive care: rehydration
- Medications: metronidazole, tinidazole, nitazoxanide if severe

Prevention includes the following:

- Wash hands, clean drinking water, wash fruits/vegetables
- Close mouth when swimming/avoid swallowing pond water
- Practice safe sex

Coronavirus Infections

A **coronavirus** is a common virus that causes cold-like symptoms, including a cough, runny nose, sore throat, and congestion. Most cases of coronavirus are not dangerous and are often given little attention or go entirely unnoticed. However, specific coronavirus strains have led to two worldwide pandemics. The first, **Severe Acute Respiratory Syndrome (SARS)**, appeared in China in 2002 and quickly spread worldwide. Presenting symptoms of SARS were fever, cough, dyspnea, and general malaise. It was extremely virulent, spreading easily from person to person through close contact by way of contaminated droplets produced by coughing or sneezing. SARS was also very deadly, with a case fatality rate of nearly 10%. High rates of infection occurred in health care workers and others in contact with infected patients, so prompt diagnosis and proper isolation were essential. By 2004, there were no longer any documented active cases of SARS.

The most recent coronavirus outbreak was the **COVID-19** strain, which first appeared in December of 2019, in the Chinese city of Wuhan, and quickly became a global pandemic. Presentation of COVID-19 was similar to that of SARS, with the notable additional symptom of acute loss of taste/smell as a unique identifier. Much is still unknown about this strain, including exact transmission methods (though droplet transmission is suspected), effective treatment protocols, and long-term effects.

Precautions to take when treating patients with pandemic coronavirus include the following:

- Contact and droplet precautions, including eye protection and appropriate personal protection equipment.
- Airborne precautions (recommended by the CDC), especially with aerosol-producing procedures (ventilators, nebulizers, intubation).
- Immediate notification of public health authorities and institution of contact tracing.
- Activity restrictions of exposed health care workers planned in coordination with public health officials.

Gram-Positive Listeria Monocytogenes Infections

Listeriosis, caused by **Listeria monocytogenes**, finds expression in encephalitis, meningitis (or meningoencephalitis), and septicemia. It is also a factor in intrauterine or cervical infections in pregnant women. (It can result in stillbirth or spontaneous abortion.) Onset to GI symptoms may take more than 12 hours, whereas the time to serious forms of listeriosis may range from a few days to 3 weeks. For infections during pregnancy, the mother usually survives. It has been associated with consuming raw or badly pasteurized milk, raw meats of all types, ice cream, and uncooked vegetables. Cheeses, raw and cooked poultry, fermented raw-meat sausages, and raw and smoked fish are thought to be other sources. Particularly concerning is the fact that it can grow in refrigerated foods.

Treatment is as follows:

- Listeriosis is effectively treated with penicillin, ampicillin, or trimethoprim/sulfamethoxazole.

Prevention includes the following:

- Date all refrigerated items and do not use past expiration/best-by dates.
- Cook meat thoroughly; wash hands before and after preparation.

Rotavirus Infections

Rotaviruses, transmitted by the fecal-oral route, are spread most commonly by dirty hands. Commonly found in day care centers, pediatric and geriatric wards, and family homes, they may also be found in uncooked food contaminated by infected food handlers. Sanitary measures adequate for bacteria and parasites seem to be ineffective in controlling rotavirus; a similar incidence of infection is observed in countries with both high and low health standards.

Those with severe diarrhea who do not get quick access to fluid and electrolyte replacement may die; otherwise, recovery from infections is usually complete. Childhood mortality due to rotavirus is relatively low in the United States, with an estimated 100 cases/year, but approaches nearly a million cases per year worldwide. Of childhood cases of severe diarrhea that require hospitalization, about half can be attributed to group A rotavirus.

Treatment includes:

- Supportive care: rehydration.

Prevention includes the following:

- Wash hands, drink clean drinking water, wash fruits/vegetables.
- Close mouth when swimming/avoid swallowing pond water.

Shigella Infections

The illness caused by **Shigella (shigellosis)** accounts for less than 10% of the reported outbreaks of foodborne illness in the United States, at an estimated 300,000 cases. Infants, elderly patients, and those in poor health are susceptible to the most severe symptoms of the disease, but all humans are susceptible to some degree. Fatalities may be as high as 10%-15% with some strains. Shigellosis is a very common malady suffered by individuals with AIDS. The organism is frequently found in water polluted with human feces. Infection, which requires as few as 10 cells, depending on age and condition of the host, is characterized by abdominal pain, cramps, diarrhea, fever, vomiting, blood, pus, or mucus in stools. The usual medium is food contamination, usually through the fecal-oral route, as a result of unsanitary food handling.

Treatment includes:

- Supportive care: rehydration.

Prevention includes the following:

- Wash hands, drink clean drinking water, wash fruits/vegetables.
- Close mouth when swimming/avoid swallowing pond water.
- Practice safe sex.

Pseudomonas Aeruginosa Infections

Pseudomonas aeruginosa is an opportunistic pathogen, exploiting breaks in host defenses to initiate urinary tract infections, respiratory system infections, dermatitis, soft tissue infections, bacteremia, bone and joint infections, gastrointestinal infections, and a wide variety of nosocomial infections. Particularly active in patients with cancer, cystic fibrosis, severe burns, or immunosuppressed AIDS, this disease has a fatality rate of 50% in these patients.

Accounting for 10% of all hospital-acquired infections, *Pseudomonas aeruginosa* is the fourth most commonly isolated nosocomial pathogen. Only the antibiotic drug classes of fluoroquinolones, gentamicin, and imipenem are effective against it, and even these drugs are not effective against all strains. *In wounds, it is infamous for the blue-green colored discharge it creates.* The futility of treating *Pseudomonas* infections with antibiotics is most dramatically illustrated in cystic fibrosis patients, virtually all of whom eventually become infected with a strain so resistant that it cannot be treated, and death is the general outcome.

Treatment includes the following:

- Intense antibiotic therapy
- Supportive treatment.

Prevention includes the following:

- Clean mop water and other solutions
- Wash hands, disinfect common areas

Vibrio Cholerae Serogroup O1 Infections

Unsanitary conditions pollute waters, providing the breeding grounds for **Vibrio cholerae**, the bacterium responsible for epidemic cholera.

Ingested viable bacteria attach to the small intestine and produce cholera toxin. Dehydration and loss of essential electrolytes bring death. While formerly responsible for mass epidemics, with today's medical advances, supportive care means the illness is generally self-limiting.

Treatment includes the following:

- Rehydration, either intravenously or orally, with a solution containing sodium chloride, sodium bicarbonate, potassium chloride, and dextrose (glucose).
- Antibiotics such as tetracycline have been shown to shorten the course of the illness.

Prevention includes the following:

- Ensure water is clean before drinking: avoid drinking stale water or water from outdoor streams/ponds
- Increased risk with seafood

Varicella Zoster Virus

Varicella zoster ("chickenpox") is a common childhood illness, though it can cause severe illness and complications such as encephalitis and bacteremia in adults. It is highly contagious, and can be spread 2 days before the appearance of a rash until the point where all lesions are crusted over.

Signs and Symptoms: Incubation 11-21 days; runny/stuffy nose, cough, sneezing, 24-48 hours later, rash with small blisters of variable size usually beginning on head and chest, spreading to limbs, reddened skin, fever.

Diagnosis: physical exam, can confirm with blood test if necessary.

Treatment includes the following:

- Patient must be kept in isolation. If the patient scratches the lesions they will spread.
- Severe cases: Acyclovir or infusion of immunoglobulin.
- Immunization available; important, because once a child has had varicella, they can develop shingles later in life. However, cannot catch varicella twice.
- Symptom management: calamine lotion, cool oatmeal or baking soda baths, trim fingernails and have child wear gloves; Tylenol or Advil/Motrin for fever (do not give aspirin, which may cause Reye syndrome).

Hepatitis A Virus Infections

Hepatitis A is a systemic viral infection (short incubation type hepatitis) that involves the liver. Hepatitis A is extremely contagious and caused by an RNA enterovirus. It is transmitted via the fecal-oral route or paternally. It is most often found in areas of poor sanitation and overcrowding, though epidemics from contaminated food and water also occur. The period of communicability extends from early in the incubation period to about a week after the development of jaundice. Most cases resolve within 3 weeks and there are seldom fatalities.

Signs and Symptoms: sudden onset of fever, malaise, nausea, anorexia, abdominal discomfort, jaundice, enlarged liver (hepatomegaly), dark urine, transient pale stools, upper right abdominal quadrant pain, and fatigue.

Diagnosis: blood work - hepatitis A antibodies

Treatment is supportive: rest, fluids, nutrition

Patient education should include education on the disease and disease process, education on hygiene, handwashing, vaccinations to prevent hepatitis A. Educate the individual to cover broken or open skin and to avoid sexual contact and food preparation.

*Hepatitis E, which has symptoms similar to Hepatitis A, has a fatality rate of 20% among pregnant women.

Pandemic Influenza

Pandemic influenza is a worldwide epidemic of influenza that causes serious respiratory illness and/or death in large populations of people. Pandemics can occur when a virus mutates, creating a new subtype that infects humans and spreads easily from person to person. Should a global outbreak and a pandemic occur, the implications for health care are profound because the potential number of infected patients will be overwhelming to the medical system.

Precautions are as follows:

- Standard precautions with careful hand hygiene.
- Contact precautions with gloves and gown for all patient contact and goggles when within 3 feet.
- Dedicated equipment.
- Airborne precautions in isolated negative pressure rooms and use of N-95 filter respirator.

Nosocomial Infections

The following are different types of nosocomial infections:

- **Exogenous infections**: Caused by microorganisms that are not found in normal flora (e.g., *Aspergillus, Salmonella*).
- **Endogenous infections**: Microorganism overgrowth causes a different area of the body to become infected (e.g., enterococci (GI) to wound site or *E. coli* (GI) to urinary tract via Foley catheter).
- **Iatrogenic infections**: Infections that are caused by procedures (e.g., UTI after Foley insertion or bacteremia after IV insertion).

Infection Control Strategies

The following are some common **infection control strategies** used by health care workers:

- **Transmission-based precautions** are appropriate for some patients, especially those who are immunocompromised.
- **Handwashing and aseptic techniques** are especially important for person-to-person transmission.
- **Central venous line precautions** include using antimicrobial/antiseptic-coated catheters, using clear dressings that do not obscure site; assess for signs of infection.
- **Cleaning equipment** used for multiple patients in between uses.
- **Temperature monitoring, full body assessments**, and questionnaires as appropriate will help identify infections early.
- **Post-discharge questionnaires** or telephone surveys of patients and physicians can identify potential problems after discharge.
- **Preoperative shaving should be replaced with clipping** and depilatories, or done immediately prior to procedures.
- **Glucose/blood sugar control** increases resistance to infection.
- **Teach medication compliance**: must take all antibiotics exactly as prescribed to decrease antibiotic resistance.
- **Protect immunocompromised patients**: no fresh flowers/fruit, wear mask, no sick visitors, dedicated equipment.

Standard/Universal Precautions

Standard/ Universal Precautions are used with all patients to prevent the spread of pathogens. They apply to blood; all body fluids, secretions, and excretions (except sweat), regardless of whether or not they contain visible blood; non-intact skin; and mucous membranes.

- Proper handwashing should be utilized at all times.
- Wear gloves when contact is possible with any body fluids/blood.
- Never recap needles, and immediately place used needles in the closest puncture-resistant container, which should be removed for disposal when about 3/4 full. Never point a needle toward any part of the body or manipulate it using both hands.
- Should mouth-to-mouth resuscitation become necessary, it must be performed only with the use of mouthpieces, resuscitation bags, or other ventilation devices.
- A patient who contaminates the environment and will not (or cannot) follow rules of proper hygiene and environmental control must be placed in a private room.

Correct Procedure for Handwashing

Handwashing is the number one way to prevent disease, if done properly. The proper technique for both is as follows:

- Soap and water:
  - Performed when hands are visibly soiled, beginning/end of shift, after using the restroom, or any other time as needed.
  - Handwashing is done under running water with soap.
  - Hands must be lathered thoroughly and scrubbed for a full 30 seconds, covering all areas of the hands and wrists with soap, and then rinsed.
  - The faucet should be turned off by using the elbow or upper forearm or holding a piece of paper towel as a barrier.
  - Hands should be dried using disposable, clean towels. Keep hands above elbows so water runs in one direction (clean to dirty).
- Alcohol-based scrub:
  - Performed when entering/exiting rooms, taking off gloves, patient contact, etc.
  - All hand surfaces should be thoroughly coated with the alcohol rub, including between the fingers, the wrists, and under the nails.
  - Hands rubbed together until the solution evaporates. Hands should not be rinsed.

Surgical Asepsis

Principles of surgical asepsis are as follows:

- A sterile object remains sterile only when touched by another sterile object.
- Only sterile objects may be placed on a sterile field.
- A sterile object or field out of the range of vision or an object held below a person's waist is contaminated.
- A sterile object or field becomes contaminated by prolonged exposure to air.
- When a sterile surface comes in contact with a wet, contaminated surface, the sterile object or field becomes contaminated by capillary action.
- Fluid flows in the direction of gravity – clean from clean-to-dirty, top-to-bottom.
- The edges of a sterile field or container are considered to be contaminated about 1 inch from the outer edge.
- When opening sterile supplies, avoid crossing over the sterile object or sterile field.

Transmission of Infection in Operating Rooms

Strategies for preventing and controlling transmission of infection in operating rooms include:

- **Preoperative surgical hand scrubs** for 3-5 minutes and aseptic techniques at all times.
- **Positive-pressure ventilation** with respect to corridors and adjacent areas.
- ≥15 air exchanges per hour (ACH*)* with at least 3 fresh air.
- *Filtering* of all recirculated and fresh air though filters with 90% efficiency.
- **Horizontal laminar airflow** or introduction of air at ceiling and exhaust near the floor level.
- **Operating room closed** except to allow passage of essential equipment and staff.
- **Clean visible soiling** with approved disinfectants between patients.
- **Wet vacuum** operating room at end of each day.
- **Sterilize surgical equipment** and avoid use of flash sterilization.

- **Perform environmental sampling** of surfaces or air as part of epidemiological investigation.
- Establish protocols for patients with airborne precautions, such as tuberculosis.

Surgical Hand Disinfection

Surgical handwashing aims to remove and kill transient flora and decrease resident flora to reduce the risk of wound contamination should surgical gloves undergo damage. Agents are the same as those used for hygienic hand washes, the primary difference being that more time is spent in scrubbing, an extra 2-3 minutes, and it includes both wrists and forearms.

Sterile disposable or nailbrushes sterilized in an autoclave may be used to clean the fingernails only, but not to scrub the hands. A brush should only be used for the first scrub of the day.

After handwashing with soap and water, a hand rub with an alcohol base formulation (70%) should be used if possible. This enhances the destruction or inhibition of resident skin flora. If an alcohol preparation is used, two applications of 5 mL each is suggested, both rubbed to dryness. Sterile towels should be used to dry the hands thoroughly after washing and before alcohol is applied.

Surgical Wound Infections

Surgical wound infections typically occur on approximately the fifth postoperative day. There may be initial symptoms present during the first 36 to 48 hours following a surgical procedure. Causative agents of surgical wound infections include, but are not limited to, *Staphylococcus aureus*, *Escherichia coli*, *Pseudomonas aeruginosa*, *Proteus vulgaris*, and *Enterobacter aerogenes*.

Signs and Symptoms: increased temperature, pulse, respirations, and blood pressure; reddened wound, purulent/foul-smelling discharge, swelling, dehiscence (opening of the wound)

Diagnosis: culture of wound, physical exam, blood work (WBCs)

Treatment includes the following:

- Medications: antibiotics (based on culture results), Tylenol
- Monitor for systemic effects
- Apply and change dressings as ordered
- *Wound Assessment:* **OREEDA**: **O**dor, **R**edness, **E**dema, **E**cchymosis, **D**rainage, **A**pproximation
- *Drainage Amount*: **C-COAL**: **C**olor, **C**onsistency, **O**dor, **A**mount, **L**ocation

Review Video: Wound Infection
Visit mometrix.com/academy and enter code: 794740

Terms Related to Surgery

Emergency	Something that must be immediately performed to save the patient's life, such as an appendectomy, traumatic amputation repair, etc.
Diagnostic	Surgical exploration, such as a biopsy or laparoscopy.
Ablative	Removal or excision or removal of a diseased part, via amputation, appendectomy, tissue, cholecystectomy, colostomy, etc.
Palliative	Reduces or relieves symptoms or pain but does not provide a cure. Examples include colostomies and debridement.
Reconstructive	Restores tissue function or appearance via scar revision, ORIF, etc.
Transplant	Replaces failing or diseased organs, such as a kidney, heart, lung, cornea, or liver.
Constructive	Restores lost or reduced function from congenital deformities, such as a cleft palate and lip.
Cosmetic/plastic	Improves appearance, for example, facelift or rhinoplasty.

PPE for Protection Against Communicable Diseases

Personal Protective Equipment (PPE) are devices and wearable items such as surgical gowns, gloves, masks and respirators that act as barriers between the infectious material and the health care provider. The use of PPE alone does not fully protect against acquiring an infection. Handwashing, isolation of patients, and care in coughing or sneezing are also important to minimize risk of infection, and protective clothing should be changed whenever torn or ripped.

- **Gloves:** worn before touching mucous membranes/nonintact skin, or other potentially infectious substances. Must be removed promptly after use without touching outside; donned last after all other PPE; removed first.
- **Goggles/Faceshield**: non-vented, worn when there is a risk of splashing/risk to face or eyes.
- **Gowns:** moisture resistant, worn when there is risk of contamination on clothes from blood/body fluids. Put on first.
- **Mask**: protect patient from droplets during sterile procedure, but also protect nurse as well. For airborne precautions, a special mask called a N95 respirator should be specially fitted to the nurse and used. Put on after gown.

PPE is listed above in the order in which it should be removed.

Isolation of Patients with Communicable Disease

Contact Precautions

Contact precautions reduce the risk of transmitting microorganisms by skin-to-skin contact, whether direct, as occurs when health care personnel perform activities requiring physical contact with a patient, or indirect via contaminated intermediate objects in the patient's environment.

- **Patient placement**: A private room when possible.
- **Gloves and handwashing**: Wear gloves, dispose of them and wash hands before leaving a patient's room.
- **Gowns**: Wear when there is any chance of clothing touching a contaminated person or surface.
- **Patient transport**: Limit movement and use barriers to prevent spread of infection.
- **Patient care equipment**: Avoid, if possible, using a piece of durable equipment with more than one patient.

Droplet Precautions

Droplet precautions are used for diseases transmitted through large droplets (larger than 5 μm in size). They infect by making contact with the mucous membranes of the nose or mouth of a target. They are contained in droplets generated from a carrier's cough or sneeze, or even talking.

- Gown/gloves worn when contact with fluids is likely, and a mask should be worn when working within 3 ft of the patient. May also need to wear a mask during suctioning.
- Have patient wear a mask during transport
- Can have door open; private room, or room with cohort
- Used for the following pathogens: **SPIDERMAN**
  - S – sepsis, scarlet fever, streptococcal pharyngitis
  - P – parvovirus B19, pneumonia, pertussis
  - I – influenza
  - D – diptheria (pharyngeal)
  - E – epiglottitis
  - R – rubella
  - M – mumps/meningitis/mycoplasma/meningeal pneumonia
  - An – adenovirus

Airborne Precautions

Airborne precautions are to be taken with infected patients to prevent transmitting disease through airborne droplets containing suspended microorganisms that can be dispersed by air currents.

1. Place infected patients in a private, closed-off room equipped with a monitored, high-efficiency air filtration system and negative air pressure system, minimum of 6 exchanges per hour.
2. If no private room is available, the patient may be cohorted – placed in a room with another patient with the same infection.
3. All personnel must wear gown, gloves, and respiratory protection when entering the room, using special N95 respirator mask or PAPR machine.
4. Limit movement and transport of patients outside the room to essential purposes only, at which time the patient must wear a surgical mask to minimize dispersal of droplet nuclei.

Body Mechanics and Home Safety

Ergonomics

Ergonomics is the study of preventing workplace injury and stress. In nursing, it refers to the way in which a nurse can prevent injury to self and others due to the stressors and strains required in the nursing field. Some important ergonomic principles include:

- **Body Mechanics:** The body should be kept in proper alignment during tasks, with a wide base of support and center of gravity low. Use larger muscles (buttocks, thighs, shoulders) for activities rather than smaller when possible. Avoid twisting or jerking movements. Maintain 90° angle in elbows and knees when sitting, elbows at the side, with back straight and looking straight ahead.

- **Lifting:** Use appropriate transfer devices; use as many people as necessary. Manual lifting should be avoided. Bend at the knees, tighten core, and keep weights close to the body – *never* bend or twist when lifting.
- **Repetition**: Avoid repetitive movements/stressors and use proper safety equipment when needed (earplugs for loud noises, etc.).

Assistive Devices

Crutches should be properly fitted before client attempts ambulation. Correct height is one hand-width below axillae. The handgrips should be adjusted so the client supports the body weight comfortably with elbows slightly flexed rather than locked in place. The client should be cautioned not to bear weight under the axillae as this can cause nerve damage but to hold the crutches tight against the side of the chest wall. The type of gait used depends on the type of injury.

A **cane** should be held in the opposite hand of the side of injury. When holding the cane in neutral position, the elbow should be bent at about a 15-degree angle and if holding the cane straight down to the side of the body, the top of the cane should be in line with the crease of the wrist.

The same is true of a **walker**, the elbow should be bent at 15 degrees when standing up straight and grasping the handles, and the handle grasps should be in line with to the crease of the wrists. The client should be able to move the walker forward without leaning over.

Modifications for Home Safety

Modifications for **home safety** may include:

- **Lighting**: Entry ways and stairwells especially must have adequate lighting to prevent falls. Lighting throughout the home should be assessed to determine if lightbulbs need to be replaced and if lighting is adequate for the client to move safely through the home.
- **Handrails**: Stairways should have handrails. Additionally, some clients may need handrails in long hallways as well. Bathrooms may need grab bars to assist clients getting onto and off of the toilet and in and out of the tub or shower.
- **Kitchen safety**: Items may be moved for convenient access as well as a sturdy step stool provided. Unsafe equipment/tools (such as knives for those with cognitive impairment) should be removed. The client's ability to safely use a gas stove should be assessed (especially older models with less safety features). The temperature of water at the sink should be adjusted so that it does not exceed 120 degrees.

Fire/Environmental Hazards in a Home Safety Evaluation

Fire and environmental hazards that may be found in a home safety evaluation include:

- Frayed cords on electrical appliances, multiple electrical cords plugged into power strips.
- Paper or other combustibles near heaters, fireplaces, or other sources or heat and/or flames.
- Gas leaks, gas stoves (especially for clients with cognitive impairment) or other appliances.
- Electric cords across walkways, space heaters.
- Clutter, especially on floors and in walkways, throw rugs.
- Inadequate lighting, stairways or steps without safety rails.
- Kerosene heaters, use of candles, matches within reach of children.
- Lack of smoke/carbon monoxide detectors.
- Furniture with sharp corners, Hazardous materials/substances within reach of children.

- Hot water heater temperature set too high (>120 degree).
- Lack of grab bars in the bathroom.

Carbon Monoxide Poisoning

Carbon monoxide poisoning occurs when people breathe in carbon monoxide, usually related to industrial or household accidents or suicide attempts. Carbon monoxide binds to hemoglobin 200 times more readily than oxygen, and once the carbon monoxide binds to hemoglobin (creating carboxyhemoglobin), the hemoglobin can no longer bind to or transport oxygen, resulting in hypoxemia.

Signs and Symptoms: Varies depending on percentage of saturation. At 10%, patients may complain of headache and nausea. At >20%, patient becomes increasingly weak and confused with alterations in mental status. At >30%, patient may have dyspnea, chest pain, and increased confusion. When the level continues to increase, patient may experience seizures, coma, and death. Skin color may be cyanotic, pink, or bright cherry red (but not a reliable sign); realize that pulse oximetry may read 100%, but patient is severely hypoxic.

Diagnosis: evaluation of symptoms and situation, carboxyhemoglobin level per CO-oximeter.

Treatment: Patient should be administered 100% oxygen with non-rebreather mask. Hyperbaric oxygen treatment is utilized for some patients with severe symptoms.

Preventive Maintenance

Preventive maintenance requires inspecting equipment for safety. Steps include:

- **Organizing**: Checklists should be prepared for different types of equipment to ensure that preventive maintenance is done consistently, following the same procedures, so that no steps are missed.
- **Cleaning/Storing**: The appropriate manner of cleaning (including the correct cleaning solution), drying, sterilizing, and storing surgical equipment should be utilized to prevent damage. Blood and body fluids should be removed within 20 minutes of surgery, if possible, to prevent corrosion of metal.
- **Inspecting/Testing**: All equipment should be examined with each use to ensure it is intact and operating correctly. Cords of all electrical equipment must be inspected and the equipment removed from service with any sign of fraying or breakage. Routine testing should be carried out. Multiple adaptors and plugs should be avoided.
- **Maintaining**: According to manufacturer's guidelines, all routine maintenance procedures should be scheduled, carried out, and documented.
- **Repairing/Reporting**: Damaged equipment should be reported to the appropriate department/person and immediately removed, repaired, or discarded if unusable. Replacement parts should be readily available to prevent extended down time.

Incident Reporting

Incident Reporting should take place anytime there is a situation in which patient/employee safety is actually or potentially compromised. While many nurses may hesitate to complete incident reports due to fear of punitive action, it is important to realize that incident reporting is a critical component of quality improvement and safety. Incident reports should be filled out as quickly as possible after the occurrence, to ensure the report is accurate and devoid of omissions. The nurse should use simple and precise language to describe what occurred, and should not include opinions or theories related to the event. When reviewing incident reports, the circumstances and precipitating factors of the incident should all be analyzed to see where the break(s) from policy occurred, or if there needs to be new policy written to avoid future incidents of the same kind.

Practice Errors and Near Misses

Situations when **reporting events** is appropriate include falls, injuries, medication errors (wrong medications, wrong dosage, missed medication), and any type of abuse, practice errors, or near misses. Many incidents include some type of injury (such as a needlestick), but all incidents must be reported following the protocol established by the organization. For example, if a client receives the wrong dosage of a medication, the usual procedure is to document the actual dosage given and the client's response and to fill out an incident report that is maintained separately from the client's record. In most cases, no mention of the incident report is made in the client's medical record. The incident report is initiated by the staff member who is involved in the incident or observed the incident but must be reviewed by a supervisor before submission. Incident reports include: names of those involved, including witnesses; other identifying information; time; date; location; and narrative description of any actions taken.

Unsafe Practices of Personnel

Unsafe practices of personnel include:

- **Substance abuse**: When personnel are expected of substance abuse (smell of alcohol, impaired cognition/judgment, diversion of drugs), this person should be immediately reported to a supervisor and removed from client care. The nurse, unless in a supervisory position, should not directly accuse the impaired staff person or intervene unless the staff person poses a risk to clients but should also not leave the staff person alone with clients or stand by while the person gives unsafe care.
- **Improper care**: If a nurse observes another healthcare provider giving improper care (contaminated sterile field, improper positioning, incorrect procedure, abusive behavior), the nurse should immediately intervene to protect the client, "Let me help you reposition the client," but should then immediately report the incident to a supervisor.
- **Improper staffing**: If staffing is inadequate according to established guidelines or state regulations, the nurse should report this to an immediate supervisor in the chain of command, explaining exactly where and how the staffing is inadequate.

Client Safety

Restraints

Types

Various **types of restraints** are available to use for client safety:

- **Electronic devices**: Often used as an alternative to traditional restraints, sound alarms, if clients try to get up or climb out of bed. An example is the Ambularm® device that fastens about the client's thigh and signals if the leg is in a dependent position. Weight-sensitive floor mats may also be used.
- **Enclosure (Posey®) bed**: Enclosed bed (soft-sided) allows the client to move freely about the bed but prevents the client from getting out of bed.
- **Physical restraints**: May be fastened about the wrists, ankles, or waist to prevent the client from getting up. Jacket or vest restraints may be utilized to help keep clients from falling out of wheelchairs.

- **Hand mitts/Soft splints**: Used to prevent clients from grabbing at or pulling out tubes.
- **Chemical restraints**: Medications used to control behavior, include antipsychotics and benzodiazepines.
- **Environmental restraints**: Alteration of the environment to reduce risks to clients.

Requirements for Use

Restraints are used to restrict movement, activity, and access. There are two primary types of restraints used with individuals: behavioral and clinical. Behavioral restraints are more commonly used in the psychiatric unit or when individuals are at risk of hurting themselves or others. More commonly, clinical restraints are used to ensure that the individual does not interfere with safe care. The federal government and the Joint Commission have issued strict guidelines for temporary restraints or those not part of standard care (such as post-surgical restraint):

- There must be a written policy.
- An assessment must be completed.
- An alternative method should be tried before applying a restraint.
- An order must be written.
- The least restrictive effective restraint should be used.
- A nurse must remove the restraint, assess, and document findings at least every 2 hours.

Physical restraints may involve the use of a person physically restraining an individual or the use of a mechanical device to restrict movement.

Falls and Fall Prevention

Risk Factors and Fall Prevention

The following are risk factors for falls and interventions:

- **Orthostatic hypotension**: Stand up and move slowly; stand stationary for a few seconds; walk a short distance
- **Urinary incontinence**: bedside commode; assistance
- **Weakness**: therapy; call for help; monitor progress and tolerance
- **Current medications**: hypnotics, sedatives, tranquilizers, diuretics, narcotic analgesics; bed set in low position, maintain half rails or side rail up on one side.
- **Monitoring devices**: employ if available

Restraints for Fall prevention

The appropriate use of restraints is discussed below:

- Need a physician's order in acute and long-term care to apply restraints; renewed every 24 hours.
- Assess patient frequently (every hour with violent/every 2 hours with nonviolent restraints) – circulation, ROM, pain, nutrition and toileting needs.
- Can be delegated to non-licensed personnel; however, nurse is responsible for monitoring.
- More restrictive guidelines with youth/adolescents.

KEY: Use least restrictive device for least amount of time

Review Video: Sedative Hypnotic Drugs
Visit mometrix.com/academy and enter code: 725645

Health Promotion and Maintenance

Normal Physiological Changes in Older Adults

With age, the human body begins to slow down, and the metabolic processes become slower and less effective at repairing age-related damage. The following are **expected changes in the physical assessment of the older adult**:

- **Neurological**: Decreased acuity of hearing/vision/smell; some mild memory loss, especially short-term memory, is common.
- **Cardiac:** Decreased elasticity of heart and blood vessels; anemia.
- **Pulmonary**: Decreased lung capacity. Weakened cough/gag reflex.
- **Gastrointestinal:** Decreased taste, peristalsis, and digestive enzyme production. Dry mouth. Increased occurrence of constipation; increase of fat-muscle ratio.
- **Genitourinary:** Decreased bladder capacity; genital atrophy.
- **Integumentary:** Decreased skin elasticity; dry skin common.
- **Musculoskeletal:** Decreased bone density, decreased balance and muscle strength. Increased fat-muscle ratio.

"Everything slows and decreases, except for fat."

Ante/Intra/Postpartum and Newborn Care

Menstrual Cycle

The **menstrual cycle** is a three-phase cycle in which a woman's body prepares for pregnancy. The days listed are based on a typical 28-day cycle, but it is important to realize that the days can vary based on cycle length and hormone levels of the individual woman.

1. **Menstruation (day 1-6)**: During the menstrual cycle, the woman experiences decreased levels of estrogen and endometrial tissue detaching, resulting in 3-7 days of vaginal bleeding.
2. **Proliferation Phase (day 7-14)**: During the proliferation phase, the woman will experience endometrial thickening, peak levels of estrogen, and decreased body temperature. This phase ends with ovulation.
3. **The Luteal Phase (day 14-28)**: The luteal phase of the menstrual cycle consists at first of increased uterine vascularity, and preparatory signs of implantation. However, if no fertilized ovum implants, the levels of estrogen and progesterone levels begin to decrease, resulting in pale endometrial tissue, vasoconstriction of the spiral arteries, rupture of the blood vessels, and the stromal cells of the uterus become filled with blood as the body prepares for menstruation.

Ovulation

Ovulation is the release of an egg (ovum) from the ovaries, generally occurring on day 14 of the typical menstrual cycle. The ovarian cycle consists of the follicular phase, during which follicle-stimulating hormone (FSH) and luteinizing hormone (LH) begin to be excreted in increasing amounts, causing the maturation of one or more of the graafian or ovarian follicles. When fully mature, the ovarian follicle ruptures and expels the ovum or female egg into the fallopian tube. This event is known as ovulation. If implantation occurs, the ovum will continue to grow and the corpus luteum will secrete estrogen and progesterone to maintain pregnancy. Otherwise, the corpus luteum disintegrates and the levels of progesterone and estrogen will steadily decrease, signaling menstruation to occur.

Some signs and symptoms of ovulation may include:

- Increased watery vaginal discharge.
- "Ferning" pattern of vaginal mucous/saliva.
- Sharp, unilateral abdominal pain (called *Mittelschmerz,* "lightning pain").
- Increase in basal body temperature (BBT).
- Slight mid-cycle spotting.

Pelvic Structures of Women

The following are various types of *pelvic structures* of women:

1. **Gynecoid pelvis:** A gynecoid pelvis is characterized by a round inlet, and is the most often seen type of pelvic structure.
2. **Android pelvis:** An android pelvis is characterized by a heart-shaped inlet, and is the normal male pelvis.
3. **Anthropoid pelvis:** The anthropoid pelvis is characterized by an oval-shaped inlet.
4. **Platypelloid pelvis:** A platypelloid pelvis is characterized by a transverse oval inlet, and is often noted as a flat pelvis.

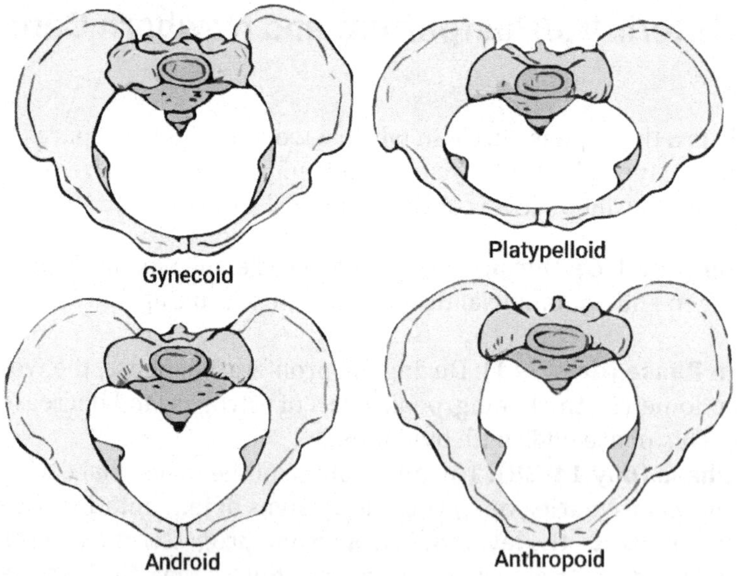

Irregularities Associated with Menses

Irregularities associated with menses include the following:

- **Amenorrhea** is characterized by a lack of or uncharacteristic pause of menses.
- **Dysmenorrhea** is characterized by painful menses.
- **Hypomenorrhea** is characterized by a menses of short duration.
- **Menorrhagia** is characterized by an extensive menses.
- **Oligomenorrhea** is characterized by infrequent menses/ cycle length greater than 35 days.
- **Polymenorrhea** is characterized by abnormally frequent menses.
- **Anovulatory cycle** is characterized by a menstrual cycle in which a woman does not ovulate.

Endometriosis

Endometriosis is the occurrence of endometrial tissue in areas other than the uterine cavity, such as peritoneal surfaces, fallopian tubes, lymph nodes, ovaries, or bowels. Endometriosis can occur in a woman at any age. It is theorized to be caused by retrograde menstruation (flow of menstrual blood backwards through fallopian tubes), but exact cause is not known. Family history, PID, abnormally shaped uterus, and woman without children are at greater risk.

Signs and symptoms: dyspareunia (painful intercourse), dysmenorrhea, dyschezia (difficult production of stool), pelvic and low-back pain (acute or chronic), premenstrual spotting, and spontaneous abortion, infertility.

Diagnosis: Pelvic US, laparoscopy, pelvic exam.

Treatment includes:

- Pain medications: NSAIDs
- Hormone Therapy: OCPs, medroxyprogesterone injection, Gn-RH agonists/antagonists, danazol (risk of birth defects)
- Surgery: to remove endometrial tissue or radical hysterectomy
- Lifestyle Modification: regular exercise, drink fluids, heating pads/warm baths

Psychosocial Responses to Pregnancy

Psychosocial responses to pregnancy vary. Many have feelings of ambivalence about the challenges of parenthood, and these feelings are normal and healthy, representing a transitional stage leading to acceptance. Areas of concern include:

- Changing body image/sexuality: Weight gain, varicose veins, growing abdomen, stretch marks, and breast changes may cause the mother to fear she is no longer attractive.
- Labile moods: Hormonal and body changes can lead to rapid mood swings and emotional outbursts that may affect relationships, especially if the partner is unprepared.
- Personality changes: Pregnancy often results in a tendency toward introversion, with the mother requiring more rest and personal time, and this can lead to conflicts.

If the pregnancy was unintended, the mother may especially resent the pregnancy and consider abortion, leading to feelings of guilt. Educating the mother and partner about pregnancy, being supportive, and addressing these issues directly are essential. These changes are less likely to cause undue concern if the woman is prepared and given tools to help cope, such as taking short naps and/or practicing relaxation techniques.

Cultural Responses to Pregnancy, Birth, and Postpartum

Pregnancy

Beliefs vary widely. Some people believe pregnancy is a natural occurrence, so they may not seek help unless a problem arises. Other people believe women are more vulnerable during pregnancy and need protection to some degree. Women may exercise caution and avoid taboos, depending on cultural beliefs and superstitions.

Birthing

While most women in the United States depend on an obstetrician during pregnancy, some cultures may prefer lay midwives, indigenous healers, or spiritualists.

Postpartum

Non-Western cultures often expect women to be quarantined, confined, or have a prolonged period of rest with assistance in caring for the home and child after delivery for periods ranging from 10 to 100 days. For example, in Mexico, women often observe the *cuarentena*, a 40-day period of rest and restricted diet and activity. Chinese women may be expected to avoid hot or cold foods and raw fruits and vegetables and to stay in bed and refrain from bathing for 30 days.

Birth Rate, Infant Mortality, and Maternal Mortality

Birth rate, infant mortality, and maternal mortality are defined below:

1. **Birth rate**: The number of babies born alive per 1,000 individuals in a population during a specific period of time (normally 1 year).
2. **Infant Mortality:** The number of babies who die per 1,000 live births in a population during a specific period of time (normally 1 year).
3. **Maternal Mortality:** Any death of a woman during pregnancy or that occurs within 42 days of the termination of a pregnancy per 100,000 live births.

Presumptive, Probable, and Positive Signs of Pregnancy

Signs and symptoms of pregnancy are as follows:

- Presumptive:
  - Delayed menstruation.
  - Nausea and vomiting; 2-8 weeks after conception.
  - Tender or swollen breasts; 1-2 weeks after conception.
  - Feeling exhausted or sleepy; 1-6 weeks after conception.
  - Backaches/headaches.
  - Food cravings.
  - Frequent urination; 6-8 weeks after conception.
- Probable:
  - *Chadwick's sign:* a bluish discoloration of the vaginal tissue, caused by venous congestion; ~6 weeks.
  - *Hegar's Sign:* softening of the uterus; ~6 weeks.
  - *Goodell's Sign:* softening of the cervix; ~6weeks.
  - Abdominal enlargement.
  - Positive pregnancy test (blood or urine).
- Positive:
  - Fetal movements felt by examiner (ballottement); 16-22 weeks after conception.
  - Doppler of fetal heart beat; 10-14 weeks.
  - Fetal outline on x-ray.
  - Ultrasound examination of fetus: 4-6 weeks.

High Risk Pregnancies

High-risk pregnancies are pregnancies in which some physiological condition causes an increased risk of injury to mother and baby. Maternal conditions that increase this risk include:

- **Diabetes mellitus:** severity of effects on infant affected by severity of disease. Hypoglycemia is one major risk in infant, and can occur in infant after birth within 1.5-4 hours.

- **Drug abuse:** narcotics readily cross placenta; will see symptoms of withdrawal in infant after birth.
- **Smoking:** Low Birth Weight (LBW) and low APGAR scores in infant; smoking in the home increases risk of SIDS, respiratory infections, and developmental delays in childhood.
- **Alcohol use:** leads to *fetal alcohol syndrome (FAS)*; infant will show cognitive and physical impairment; facial dysmorphia. *This is a leading cause of preventable intellectual disability.*
- **Maternal infection** – especially in early pregnancy.

**TORCH is a helpful mnemonic to remember the infections that can be vertically transmitted from mother to fetus/embryo, causing marked birth defects.*

- **T**oxoplasmosis
- **O**ther viruses
- **R**ubella
- **C**ytomegalovirus
- **H**epatitis A and B

Review Video: TORCH Syndrome
Visit mometrix.com/academy and enter code: 734704

Nagel's Rule

Nagel's rule is a method used to calculate a woman's due date, or Estimated Date of Delivery (EDD). It is crucial to remember that the steps of this rule must be completed in order for the result to be accurate.

EDD = 1st day of last menstrual period + 1 year - 3 months + 7 days

Weight Gain Related to Pregnancy

Proper diet and adequate weight gain during pregnancy are essential for good health of the mother and optimum development of her baby. The appropriate total weight gain during a pregnancy depends on several factors, including mother's pre-pregnancy weight and age. A woman who is of average weight is encouraged to gain somewhere between 25-30 pounds during pregnancy. Underweight women need to gain a bit more weight, and overweight women will need less. It is generally not advised for an overweight woman to try to lose weight, especially late in the pregnancy, as this could harm the baby.

For a pregnant woman of a healthy weight, the expected weight gain should be approximately 2.5-5 lb in the first trimester (12 weeks), and then approximately 1 lb/wk. in the second and third trimesters.

Fetal Development

Fetal development takes 40 weeks from fertilization to birth.

- **Pre embryonic phase**: Fertilization – Week 2: rapid growth and cellular replication to form embryonic membranes and germ layers.
- **Embryonic phase**: Week 3-12 - Embryo developing tissue that will distinguish the various organs, development of external features.
- **Week 8**: Embryo has the appearance of a human.
- **Week 13-16**: Fetal heartbeat and movements discernible.

- **Week 16-20**: Fetal movements felt by mother ("quickening"); gender discernible at this time.
- **Week 24**: Development of alveoli in the lungs.
- **Week 25-28**: Fetal lungs can facilitate gas exchange.
- **Weeks 29-32**: Fetal bone and central nervous system development.
- **Week 37**: The fetus is considered to be full term at 37 weeks.

Fetal Lung Development

Embryonic and fetal lung development is a continuous process that begins during the embryonic stage:

- **Embryonic stage (weeks 3-7)**: Two lung buds develop from endoderm of the foregut, and the trachea and main bronchi begin to form.
- **Pseudoglandular stage (weeks 7-16)**: Airway branches form until they reach a pattern similar to those in the adult by the end of the period. Cartilage and smooth muscle also begin forming about the airways. Primitive lung lobules are evident.
- **Canalicular stage (weeks 16-24)**: Capillary networks form. Gas exchange units form. Epithelial cells differentiate. Pulmonary arteries and veins develop along the branching airways. The air-blood barrier forms that could support air exchange.
- **Saccular stage (weeks 28-35)**: Epithelial cells thin, terminal saccules form, and surfactant production occurs.
- **Alveolar stage (weeks 36-40 weeks)**: Alveolar formation begins (and continues after birth) and air spaces expand. Lungs support gas exchange.

Amniocentesis

Amniocentesis is the removal of some of the fluid surrounding the fetus for analysis. Fetus location is identified by US prior to the procedure. Using ultrasound, a long needle is inserted into the woman's abdomen, and some fluid is aspirated and sent to a laboratory for testing. Results may take up to a month to come back.

Used to Diagnose: spina bifida, Rh compatibility, immature lungs, Down syndrome

Potential Complications: Infection, miscarriage, bleeding, fetal harm, oligohydramnios

Chorionic Villus Sampling

Chorionic villus sampling is the removal of placental tissue from the uterus for analysis during early pregnancy. The advantage of chorionic villus sampling is that it can be performed earlier than amniocentesis, and is used to diagnose Tay-Sachs disease, Down syndrome, and other genetic disorders.

Considerations: Ensure woman is well hydrated and able to lie completely still during test. Contraindicated rarely in conditions such as retroverted uterus or poor fetal positioning. Possible complications include infection, miscarriage, and bleeding. May want to have support person with her during procedure.

Procedure: The woman is supine and abdomen is cleansed and prepped with a sterile drape. Using ultrasound, a long needle is inserted into the woman's abdomen, and cells are aspirated to be sent to the lab. Risks include infection, miscarriage, and bleeding; this test can also be performed transvaginally. The woman may experience some cramping during the procedure.

Gestational Diabetes

Gestational diabetes (GDM) is defined as glucose intolerance of variable degree with onset or first recognition during the present pregnancy. Pregnancy results in an elevation in serum estrogen, progesterone, and many other hormones. These hormones form as a catalyst for insulin production, causing an increase in insulin during the early months of pregnancy. However, during the last months of pregnancy, there is a rise in cortisol and glycogen. This will cause insulin resistance to occur. The result of all this is hypoglycemia in early pregnancy, followed by hyperglycemia in later months. It can be screened by drawing a 1-hour glucose level following a 50 g glucose load, but is definitively diagnosed only by an abnormal 3-hour oral glucose tolerance test (OGTT) following a 100 g glucose load. Mothers with GDM have a higher risk of urinary tract infections, hypertension and preeclampsia, cesarean section deliveries, and future diabetes. Many of the same problems associated with overt diabetic pregnancies are seen in infants born from gestational diabetic pregnancies, including macrosomia, neonatal hypoglycemia, neural tube defects, hyperbilirubinemia, hypocalcemia, hypomagnesemia, birth trauma, prematurity issues, and subsequent obesity in childhood and adolescence.

Hyperemesis Gravidarum

Hyperemesis gravidarum refers to severe and intractable nausea and vomiting during pregnancy. It is a diagnosis of exclusion. It can result in nutritional deficiencies, weight loss, and abnormalities in fluid levels, electrolyte concentrations, and acid-base balance. The peak incidence is between eight and twelve weeks of pregnancy. Normally, symptoms resolve by week 16 of gestation. Interestingly, pregnancy-related nausea and vomiting is typically associated with lower miscarriage rates. Severe nausea and vomiting may be associated to elevated estrogens or human chorionic gonadotropin levels. These patients need to be monitored, as severe dehydration and metabolic imbalances can develop.

Signs/Symptoms include: weight loss, dehydration, postural changes in blood pressure and pulse, decreased skin turgor

Diagnosis is based on physical exam, CMP, and tests to rule out other causes. Treatment includes:

- **Medications**: oral/IV antiemetics: ondansetron, promethazine (off-label), Diclegis, etc.; IV fluids/electrolyte replacement for dehydration.
- **Lifestyle Modification**: frequent small meals and sips of fluid, increased protein may help, eating before getting out of bed.

Preeclampsia

Preeclampsia is a condition characterized by an increase in blood pressure caused by pregnancy. If not promptly recognized and treated, it can lead to *eclampsia*, a condition that is very dangerous for mother and baby. Risk factors include first pregnancy/pregnant with multiples, history of previous preeclampsia, obesity, increased maternal age, and history of other conditions such as diabetes, HTN, or renal disease.

Symptoms: Abnormal and rapid weight gain, hypertension, protein in the urine (common though not required for diagnosis), headaches, peripheral edema, nausea, anxiety, decreased urine output.

Tests: Urinalysis, blood pressure, daily weight, complete blood cell count.

Treatment includes the following:

- Medications: antihypertensives may be used.
- Frequent monitoring: worsening preeclampsia will indicate need for hospitalization and possible delivery.
- NOTE: **HELLP** syndrome is an acronym/syndrome that indicates preeclampsia is worsening and/or leading to eclampsia. The acronym discusses the main symptoms of this disorder:
  - **H** - hemolysis
  - **EL** - elevated liver enzymes
  - **LP** - low platelet count

Eclampsia

Eclampsia is a condition in which seizures occur during pregnancy due to abnormally high blood pressure, which can result in severe neurological compromise and death. It is a progression of untreated/uncontrolled preeclampsia. See preeclampsia card for risk factors.

Signs and symptoms: Severe hypertension, upper right quadrant pain, sudden weight gain, vision changes, severe headache, seizures, abdominal pain, proteinuria; progression of signs and symptoms of preeclampsia.

Diagnosis: Elevated liver function tests (AST/ALT), vital signs, urinalysis.

Treatment includes the following:

- Medications: Magnesium sulfate IV*, antihypertensives
- Seizure precautions, bedrest; immediate delivery of infant may be only cure
- ***NOTE**: **BURP** is a helpful mnemonic to assist you to remember the symptoms of magnesium sulfate toxicity:
  - **B**lood pressure – decreased.
  - **U**rine output – decreased.
  - **R**espiratory rate – decreased.
  - **P**atellar reflex – absent.

Umbilical Cord

The **umbilical cord** is a maternofetal vessel that serves as a pathway for oxygen and nutrients to be passed between the fetus and mother during the intrauterine period. The umbilical cord should measure 55 cm in length and contain two arteries and one vein; the acronym "AVA" is often used to remember this (artery-vein-artery). The nurse should be aware of the following anomalies that can occur during birth related to the umbilical cord:

- **Prolapsed cord**: The cord is delivered prior to the presenting fetal part. May result in cord compression.
- **Cord compression**: A cease in flow of blood and oxygen between the mother and fetus.
- **Missing vessels**: Congenital artery absence can cause fetal anomalies and problems with gestational age.
- **Rips or tears in the cord**: Due to lack of Wharton's jelly (the natural protective mechanism of the cord). Causes hemorrhages and fetal heart rate irregularities.
- **Shortened cord**: May lead to umbilical hernia, abruptio placenta, and cord rupture.

- **Extensive cord**: Increased risk of nuchal cord and knots in the cord that decrease blood and oxygen supplies.
- **Nuchal cord**: Cord wrapped around baby's neck. May require emergency cesarean delivery to prevent strangulation if severe.

Placenta

The **placenta** is a *fetomaternal organ,* meaning that it is an organ that is shared by mother and child. The function of the placenta is the exchange of nutrients, waste, blood, and oxygen between the blood of the fetus and the mother. The placenta continues to function throughout the birthing process until the umbilical cord is cut and/or the baby takes his first breath. However, there are certain complications that happen in relation to the placenta of which the nurse should be aware:

- **Abruptio Placenta**: An early and unexpected break of the placenta from the intrauterine wall during pregnancy or labor. This causes blood flow/oxygenation to the baby to cease, causing fetal demise and possible maternal hemorrhage if not caught early. (See below for more information).
- **Placenta Previa**: Placenta previa is an altered position of the placenta, traditionally on the lower uterine wall or covering the cervical os. This can cause the placenta to be delivered before the child, resulting again in hemorrhage and fetal demise. The treatment is cesarean delivery and no vaginal exams.
- **Retained Placenta**: After birth, parts of the placenta may still be retained inside the uterus. This places the mother at a greatly increased risk of hemorrhage and infection, and must be dealt with immediately if caught.

Abruptio Placenta Classification

The most common cause of **abruptio placenta** is maternal hypertension, as it is the cause of approximately 44% of all abruption cases. It is **classified** based on the following:

- **Class 0**: Abruption asymptomatic. It is diagnosed retrospectively by examining the delivered placenta and finding a depressed area or an organized blood clot on it.
- **Class 1**: Representing approximately 48% of all placental abruption cases, is mild. There is either mild or no vaginal bleeding. The uterus may be slightly tender but there is no fetal distress. The mother's blood pressure and heart rate are normal and there is no coagulopathy.
- **Class 2**: Representing approximately 27% of all abruption cases, is considered moderate. There is moderate vaginal bleeding (or mild or none). Uterine tenderness may be moderate-to-severe but there is fetal distress. The mother's heart rate is elevated (tachycardia) and there are orthostatic changes in blood pressure.
- **Class 3**: Representing approximately 24% of all abruption cases, is severe. Vaginal bleeding may be heavy and the mother has a very painful tetanic uterus. She may be in shock and have coagulopathy. This class results in fetal death.

Signs and symptoms: Sharp, stabbing pains in uterus, tender on palpation, rigid/board-like uterus, drop in H&H

Diagnosis: Physical exam of abdomen/uterine palpation, CBC, ultrasound

Treatment: Oxygen, fluids, lateral position, bedrest, emergency C section for fetal distress. **NO PELVIC EXAMINATIONS.**

Oligohydramnios/Polyhydramnios

Oligohydramnios is a condition in which there is a lack of sufficient amniotic fluid in the placenta surrounding the baby. This is concerning, as low levels of amniotic fluid can cause fetal abnormalities, miscarriage, and labor complications. Oligohydramnios can be caused by fetal kidney disorders, a ruptured amniotic sac, and possibly NSAID use; however, it is generally unknown as to what causes the condition. Treatment may include amniotic fluid infusions, fluids for the mother, and bedrest.

Polyhydramnios is an abnormally high level of amniotic fluid that can cause premature labor/rupture of membranes, fetal abnormalities, and fetal death. It can be caused by hydrops fetalis, multiple fetus development, anencephaly, or other problems that would cause the fetus to have swallowing difficulty/excess urination. The treatment could include medication to reduce fetal urination, removal of fluid, along with bedrest/symptom management. However, treatment is often not indicated.

Rh Incompatibility

Rh is a component of the blood, generally expressed as "positive" and "negative" blood type. Rh compatibility comes into play when an Rh-negative woman is carrying the child of an Rh-positive man. Since the woman is Rh negative, her body will develop RhD antibodies if exposed to the RhD antigen. This is known as *sensitization*. Because of genetics, there is a 50% to 100% chance that the baby of an Rh-positive man will be Rh positive, depending on if he is homozygous or heterozygous Rh positive.

If the baby is Rh positive, then the mother will develop anti-D antibodies when the baby's blood is mixed with hers during placental separation. The first child would remain unharmed; however, during subsequent pregnancies, the mother's anti-D antibodies can cross the placenta to the fetal blood, causing agglutination and hemolysis of fetal cells to a varying degree. This could result in fetal demise, erythroblastosis fetalis, icterus gravis neonatorum, hemolytic anemia, kernicterus, or liver damage of the fetus.

Treatment: Screening pregnant woman for Rh status is critical to prevent Rh sensitization. If Rh negative, the woman will be required to take a medication known as RhoGAM. This is an IM injection given throughout pregnancy that prevents sensitization in the woman. RhoGAM will not work if sensitization has already occurred.

Induced Labor

While formerly common practice, today it is rare that a doctor will choose to induce labor unless it is considered medically necessary for the health of mom and baby. **Induced labor** may occur in the following situations:

- Eclampsia/HELLP syndrome
- High serum creatinine levels
- Premature rupture of membranes (PROM)
- Thrombocytopenia
- Abnormal fetal growth
- 2 weeks past due date

Impending Labor

The following are some of the signs and symptoms of *impending labor:*

- **Lightening:** Also called engagement. Occurs when fetus moves into position for birth. Maternal breathing is easier after lightening, since it relieves pressure on the diaphragm. Other symptoms include lower extremity pain, pressure and leg cramping, a noted increase in the amount of pelvic discomfort and pressure felt, bilateral lower extremity edema related to the decreased return of blood flow to the heart.
- **Nesting**: A subjective sign; the mother to be may experience a renewed energy. She may begin to clean and organize the baby's things, and have a sense of urgency to accomplish tasks before the baby arrives.
- **Braxton Hicks contractions**: Consist of the irregular, discontinuous uterine contractions that should subside with rest. Braxton Hicks are termed "false labor" if the contractions are consistent. A vaginal exam may be required to differentiate between Braxton Hicks and true labor.
- **Cervical changes**: As labor approaches, the cervix thins (called *effacement)* and the cervical os will begin to dilate.
- **Bloody show:** The mucus plug that develops over the length of the pregnancy is released as the cervix thins. Once the presence of bloody show is evident, labor will proceed within 24 to 48 hours.
- **Rupture of membranes**: When the bag of amniotic fluid that contains the fetus ruptures, labor traditionally results within 24 hours.

Stages of Labor

The stages of labor are described below:

- **Stage I:** Starts with the beginning signs of labor and concludes at the time the cervix reaches a dilatation of 10 cm. Stage I labor consists of the latent phase, the active, and the transition phases.
    - **Latent phase** (cervix 1-3 cm; contractions 30-45 seconds/5-30 minutes apart): characterized by routine contractions and rupture of the membranes.
    - **Active phase** (cervix 4-7 cm; contractions 45-60 seconds/3-5 minutes apart): characterized by increased strength and frequency of contractions.
    - **Transition phase** (cervix 8-10 cm; contractions 60-90 seconds/ 30 seconds-2 minutes apart): characterized by strong, frequent contractions and pressure in pelvis; anxiety and a sense of helplessness may be present.
- **Stage II:** Begins with complete dilatation and concludes with the birth of the baby. Fetal descent and *crowning* (baby's head becomes visible) takes place. As this stage progresses, the fetus changes position to accommodate birth. These changes of position are known as flexion, internal rotation, extension, restitution, external rotation, and expulsion.
- **Stage III:** Placenta separates from the uterine wall / delivery of the placenta.
- **Stage IV:** Includes the first 4 hours post labor, in which the mother's body begins to return to its pre-pregnant state.

Variations in Fetal Heart Rate Monitoring

During labor and delivery, it is common practice to monitor the fetal heart rate (FHR). The heart's rate and rhythm give the practitioner key information about the condition of the fetus. The following **variations** may be heard during fetal heart rate monitoring:

- **Accelerations**: The heart rate jumps up at random times during labor; also known as "variability" and is a normal and reassuring sign.
- **Early decelerations**: Slight dip in FHR at the beginning of contractions; due to head compression and is a reassuring sign.
- **Late decelerations**: U-shape and have both a gradual onset and return. They are typically shallow (around 10-30 beats per minute), and after the contraction' speak, they reach their nadir. They occur when the mother's uterine contractions decrease fetal oxygenation. In milder cases, late decelerations can result from CNS hypoxia. In cases that are more severe, they may result from direct myocardial depression. As the hypoxia becomes more severe, late decelerations usually become deeper. It is not uncommon for mothers to have occasional or intermittent late decelerations during labor.
- **Variable decelerations** are characterized by an abrupt FHR slowing and return. Frequently, they are followed by small FHR accelerations. Their depth, duration, and shape can vary. It can be non-reassuring to experience variable deceleration that are persistent, deep, and long-lasting. Those variable decelerations dropping to less than 70 bpm and lasting more than one minute are concerning.

The following are interventions for late and variable decelerations:

1. Turn mother on her left side and apply manual pressure to baby's head.
2. Apply 10L oxygen via facemask and stop oxytocin if infusing.
3. Call the MD.

Causes of Fetal Tachycardia

The following are potential causes of fetal tachycardia:

- Fetal hypoxia
- Maternal fever
- Hyperthyroidism
- Maternal or fetal anemia
- Drugs: atropine, hydroxyzine, terbutaline
- Chorioamnionitis
- Fetal heart arrhythmias
- Prematurity

Rubin's Theory of the Stages of Postpartum

Reva Rubin discusses and theorizes the biopsychosocial experience of childbirth. The postpartum phases according to Rubin include:

1. **Taking in**: First 2 to 3 days following labor. This is a time in which the mother begins to claim her baby, and regenerate herself from childbirth. This is a period of rest and acquaintance for the neonate and the mother. The nurse should encourage the mother to reflect and verbalize her labor and delivery experience during this time.

2. **Taking hold**: Day 3 to Week 2. The mother begins to feel more autonomous and require less assistance from those around her, dominating the care of the infant. The mother's own bodily functions should be returning to normal during this period. Mothers in the "taking hold" phase are very sensitive to the care of the infant and insist they want everything to be done right. The nurse should praise the mother during this phase if they have the opportunity, and should educate the family on offering praise to new mothers.
3. **Letting go**: ~ Week 2-3. The mother begins to see the infant as a separate entity from self. Until this point the mother may have felt guilt when separated from her infant and may grieve over this separation. The "letting go" phase is a time of returning to pre-pregnancy norms.

POSTPARTUM HEMORRHAGE

Postpartal hemorrhage may be early (≤24 hours) or late (≤6 weeks). Normal blood loss with vaginal delivery is about 500 mL and with Caesarean about 1000 mL. The formal definition of postpartum hemorrhage, according to the ACOG, has been changed to required ≥1000mL blood loss with signs/symptoms of hypovolemia within the first 24 hours after birth, regardless of the mode of delivery. Blood loss is difficult to estimate because it is mixed with amniotic fluid and mucus, and hemorrhage may be internal and not obvious on examination. Usual indications of hemorrhage, such as increased pulse, decreased blood pressure, and decreased output of urine may be delayed until about 2 L of blood loss. A significant drop in hematocrit (10 points) is indicative of hemorrhage. Early hemorrhage poses more risk of mortality than late hemorrhage. When hemorrhage is suspected, such as with steady flow of lochia rubra, then the woman's vital signs should be checked every 5 to 15 minutes and perineal pads weighed (1 mL of blood weighs about 1 g). A soft boggy uterus should be massaged frequently to maintain firmness, with clots expressed. IV access should be maintained. Urinary output <30 mL/hr. should be reported to physician.

CAUSES

The following are causes of postpartum hemorrhage:

- Early Causes:
  - Uterine atony: Most common with multiple gestations, prolonged labor, labor induction, anesthesia, pre-eclampsia, and placenta previa. Uterine contractions necessary to occlude blood flow to placenta.
  - Genital lacerations: Lacerations may be undetected, or the episiotomy may continue to slowly ooze blood.
  - Hematomas: Trauma to blood vessels may occur, especially with pudendal anesthesia, forceps or vacuum-assisted delivery, macrosomia, and prolonged second stage of labor.
  - Inversion of uterus: This is rare but may occur with weak uterine muscles, extended labor, anesthesia, magnesium sulfate, and manual removal of placenta with excess traction.
  - Rupture of uterus: This is also rare but can occur with previous C-section, multiparity, and induction (oxytocin).
  - Abnormal implantation of placenta.
  - Coagulopathies: DIC may occur in response to blood loss or cause blood loss.
- Late Causes:
  - Subinvolution of placental implantation site (failure of implantation site to shrink and heal): Leaves open tissue that may bleed.
  - Retained placental tissue: Bleeding occurs when it sloughs from implantation site.

Postpartum Infections

Metritis (endometrial inflammation) may result from C-section, PROM, repeated vaginal examination, fetal scalp electrode, instruments (forceps or vacuum), high-risk status of mother (drug use, smoker, poor nutrition), pre-existing vaginal infection, and aseptic techniques.

Indications include foul or scant lochia (depending on organism), uterine tenderness, temperature elevations (sawtooth pattern) 38.3-40 °C, tachycardia, and chills.

Parametritis (pelvic cellulitis/peritonitis) is an infection of connective tissue of broad ligament or all pelvic structures may result from bacterial invasion of cervical laceration or pelvic vein thrombophlebitis. Abscess may form.

Indications include chills, high fever (38.9-40°C), abdominal pain, uterine subinvolution, local and rebound tenderness, tachycardia, abdominal distention, nausea and vomiting.

Urinary infection may result from birth trauma, urinary retention, and contamination (catheter).

Indications include dysuria, fever, and urinary retention.

Wound infection may result from contamination of lacerations, episiotomy, and C-section incisions.

Indications include erythema, local pain, purulent discharge, edema, and (rare) dehiscence.

Lochia

After labor, a woman will have continuous discharge as the uterus sheds the pregnancy lining and returns to its original state. This discharge is known as **lochia**, and may last 5 to 6 weeks. The phases are as follows:

- **Lochia Rubra**: Occurs 1-3 days postpartum; heavy flow, bright red and may have clots.
- **Lochia Serosa:** Occurs 3-10 days postpartum, appears brown-pink.
- **Lochia Alba:** Starts around postpartum day 10, lasting for 2-6 weeks; it is yellow in color.

Sheehan Syndrome

Sheehan syndrome is hypopituitarism caused by uterine hemorrhage during childbirth. The blood loss, hypotension, and resulting hypoxemia cause the pituitary gland to cease to function. The onset of symptoms may be rapid, or take years to develop. Sheehan syndrome is more commonly seen in underdeveloped countries.

Signs and symptoms: amenorrhea, fatigue, unable to breastfeed baby, anxiety, decreased BP, hair loss, hypothyroidism, decreased libido.

Diagnosis: CT/MRI scan of pituitary gland, blood levels, pituitary hormone stimulation test.

Treatment: Life-long hormone therapy to replace lost hormones; may include levothyroxine, estrogen, growth hormone, and corticosteroids.

Prevention: early recognition and treatment of blood loss in post-partum period.

Mastitis

Mastitis is a common infection and inflammation of the breast due to bacteria, often *S. aureus.* Risk factors for mastitis include sudden cessation of breastfeeding, poor hygiene, prior colonization with

S. aureus, and broken skin on the breast. It is important to note that doctors often recommend that a mother continue to breastfeed, despite the infection.

Symptoms: fever, nipple pain/discharge, breast pain/swelling, pain with breastfeeding.

Diagnosis: Physical examination, culture of human milk, rarely mammogram to rule out more serious cause of inflammation (breast cancer).

Treatment includes:

- Medications: oral antibiotics, pain relievers (Tylenol/Ibuprofen).
- Lifestyle Modification: moist heat, breastfeed often/change positions frequently, rest, increase fluids, wash nipples with plain water and allow to air dry to prevent cracking/drying.

Postpartum Depression

Postpartum depression (PPD) is an episode of depression related to the birth of a child. PPD may begin during pregnancy, but onset is most common within the first 2 weeks to 3 months after delivery, although it may occur up to 1 year after. The cause is not clear but risk factors include first pregnancy; history of depression, alcoholism, or mental disorder; low self-esteem; hormonal imbalances, marital difficulties; lack of sleep; and chronic stress.

Signs and symptoms: depressed mood with loss of emotional response and inability to respond with pleasure to the infant. Some patients may express dislike or hatred for the infant. Sleep disturbance and fatigue is common. Patients may feel anger, anxiety, or shame.

Treatment: Ensure safety of infant even if that means removing the infant from the mother's care. Patients may need psychotherapy and medications, such as SSRIs or TCAs, as well as emotional support of family and friends.

Hospitalization of Infants and Children

Hospitalization is a stressful time for infants and young children. It is not uncommon for them to experience stress and **regression**, a coping mechanism in which the child returns to previous developmental stage. The nurse needs to be cognizant of the child's specific needs to better anticipate problems arising from loss of control and to mitigate its effects.

- Infants' Needs
  - Trust, consistent loving caregivers, daily routines.
  - Loss of Control: agitation, malaise/failure to thrive (FTT).
- Toddlers' Needs
  - Autonomy, daily routines and rituals.
  - Loss of control: regression, negativity, temper tantrums.
- Preschoolers' Needs
  - Egocentric and magical thinking, imaginative play, creativity.
  - Loss of control: May view illness/hospitalization as punishment for misdeeds; fear mutilation.
- School Age' Needs
  - Independence and productivity, feeling of control over self.
  - Loss of Control: Fears of death, abandonment, boredom.

- Adolescent Needs:
  - Independence/ liberation, connection with peer group, information about condition (talk to as an adult).
  - Loss of Control: anger, frustration, feelings of isolation.

Apgar Score

The **Apgar score** is a universal tool used to determine the condition of the newborn at the time of birth. The Apgar score is taken 1 minute and 5 minutes after birth, with scores ranging from 0-10. Infants delivered by cesarean birth (C-section) will get an additional score 15 minutes after birth. The factors that make up the Apgar score include:

A. **Heart rate**: 0, absent; 1, slow or below 100; 2, >100

B. **Respiratory effort**: 0, absent; 1, slow and irregular; 2, good, vigorous crying

C. **Muscle tone**: 0, flaccid; 1, some extremity flexion; 2, active motion

D. **Reflex irritability**: 0, none; 1, grimace; 2, vigorous cry

E. **Color**: 0, pale blue; 1, body pink, extremities bluish; 2, completely pink

Can be remembered by* **APGAR*: **A**ppearance (color),* **P***ulse (heart rate),* **G***rimace (reflex),* **A***ctivity (muscle tone), and* **R***espirations.*

Changes in Neonatal Cardiovascular System

The birthing process brings about a marked change in the **circulatory system of the newborn**. During fetal development, blood is routed from the mother to the infant through the placenta. Upon birth, however, the first breath of the infant causes maximum inflation of the lungs. The resulting resistance stimulates increased blood flow to the pulmonary veins. Then, as blood begins to return from the pulmonary veins into the left atrium, the pressure in the right atrium decreases. The pressure in the right atrium is additionally decreased related to a marked drop in blood supply after the clamping of the umbilical cord. The clamping of the umbilical cord also causes the *ductus venosus* to close, resulting in the circulation of blood to the liver. The resulting change in arterial pressure will cause the *foramen ovale* (a hole between the left and right atria) to close within the first 2 hours following birth. The *ductus arteriosus* then closes as the flow of blood is rerouted into the pulmonary artery instead of the aorta.

Variations of Coloring in Newborns

Healthy newborns have a characteristic pink flush to the skin. Any variation of this **coloring** may indicate problems within the body.

- **Ruddy (red) hues**: increase in red blood cell concentration to the area; decreased amount of subcutaneous fat.
- **Cyanotic at rest/pink during activity:** may have a congenital defect known as choanal atresia (a blockage between the nose and pharynx).
- **Cyanosis when crying:** may signal cardio or pulmonary problems.
- **Pale**: anemia; decreased fluid volumes.
- **Acrocyanosis:** transient, not normally a cause for concern; indicates normal pink coloring with bluish hands and feet.

- **Harlequin sign:** one side of the newborn's body red, other white; the result of vasodilatation, usually dissipates within a few hours.
- **Jaundice**: yellowish color noted at birth; caused by breakdown of red blood cells. Dissipates within the first 24 hours of birth; prolonged jaundice indicates liver dysfunction.

Newborn Reflexes

Common newborn reflexes include:

- **Babinski**: Toes should hyperextend if side of sole of foot stroked from heel to ball of foot.
- **Blinking**: Eyes should close if light flashed in eyes.
- **Moro** (startle): Infant should extend limbs and neck symmetrically and then pull back in response to loud noise or jolt.
- **Palmar grasp**: Infant should grasp finger if palm stroked.
- **Rooting**: Infant should open mouth and turn to the side of touch when the infant's cheek is stroked.
- **Sucking**: Infant should suck if mouth touched. Reflex may be weak in premature infants.
- **Tonic neck** (fencing): With infant lying flat and the head turned to one side, the infant should flex limbs on opposite side and extend limbs on the side to which head is turned.
- **Trunk incurvation**: With infant prone, stroking down one side of spine (1 inch from spine) should result in the pelvis turning to stroked side.
- **Tongue extrusion**: Infant should push tongue out of mouth if tip of tongue touched.

Review Video: Tonic Neck Response
Visit mometrix.com/academy and enter code: 421866

Prophylactic Measures for Newborns

According to many state's laws, there are two different **prophylactic (preventative) treatments** that are given to all newborns delivered in the hospital setting:

1. **Vitamin K shot**: This is an intermuscular injection that provides a boost of vitamin K to the infant to prevent hemorrhage. At birth, the infant has little or no bacterial flora within the gastrointestinal tract that produce vitamin K, thus most newborns are deficient. Vitamin K is crucial to blood clotting, so this injection helps prevent hemorrhage and the resulting injury.
2. **Antibiotic Eye Ointment**: Newborns are also given prophylactic eye ointment to prevent blindness caused by exposure from the mother's vaginal tract to *Neisseria gonorrhoeae*. This ointment is given even if previous STI screening of the mother is clear. In order to be most effective, the ointment should be deposited directly in the lower conjunctival sac of both eyes shortly after birth.

Head-to-Toe Assessment of Newborns

Newborn assessment consists of the following:

- **Head/Face**: Circumference 32-38 cm. Sutures palpable with small separations noted. Anterior fontanel diamond-shaped and 4-5 cm and soft. Posterior fontanel triangle-shaped 0.5-1 cm. Molding may result in overriding sutures. Note caput succedaneum (crosses suture lines) or cephalhematoma. Facial features symmetrical.
- **Chest**: Circumference 2-3 cm less than head circumference. Chest movements during respirations symmetrical. Note sternal retraction, periods of apnea.

- **Abdomen**: Rounded and soft with bowel sounds. Note distention, masses, and abdominal wall defects. Umbilical cord should have 3 vessels.
- **Genitalia**: Females—labia majora cover clitoris and labia minora. Male—testes should be within scrotal sac, rugae on scrotum, and urinary meatus at the end of the penis.
- **Back**: Anus present and open. Back closed and no abnormalities felt in vertebral column.
- **Extremities**: Equal in size and shape, bilateral movements, flexed, good muscle tone, gluteal and thigh creases equal, two transverse palm creases, and feet in normal position.
- **Vital signs**: Axillary 36.5 °C to 37.3 °C, heart rate 120 to 160 bpm when awake and not crying, respirations 30 to 60 per minute with symmetric chest movement and clear breath sounds, BP 65-95/30-60 mm Hg.

Benefits of Breastfeeding

The following are **health benefits of breastfeeding for mother and baby**:

- Bolstered immune system and infection resistance.
- Human milk contains antibodies that help protect infants from different viruses and bacteria.
- Because babies fed with human milk are less frequently sick, they have fewer pediatrician visits.
- The immune systems of breastfed babies respond more favorably to immunizations such as polio, tetanus, Haemophilus influenzae, and diphtheria, and to the common infantile respiratory infection.
- Direct human milk is always sterile.
- A mother's milk has exactly the amount of fat, water, protein, and sugar that the baby needs for growth and development. Moreover, it is easier for most babies to digest human milk than formula.
- Nursing expends calories, making it easier for the mom lose the pounds gained during pregnancy. It also helps the uterus return to its normal size and lessens any post-birth maternal bleeding.
- Breastfeeding reduces the risk of developing breast and ovarian cancers.

Circumcision

Circumcision is the surgical removal of the prepuce (epithelial tissue sometimes termed "foreskin") from the tip or head of the penis. It is also a religious practice of the Jewish culture, being performed by their priest on the eighth day following birth. However, in the hospital, circumcision is an optional procedure, and usually takes place a few days after birth. The AAFP believe that the benefits of male circumcision outweigh the risks, but does not have a policy for or against it. Instead they recommend that the parent(s) be educated on the risks and benefits of the procedure so that they can make an informed personal decision.

Considerations

This procedure should not be performed in infants with an increased risk of bleeding, those with hypo/hyperspadias, or medically unstable/premature infants. There is a small risk of infection or bleeding.

Procedure

The head of the penis is anesthetized and the child is restrained. A ring/clamp is attached to the end of the penis, and the foreskin is removed. The penis is coated with petroleum jelly and wrapped in loose gauze. It should heal within a week. The nurse should educate the parents that while some bleeding should be expected, any increased redness, foul-smelling or purulent discharge, or fever in the infant should be reported immediately.

Meconium Aspiration Syndrome

Meconium Aspiration Syndrome (MAS) is a syndrome caused by fetal asphyxia or intrauterine stress. It occurs when stress causes the relaxation of the anal sphincter of the infant, resulting in passage of meconium into amniotic fluid. This fluid is then breathed in by the infant, causing respiratory distress and compromise.

Signs and symptoms: green-tinged skin/mucus of newborn; tachypneic; hypoxic; depressed; grunting; retractions; nasal flaring; hypothermic; hypoglycemic; hypocalcemic, *quickly leads to respiratory failure*.

Treatment includes:

- Immediate suction, intubation and ventilator likely
- Broad-spectrum antibiotics to prevent infection likely
- Immediate transfer to Neonatal Intensive Care unit for monitoring.
- Surfactant replacement therapy

KEY PREVENTION MEASURES – Close monitoring for signs of fetal distress; caesarean delivery if indicated; suctioning as soon as head is through birth canal and chest still compressed to prevent inspiration of meconium may be effective, though not currently recommended.

Hypothermia in Infants

When infants are born, their thermoregulation system is still immature. This means that infants are especially susceptible to heat loss and subsequent **hypothermia**. There are generally four different types of heat loss that an infant can experience:

1. **Conduction** is the flow of heat energy through direct contact from regions of warmer temperature (infant) to regions of cooler temperature (cold surfaces touching skin)
2. **Convection** is the movement of heat by currents in the medium (such as wind [draft blowing over child's skin])
3. **Radiation** is when heat is lost to cool objects near but not in contact with the infant (walls of crib, nearby objects)
4. **Evaporation** occurs after bathing the infant or other times when water on the infant's skin evaporates, taking heat with it

Prevention of hypothermia includes the following:

- Do not place the infant's bare skin in contact with cool surfaces such as an uncovered table or tile flooring.
- Protect infant from drafts from windows/air conditioning vents.
- Keep temperature in nursery reasonably warm.
- Dry infants thoroughly and quickly after baths/when wet.
- Skin-to-Skin contact is encouraged to promote heat regulation.

Note: Never cover infants with blankets during sleep (increased risk of SIDS).

Jaundice/Icterus

Jaundice/Icterus (physiologic) is common in neonates after 2 days and is evident when bilirubin reaches 5 to 7 mg/dL. Jaundice should be assessed with transcutaneous or serum bilirubin measurements.

- **Early onset/Breastfeeding-associated**: Occurs within 1 week and relates to insufficient intake—the infant does not ingest enough colostrum, which helps expel meconium because of its laxative effect.
- **Late-onset milk jaundice**: Occurs after days 3 to 5 and may last up to 3 months. Cause is unknown but treatment is at least 8-12 feedings per day.
- **Non-physiologic hyperbilirubinemia**: Usually evident within first 24 hours and may result in acute bilirubin encephalopathy, leading to kernicterus (brain damage resulting from bilirubin in brain tissue). May result from hemolytic disease, infection, hypothyroidism, biliary atresia, and other congenital abnormalities.

The most common treatment for jaundice is phototherapy with the infant placed under fluorescent lights with eye coverings in place and wearing only a diaper. The bilirubin in the skin absorbs the light and converts into a water-soluble form that can be excreted in the urine.

Review Video: Jaundice/Icterus
Visit mometrix.com/academy and enter code: 339680

Neonatal Infection

Newborns are born with lower levels of immunity than typical adults. The alterations of the newborn's immune system make him/her vulnerable to infection and disease processes because the immune system does not readily recognize insidious bacteria. This is related to decreased levels of immunoglobulins and a decreased reaction of the complement system. Overall, this means that the newborn will not have the signs and symptoms of an infection found in an adult. The following are signs a newborn may exhibit that indicate possible **infection**:

- The most reliable sign of infection or an infectious process in the neonate is hypothermia or an abnormally low body temperature.
- Poor feeding.
- Difficulty breathing/periods of apnea.
- Low heart rate.
- Malaise.
- Increased irritability, relentless crying.
- Changes in skin color/jaundice.

Coarctation of the Aorta

Aortic coarctation is a birth defect in which the aorta has a narrowed point of variable severity. This leads to serious reduction in cardiac output, and can cause complications if not recognized and treated. These patients are at a greatly increased risk of stroke, heart failure, aortic or cerebral aneurysm, and aortic dissection.

Signs and symptoms:

- Infants: irritability, poor feeding, signs and symptoms of heart failure, diaphoresis.
- Adults: nose bleeding, fainting, dyspnea on exertion, headaches.

Diagnosis: Marked blood pressure difference between arms and legs, ultrasound, echocardiogram, CT, MRI, ECG, chest x-ray, cardiac catheterization.

Treatment includes:

- Infants only: prostaglandin E to keep ductus arteriosus open (allows bypass of the narrowed areas).
- Blood pressure medications (before surgery).
- Balloon angioplasty/stenting.
- Open heart surgery.

Down Syndrome

Down syndrome, also sometimes referred to as *trisomy 21 syndrome*, is an abnormality with chromosome 21 that results in an individual having 47 chromosomes instead of 46. This results in several physiological and cognitive abnormalities. Maternal age greater than 35 years, family history, and a previous child with Down syndrome are all known risk factors for this condition. Infants with Down syndrome will have difficulty feeding and develop frequent respiratory infections. Many children with Down syndrome also have heart defects, and have an increased risk of Alzheimer disease and leukemia later in life.

Signs and symptoms: intellectual disability, slanted eyes, flattened nasal bridge, small low-set ears, thick, fissured tongue, low muscle tone, short fingers, Brushfield spots on the iris.

Diagnosis: physical exam, karyotype test, neonatal screening -not definitive.

Treatment is as follows:

- No cure; ensure family has adequate support.
- Education on health risks – ensure early recognition and treatment of infections.
- Education: many people with Down syndrome can live normal lives.

Hypocalcemia in Newborns

Hypocalcemia is defined as a serum calcium level of less than 7.0 mg/dL in an infant. The normal range is 7.0-8.5 mg/dL. It can be of either early or late onset; either way, hypocalcemia should be recognized and treated immediately to prevent potential complications. High levels of phosphate can also cause hypocalcemia, due to the inverse relationship of phosphorus and calcium in the body.

- **Early-onset hypocalcemia** – appears in first 24-48 hours. Generally temporary and resolves on its own. It is most common in preterm/SGA infants, hypoxic infants, or infants born to a diabetic mother.
- **Late-onset hypocalcemia** – appears after 3-4 days of life; also known as *cow's milk-induced hypocalcemia* or *neonatal tetany*. Common with intestinal malabsorption, hyperinsulinemia, hypoparathyroidism, hypomagnesemia, or with phosphate enemas.

Signs and symptoms: jittery, long QT interval, apnea, cyanosis, high-pitched cry/ neuromuscular irritation, abdominal distension

Treatment includes the following:

- Correction of underlying cause: switch formula, treat hypoparathyroidism or hypomagnesia, and feed often
- IV calcium gluconate 10%—very slowly
- Monitor for signs of hypercalcemia such as vomiting or bradycardia

Developmental Stages and Transitions

Developmental Theories

Freud

Three forces in humans: 1) *Id:* unconscious/pleasure; 2) *Ego*: conscious/ reality; 3) *Superego*: conscience/ideals

Freud's psychosexual stages of development are as follows:

- Oral: Birth to 18 months: Weaning
- Anal: 18 months – 3 y: Potty Training
- Phallic*:* 3-6 y: Sexual discovery
- Latent: 6 y - puberty: Learning/pause in sexual learning
- Genital: Puberty through adulthood: Sexual Relationships

Erikson

Erik Erikson's stages of psychosocial development are as follows:

- Trust vs Mistrust (birth - 1 y)
- Autonomy vs Shame and doubt (1 - 3 y)
- Initiative vs Guilt (3 - 6 y)
- Industry vs Inferiority (~6 - 12 y)
- Identity vs Role confusion (~12 - 18 y)
- Intimacy vs Isolation (~19 - 35 y)
- Generativity vs Stagnation (~35 – 65 y)
- Ego Integrity vs Despair (~65 – death)

Piaget

Jean Piaget's stages of cognitive development are as follows:

- Sensorimotor/Intuitive (birth to 2 y)
- Pre-operational (2 - 7 y)
- Concrete operational (7 - 11 y)
- Formal operational (12 y - adulthood)

Pediatric Vital Signs

Pediatric vital signs vary according to the age of the child:

- **Temperature**: rectal, axillary, or tympanic temperatures should be taken on small children, with oral temperatures reserved for older children and adolescents. Temperatures vary from about 36.3 °C to 37.6 °C (oral). Axillary temperatures run about 1 degree less and rectal temperatures 1 degree more.

- **Blood pressure**: An appropriately sized cuff is essential to accuracy, and auscultation should be used for assessment. The pulse may remain audible from the systolic reading to 0, so the diastolic reading is the point the sound changes. BP varies widely by age and gender, increasing as the child ages. The nurse should refer to a BP chart.
- **Heart rate**: Heart rate should be assessed by auscultation with the child at rest if possible; heart rate increases in response to stress. Newborns, 100-150; infants to 2 years, 80-120; ages 2-6, 70-110; ages 6-10, 60-95; and age 10-16; 60-85.
- **Respirations**: Newborns, 30-55; 1 year, 25-40; 3 years, 20-30; 6 years, 16-22; 10 years, 16-20; and 17 years, 12-18.

Developmental Milestones in Fine and Gross Motor Skills

Age	Fine motor skills	Gross motor skills
By 2 years old	Able to build a block tower to height of at least 4 blocks, able to hold a crayon or pencil and scribble on paper, and able to throw a ball. Able to remove clothes.	Able to run and climb and descend stairs.
Ages 2 to 3 years	Able to draw rudimentary forms, such as circles, and can pour liquids and start to dress self.	Able to kick, jump, and throw ball overhand.
Ages 3 to 6 years	Able to use scissors, draw multiple shapes, and draw a 6-part human (stick figure). Learning to tie shoes and can button clothes and brush teeth. Enjoys doing arts and crafts projects.	Can climb, ride tricycle, and throw overhand.
Ages 6 to 12 years	Does more complex craft project, plays cards and board games.	Rides 2-wheel bicycle and can jump rope, roller skate/ice skate.
Ages 12 to 18 years	Can write, draw, and manipulate tools easily.	Engages in sports activities, such as team sports.

Pain Response in Infants and Children

Because of communication barriers, infants and young children respond differently to **pain** than adults. The nurse needs to be aware of these variations in order to effectively care for this population:

- Young Infant's Response to Pain
  - Generalized response of rigidity, thrashing.
  - Loud crying/ facial expressions of pain (grimace).
  - Do not understand stimuli-pain relationship; FLACC scale.
- Older Infant's Response to Pain
  - Withdrawal from painful stimuli.
  - Loud crying /facial grimace.
  - Physical resistance; FLACC.
- Young Child's Response to Pain
  - Loud crying, screaming.
  - Verbalizations: "Ow," "Ouch," "It hurts"; Faces scale.
  - Thrashing of limbs/attempts to push away stimulus.

- School-Age Child's Response to Pain
    - Stalling behavior ("wait a minute"); Faces or Numerical scale.
    - Muscle rigidity.
    - May use all behaviors of young child.
- Adolescent
    - Less vocal protest/motor activity; increased muscle rigidity.
    - Verbalizes pain ("it hurts" or "you're hurting me"); Numeric scale.

Best Toys for Different Ages of Children

The **best toys** for different ages of children are discussed below:

- 0 to 3 months: Infants enjoy mobiles, mirrors, and music players.
- 3 to 6 months: Infant begins grasping toys, such as rattles and small stuffed animals.
- 6 to 9 months: Infant begins to mouth items, so enjoys teething toys and soft stuffed animals.
- 9 to 12 months: Infant starts to enjoy blocks, pop-up toys, push and pull toys, toys that make noises.
- 2 to 3 years: The child is more engaged in play and enjoys heavy paper or cloth books, stuffed animals, dolls, toy cars and trucks, large wooden puzzles, toys they can manipulate, paper and large crayons, and household items (pans, spoons, dishes).
- 3 to 5 years: The child enjoys manipulating things such as dolls, cars and trucks, doll houses, building materials (such as Legos) and blocks, pens, paper, glue, balls, and dress-up materials.
- 6 to 12 years: The child enjoys bicycles, jump ropes, puzzles, board games, craft projects, roller skates, skateboards, and electronic games.

Developmental Stages of the Infant

The developmental stages of the infant are described below:

- Infant (0-12 months)
    - Period of intense cognitive and physical development
- Biologic Development:
    - Weight Gain: tripled since birth
    - Height: birth length increased by 50%
    - Growth: Head-to-toe development (termed *cephalocaudal*)
- Motor Development:
    - 2-3 months: grasping objects, lift head (prone), social smile.
    - 4-6 months: rolling over, sitting up alone, bringing object to mouth; holding own bottle; recognizes mother, likes/dislikes.
    - 6-7 months: crawling, transfer objects between hands; may begin to imitate sounds; stranger anxiety, responds to name.
    - 9-10 months: "creeping," pincher grasp, prone to sitting; hand preference; says "mama" and "dada"; waves "goodbye."
    - 11-12 months: block tower of 2, walking, removing objects from containers; shakes head yes/no, 5-word vocabulary.

- Cognitive Development:
  - *Piaget:* Sensory Motor / Intuitive thought: only aware of what is happening directly around them. No understanding of relationship between events.
  - *Erikson:* "Trust vs Mistrust."
  - *Freud*: Oral – Nursing/Weaning.

Vision Development in Infants

Vision development in infants is described below:

- **Birth to 4 months**: Able to see patterns of light, dark, and shades of gray. Focus is mere 8 to 12 inches, resulting in mostly blurred vision.
- **4 to 6 months**: As babies learn to push themselves up, roll over, sit, and scoot, eye/body coordination develops as they learn to control their own movements in space. Normal visual acuity, or a child's sharpness of vision, has *usually developed to 20/20 by the time the child reaches 6 months.*
- **6 to 8 months**: Most babies start crawling during this time, further developing eye/body coordination. They learn to judge distances and set visual goals, seeing something and moving to get it. Depth perception should be developing around this time
- **8 to 12 months**: Babies can now judge distances well. Eye/hand/body coordination allows them to grasp and throw objects fairly accurately.

Developmental Stage of the Toddler

The developmental stage of the toddler is described below:

- Toddler (12-36 months)
  - Intense period of exploration using all senses; temper tantrums; fierce independence (prefer finger foods to feed themselves; give choices); ritualistic (need routine).
- Biologic Development
  - Weight Gain: slows to 4-6 lb/year (4x birth weight by 2 years)
  - Height: 3 inches per year
  - Growth is "step-like" rather than "linear"
- Maturation of Systems
  - Physiologic systems relatively mature at end of toddlerhood
  - Upper respiratory infections, otitis media, and tonsillitis are common among toddlers
  - Sphincter control - age 18-24 months (anal – potty training)
  - Locomotion - improved coordination, between ages 2-3, fine motor development. Learns spatial relationships
  - Improved manual dexterity, throws ball by age 18 months; push/pull toys the best; parallel play seen
- Cognitive Development
  - *Piaget*: sensorimotor and preoperational phase = awareness of causal relationships between two events; trial and error.
  - *Erikson*: "Autonomy vs Shame and Doubt."
  - *Freud*: Anal Stage – Potty Training.

Developmental Stage of the Preschool-Aged Child

The developmental stage of the preschool-aged child is described below:

- The Preschooler (3-5 years)
  - Exhibits increased attention span and memory; is highly literal (uses language for mental symbolization).
  - Greatest fear is body mutilation, and has poorly defined body boundaries; fear that if skin is "broken" all blood and "insides" can leak out. Use dolls and play therapy to explain procedures.
- Biologic Development
  - Weight: 4-5 lb/year.
  - Height: 2-3 inches/year.
- Motor Development
  - Fine motor: refinement in eye-hand and muscle coordination, drawing, art work, skillful manipulation.
  - Gross motor: walking, running, climbing, and jumping well established.
  - Associative/cooperative play; imaginative playmates, enjoys dress up, imitation; dramatic play without rules.
- Cognitive Development
  - *Piaget*: Preoperative; no concept of time/conversation. Egocentric.
  - *Erikson*: "Initiative vs Guilt."
  - *Freud*: Phallic - Oedipus (male)/Electra(female) complex (attached to parent of opposite sex).

Developmental Stage of the School Aged Child

The developmental stage of the school aged child is described below:

- School Age (6-11 years)
  - Developing sense of self-worth; praise is vital to avoid feelings of inferiority. Detail-oriented. Wants to get things "right."
  - Enjoy competitive games, physical activities (bike riding, etc.). Often plays with same sex, creates "clubs."
  - Inquisitive: Asks many questions, wants to know how things work. Enjoys memorization.
- Biologic Development
  - Weight: gain ~5 lb/year.
  - Height: increase ~2 inches/year.
  - Adult teeth come in; muscular strength and physical skills increase.
- Motor Development
  - Fine motor skills refined; can complete arts/craft projects without difficulty – adult level ~12 years. Dressing self/completely capable of self-care.
  - Gross motor –rapid increase in coordination/motor control.
  - Verbal: Can read simple sentences. Vocabulary – 2500 words.

- Cognitive Development
  - *Piaget:* Concrete Operational – literal thinkers, but able to see other's viewpoints and discern different tenses; able to organize.
  - *Erikson:* "Industry vs Inferiority."
  - *Freud:* Latent – focus on cognitive learning, pause in sexual exploits.

Developmental Stages of Adolescents

The developmental stages of adolescents are described below:

- Adolescents (12-18 years)
  - Time of sexual maturation and social development.
  - Emphasis on social events: enjoy team sports, social outings, and connection with peers. Biggest fear is social rejection.
  - Begin to view self as separate from parents, values autonomy; may manifest in periods of rebellion of parents' rules.
- Biologic Development
  - Weight: gain 15-60 lb by end of adolescence.
  - Height: 2-12 inches of increase by age 18.
  - Maturation of sexual organs: females - develop breasts and begin menses; males - enlargement and maturation of penis and testes. Other secondary sexual characteristics develop.
  - Body image highly important to adolescents.
  - Increased activity of sebaceous glands produces acne.
- Motor Development
  - Emphasis on physical activities; may have some clumsiness in early teenage years; adult-level motor control ~15 years of age.
- Cognitive Development
  - *Piaget:* Formal operational: adult level reasoning, able to handle abstract thoughts; can hypothesize and use inductive and deductive reasoning.
  - *Erikson:* "Identity vs Social Isolation."
  - *Freud:* Genital – sexual relationships developed.

Tanner Staging for Preadolescents and Adolescents

Tanner Staging is used to describe sexual maturation.

Males: Stages of pubic hair and external genital development include:

1. Preadolescent: no changes.
2. Scrotum and testes begin to enlarge, pubic hair at base of penis.
3. Penis lengthens, scrotum enlarges, and more darkly pigmented pubic hair.
4. Penis continues to grow, pubic hair more extensive, scrotum more pigmented.
5. Pubic hair spreads to thighs, scrotum enlarges, and penis extends to bottom of scrotum.

Females:

Stages of Breast Development	Stages of Pubic Hair
1. Only nipple raised above chest.	1. No pubic hair.
2. Breast budding.	2. Soft downy hair along labia majora.
3. Breast and areola enlarge.	3. Sparse dark hair along the labia majora.
4. Areola enlarges and may form a secondary elevation.	4. Heavy coarse pubic hair about labia majora.
5. Full breasts with pigmented areola and projecting nipples.	5. Adult distribution of pubic hair extending laterally and superiorly.

Sexual Maturation in Adolescent Females

Sexual maturation in girls begins between the ages of 9 and 13. During this time, a woman will reach her peak height. The first sign of puberty in girls is the development of breast tissue. Other signs include:

- Appearance of pubic hair.
- Increase in vaginal discharge (physiologic leukorrhea).
- Menarche: occurs approximately 2 years after breast buds. The average age of menarche is about 12½ years, but can occur any time between the ages of 10 and 15. While it is still unknown what exactly causes menstruation to begin, it is theorized that it is related to body fat percentage, with some genetic and nutritional components.

Nursing interventions include the following*:*

- Sexual education, with stress on birth control methods and normal menstruation.
- Nurse should suspect the need for further follow-up if no breast development by age 13 or no menarche within 4 years of onset of puberty.
- Ensure proper nutrition, emphasizing iron to prevent menarche-related anemia and calcium for bone health.

Sexual Maturation in Adolescent Males

Sexual maturation and puberty begin in boys between the ages of 10 and 14. During this time, a male will reach 20% to 25% of lean body mass and gain up to 50% ideal adult body weight. Boys often experience "growth spurts," which refer to general increase in growth of skeletal, muscles, and internal organs, which reaches peak at ~14 years of age. The first noted change signaling the beginning of sexual maturation is testicular enlargement accompanied by thinning, reddening, and increased looseness of the scrotum. Other signs include:

- Appearance of pubic and facial hair
- Voice changes
- *Gynecomastia:* temporary breast enlargement and tenderness may occur, ceasing after 2 years
- Ejaculation occurs more frequently, either spontaneously as a "wet dream" or via self-stimulation

Nursing interventions include the following:

- Sexual education, including ejaculation to allay embarrassment and fears regarding newfound sexuality
- Ensure proper nutrition, emphasizing protein for increased rate of growth

Body Image Changes Related to Aging and Pregnancy

Body image changes that the nurse must be sensitive to include:

- **Aging**: Clients must deal with physical changes (wrinkles, health problems, gray hair, weight gain, impaired mobility, skin changes, changes in metabolism), psychological changes (fear of dependency, feelings of inadequacy, lack of respect from others, depression), and social inequities and concerns (low income, job insecurity, housing issues). Clients often experience cultural biases against aging and may begin to feel that they are less attractive and a burden to others.
- **Pregnancy**: Clients experience weight gain, breast enlargement, abdominal expansion and stretch marks, and often acne, fatigue, backache, urinary frequency, nausea, hair loss, and hemorrhoids. Some women may maintain a positive image, but many may feel that they are less attractive and "fat" and may suffer from low self-esteem and a lack of control, especially if they feel they should be able to maintain the same activities as before pregnancy. Some may develop pregorexia (anorexia associated with pregnancy).

Attachment to a Newborn and Parenting

Facilitating **attachment to newborn** begins before delivery by educating the mother about bonding and the importance of early and close contact with her infant. Ensuring skin-to-skin contact within the first hour is especially important, but different approaches are used:

- If the neonate appears stable at delivery, he/she should be placed on the mother's abdomen for drying and initial assessment and then placed between the mother's breasts and covered with a blanket to prevent temperature loss. Weighing, measuring, and bathing the infant is deferred.
- The neonate may be assessed in a warmer, dried, diapered, weighed and measured and then placed between the mother's breasts.
- After delivery, the neonate should be held with skin-to-skin contact as soon as possible and as often as possible.
- If the mother is breastfeeding, the neonate should start nursing within 30 to 60 minutes of delivery.

Providing the parents with information and resources about **parenting**, encouraging them, asking them what kind of parents they want to be and how much they know about childrearing as a basis for discussion, and answering their questions may help parents gain confidence.

Developmental Tasks of the Older Adult According to Erikson

Erikson's Psychosocial Theory of Development states that the older adults (65 years and older) are in the stage of "Ego Integrity vs Despair." The older adult is adjusting to new situations including economic, social, familial, and sexual changes that occur with age. If the older adult comes to a place of accepting the aging process and looking back on their life with a feeling of accomplishment and gratefulness, they have completed the task of ego integrity. However, if he/she fails to accomplish this task, the person will experience despair. Common fears of the older adult include death, becoming a burden to their family, inability to care for themselves, and loss of self among others.

Menopause

Menopause is the permanent termination of the menstrual cycle, considered a normal process of aging. Menopause may also be caused by ovarian failure or hysterectomy; however, traditionally menopause begins on its own around age 50 for most women.

Signs and symptoms: cessation of menstruation, insomnia, hot flashes/night sweats (vasomotor instability), and mood changes such as nervousness, irritability, anxiety, and depression. Due to the lack of estrogen production, women also often experience atrophy of the urogenital epithelium and surrounding skin.

Diagnosis: age/physical exam, blood hormone levels.

Treatment includes:

- Medications: hormone replacement therapy (HRT) if desired.
- Symptom management: fans/light clothing for hot flashes, counseling for mood swings, vaginal lubricant for painful coitus.

Retirement and the Loss of a Loved One

Life transitions include:

- **Retirement**: Clients who have strongly identified with their role at work may find retirement difficult. They may benefit from discussing their feelings and their options. Clients may be encouraged to list their skills and attributes and to consider volunteering for an organization in need of those skills, working part time, and/or becoming active in community organizations.
- **Loss of a loved one**: Providing support and acceptance is essential as is recognizing that individuals grieve in different ways. The client should be encouraged to talk about the loved on and share memories as this can help in the healing process. Some clients may benefit from support groups. For example, there are support groups for parents who have lost children and others for those who have lost spouses/partners. Discussing the grieving process and stages of grief may help clients understand that their feelings are part of a normal continuum.

Health Promotion and Disease Prevention

Health Education Methods

Health education includes:

- **Community health education**: Focuses on issues of concern to the community as a whole or to a target group within the community, including the need for immunizations, alcohol and drug abuse, homelessness, communicable diseases, chronic disease, tobacco use, nutrition, violence prevention, mental health, and environmental quality. Methods utilized may include lectures, community workshops, posters, classes, pamphlets, TV interviews/programs, websites, and radio announcements. Community organizations often collaborate in efforts to improve outreach.

- **One-on-one client education**: Focuses on more narrow areas of concern to the individual, such as a need for the client to lose weight and increase exercise or to stop abusing drugs or alcohol. The education is geared toward the individual's needs and should be a collaborative effort between the nurse and the client to improve the chance of success. One-to-one coaching may be done in person, through the telephone, or though video chat.

Education: Smoking Cessation

Health and Human Services Guidelines for Smoking Cessation	
Ask	Ask every adolescent/adult at every visit about smoking and record response.
Advise	Advise all smokers to quit and explain smoking's effect on health and benefits of quitting.
Assess	Assess general readiness to quit smoking by asking if the person is willing to try to quit, and provide resources and information. If client is unwilling to quit, provide support and try to motivate the client to quit.
Assist	Assist the smoker with a plan to quit smoking, including a target date (within 2 weeks), removal of cigarettes, enlistment of family and friends, review of past efforts, and anticipation of challenges the person will face during withdrawal (nervousness, craving). Advise the smoker about the need for abstinence and the association between smoking and drinking. Provide aids (nicotine replacement products or other prescription drugs).
Arrange follow-up	Monitor, encourage, and reinforce to evaluate progress.

Education: Exercise Needs

Daily **exercise** is an important component of good health practices but should be age-appropriate, and some health conditions may pose restrictions. Toddlers and young children usually get exercise by running and playing and do not need organized activities, but others benefit from planned exercise:

- **4-5-year-olds** may participate in dancing, skating and other supervised activities but lack coordination and judgment about safety.
- **6-12-year-olds** are still growing and muscles are short, so they do best with non-competitive sports, such as bicycling and swimming, until about age 10. Team sports should be supervised to ensure children are not straining muscles. Weight lifting may be done at 11 to build strength. Gymnastics may begin but children should be monitored for eating disorders.
- **12-18-year-olds** can participate in any sports activity unless limited by illness or disability. Exercise should be done at least 3 times weekly for 30 minutes.
- **Adults**: Exercise should be done at least 30 minutes daily or 150 minutes/week.

Education: Complementary Therapies

Complementary therapies used as well as conventional medical treatment should be included if this is what the client/family wants, empowering the family to take some control. Complementary therapies vary widely and most can easily be incorporated into the plan of care The National Center for Complementary and Alternative Medicine recognizes the following:

Whole medical systems	Include homeopathic, naturopathic medicine, acupuncture, and Chinese herbal medications
Mind-body medicine	Can include support groups, medication, music, art, or dance therapy.
Biologically-based practices	Include the use of food, vitamins, or nutrition for healing.
Manipulative/ body-based programs	Include massage or other types of manipulation, such as chiropractic treatment.
Energy therapies	May include biofield therapies intended to affect the aura (energy field) that some believe surrounds all living things. These therapies include therapeutic touch and Reiki.
Bio-electro-magnetic-based therapies	Include use of a variety of magnetic fields (pulsed, magnetic, direct current).

Educational Points for Patients with CAD

The following are crucial educational points to discuss with patient diagnosed with **coronary artery disease (CAD)** and their families:

- Definition and causes of CAD
  - A buildup of plaque causing narrowing of vessels in heart
  - Modifiable vs Nonmodifiable Risk Factors: genetics, family history, diet, exercise, smoking.
- Signs and symptoms of an impending MI
  - Chest pain/pressure, radiating to neck/jaw, shortness of breath, sweating, nausea/vomiting – go to ER!
- Signs of Heart Failure
  - Report swelling in legs, sleeping in recliner, difficulty breathing with activity – could be signs of heart failure.
- Prescribed Medications
  - Take all medicines as prescribed! Medications for blood pressure, cholesterol, clot prevention, and aspirin common.
- Cardiac Diet
  - Limit salt (canned and processed foods) and high-fat foods.
- Lifestyle Modification.
  - Immediately stop smoking and use of any illegal drugs.
  - Low-impact exercise routine (30 minutes a day of an activity such as walking.)

Review Video: Coronary Artery Disease
Visit mometrix.com/academy and enter code: 836940

Education Points for Patients with COPD

While chronic obstructive pulmonary disease (COPD) is a chronic disease, the quality of life of these patients can be greatly impacted by their adherence to the medical regimen. Crucial teaching points for these patients and their families are:

- Smoking Cessation
  - Cause of disease, constricts bronchioles, and damages lungs further.
  - Support group, nicotine patch, and other helpful therapies.
- Nutrition
  - Increased caloric needs since work of breathing in increased.
  - Frequent small meals throughout the day work best to decrease fatigue.
- Breathing exercises
  - *"Cough and Deep Breath"*- Take 2-3 deep breaths into abdomen, and while exhaling the third, cough 2-3 times. This helps open lungs/move secretions.
  - *"Pursed Lip Breathing"*- Have patient take deep breaths in through nose, and force air out through pursed lips. This opens alveoli – "smell the cake, now blow out the candles!"
- Signs and symptoms of infection
  - Report increase in sputum, green/brown/rust-colored sputum, increased dyspnea, fever, chills, and racing heartbeat right away.
- Oxygen safety
  - Never smoke in home with oxygen tank; replace before empty. Do not use more than 2-3 liters due to hypoxic drive to breathe.

Education Points for Patients with Diabetes Mellitus

The severity of the effects of diabetes is greatly impacted by the care these patients take in managing their disease. The following are crucial educational points to discuss with the diabetic patient and their families:

- Signs and symptoms of hypoglycemia/hyperglycemia:
  - "Cold & Clammy? Get some candy!"; irritability is often first sign.
  - "Hot & Dry? Sugar is high!"
- Sick Day rules:
  - Check sugar more often, stay hydrated.
- Procedure for giving insulin injections:
  - Injection Sites: arm, abdomen, inner thigh: must rotate!
  - Use of syringe: ensure no air bubbles, use sharps container
- Proper medication storage:
  - Do not store insulin in the refrigerator
  - Label with date/time; expiration date (generally 28 days)
- Diabetic Diet:
  - Count carbohydrates, avoid excess simple carbs/ add protein.
  - Refer to registered dietitian if needed
  - Check sugar before meals; eat more carbs if increased activity

- Proper care of skin and feet:
  - Inspect feet daily with mirror, always wear diabetic shoes.
  - Do not cut own nails - go to podiatrist.

Recommendations Regarding Physician Visits

For health promotion and maintenance, clients should make routine **visits to a physician** for assessment. Frequency varies according to age and condition. Those with risk factors, such as smoking, excessive drinking, and chronic disease often must visit physicians more frequently. Typical frequency:

- Infant ≤3 years: Visits at 3-5 days, 1, 2, 4, 6, 9, 12, 15, 18, 24, 30, and 36 months for assessment of growth and development and immunizations.
- ≥3 years to 18: Annual physician visits for assessment of growth and development as well as immunizations (such as HPV near age of puberty).
- 21 years: Females should have a baseline Pap smear (earlier if sexually active, especially with multiple partners) and then repeat Pap smears every 1 to 2 years.
- 18 to 30 years: Physical exam every 2 to 3 years or more frequently if presence of risk factors.
- 30 to 40 years: Physical exam every 2 years. Females should have a baseline mammogram at age 40 and then repeat every 1 to 2 years. Males should have annual prostate exams beginning at age 40.
- 40 to 50: Physical exam every 1 to 2 years. ≥50: Both males and females should have baseline colonoscopy at age 50 with repeat every 10 years until age 80 or more frequently if precancerous lesions detected. Physical exam every year. Females should have osteoporosis screening at age 65 or younger with risk factors.

Levels of Disease Prevention

Levels of disease prevention include:

- **Primary**: The goal is to prevent the initial occurrence of a health problem, such as a disease or injury, through activities such as immunizations, smoking cessation, fluoride supplementation of water, promotion of seat belt use, and use of child car seat restraints. Interventions are often aimed at the general public or large groups of people.
- **Secondary**: The goal is to identify diseases or conditions quickly and provide prompt intervention for treatment and prevention of further disability through such activities as BP screenings, breast and testicular self-examinations, hearing and vision screenings, mammography, and pregnancy testing.
- **Tertiary**: The goal is to assist those who already have disease or disability to prevent further progress of the disease and to allow people to achieve the maximum quality of life through activities such as support groups, counseling, diet and exercise, stress management, and supportive services.

Childhood Immunization Schedule

Vaccines are one of the first lines of defense against infectious diseases in the community. Study the following graph carefully to understand the current vaccine schedule recommended for all children in the U.S by the CDC.

Note: Remember that live vaccines should never be given to those that are immunocompromised, and an egg allergy is a contraindication to the flu vaccine.

Vaccine	Birth	1 mo	2 mos	4 mos	6 mos	9 mos	12 mos	15 mos	18 mos	19–23 mos	2-3 yrs	4-6 yrs	7-10 yrs	11-12 yrs	13–15 yrs	16–18 yrs
Hepatitis B[1] (HepB)	1st dose	←2nd dose→			←3rd dose→											
Rotavirus[2] (RV) RV1 (2-dose series); RV5 (3-dose series)			1st dose	2nd dose	See footnote 2											
Diphtheria, tetanus, & acellular pertussis[3] (DTaP: <7 yrs)			1st dose	2nd dose	3rd dose			←4th dose→				5th dose				
Tetanus, diphtheria, & acellular pertussis[4] (Tdap: ≥7 yrs)														(Tdap)		
Haemophilus influenzae type b[5] (Hib)			1st dose	2nd dose	See footnote 5		←3rd or 4th dose, See footnote 5→									
Pneumococcal conjugate[6] (PCV13)			1st dose	2nd dose	3rd dose		←4th dose→									
Pneumococcal polysaccharide[6] (PPSV23)																
Inactivated poliovirus[7] (IPV: <18 yrs)			1st dose	2nd dose	←3rd dose→							4th dose				
Influenza[8] (IIV; LAIV) 2 doses for some: See footnote 8					Annual vaccination (IIV only) 1 or 2 doses						Annual vaccination (LAIV or IIV) 1 or 2 doses		Annual vaccination (LAIV or IIV) 1 dose only			
Measles, mumps, rubella[9] (MMR)					See footnote 9		←1st dose→					2nd dose				
Varicella[10] (VAR)							←1st dose→					2nd dose				
Hepatitis A[11] (HepA)							←2-dose series, See footnote 11→									
Human papillomavirus[12] (HPV2: females only; HPV4: males and females)														(3-dose series)		
Meningococcal[13] (Hib-MenCY ≥6 weeks; MenACWY-D ≥9 mos; MenACWY-CRM ≥ 2 mos)			See footnote 13											1st dose		Booster

From: http://www.cdc.gov/vaccines/schedules/downloads/child/0-18yrs-schedule-bw.pdf

Nutrition Screening

NUTRITIONAL ASSESSMENT

Nutritional assessments are the first step in determining a well-balanced diet that will promote optimal nutrition, body function, and healing processes. A nutritional assessment is performed for patients when there is a suspicion of nutritional imbalance/a change in health status that will require a change in dietary habits. If done correctly, a nutritional assessment will provide information on the quantity of vitamins and minerals an individual is consuming on a routine basis; this information is then evaluated and compared with what is required to function with or without the individual disease processes the patient has.

Nutritional assessments can be done quickly by reviewing a client's history during the initial assessment. If a more in-depth nutritional history is required, a practitioner may ask the individual to track dietary intake over a period of several days with a food diary or other tool, then go over the information with the client at a subsequent visit.

If further evaluation is desired, a blood test may give a better clinical picture. *Serum albumin (not weight) is the best clinical indicator of nutritional status (malnourishment).* This means a person can be overweight/obese and still be considered malnourished.

DIETARY STANDARDS

Dietary standards are a set of guidelines in which an individual can understand essential nutrients, food consumption, and the relationship they possess. Not only do dietary standards increase understanding of foods and their nutritional values, they offer a mechanism of comparison. The *Recommended Dietary Allowances (RDAs)* are a set of standards the federal government mandates that each individual needs on a daily basis to maintain balanced and adequate nutrition. *Reference Dietary Intake (RDI)* is a combination of recommended daily allowances and mechanisms of risk reduction for diseases such as coronary artery disease, obesity, cancer, and osteoporosis. The dietary standards of RDA and RDI are used today with meal preparation for military personnel, groups such as WIC (Women, Infants, and Children), and meals on wheels programs throughout the country.

USDA'S MYPLATE AND DIETARY GUIDELINES

In 2011, the **USDA's Food Pyramid** was replaced with **MyPlate**. MyPlate consists of a picture of a dinner plate divided into four sections. Vegetables and grains each take up 30% of the plate, while fruits and proteins each constitute 20% of the plate. There is also a representation of a cup, marked Dairy, alongside the plate.

The USDA's guidelines can be easily summarized:

- To maintain or improve weight, individuals need to preserve a balance between exercise and food consumption.
- Individuals should choose to consume a diverse diet high in grains, fresh fruits, and vegetables.
- Diets that minimize the consumption of sodium, sugars, fats/cholesterol, and alcohol are recommended.

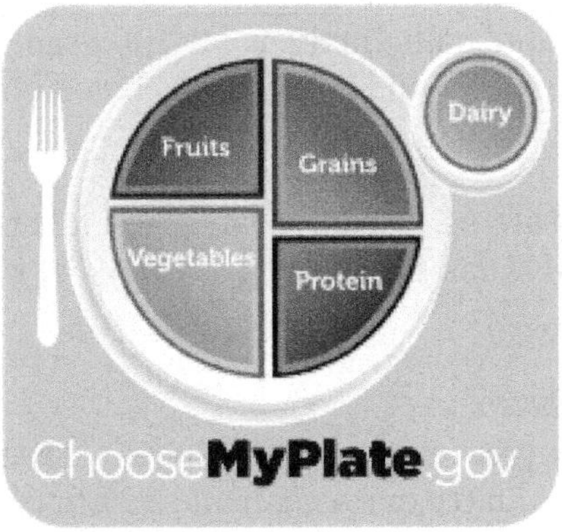

MyPlate Recommended Daily Servings

The following are the **five main food groups** and the recommended daily serving for each, according to www.chooseMyPlate.gov:

- Grains (3-5 oz/day for children; 6 to 8 oz/day for adolescents and adults; at least half of grains eaten should be whole grains)
    - Foods found in this category include breads, rice, cereals, and pasta and are divided into two subgroups: whole grains and refined grains.
- Fruits (1-2 cups daily depending on age and sex)
    - Foods found in this category include any fruit and 100% fruit juice.
- Vegetables (1-3 cups daily depending on age and sex)
    - Foods found in this category are broken down into dark green vegetables, starchy vegetables, red and orange vegetables, beans and peas, and other vegetables.
- Protein (2-4 oz/day for children, 5-6 oz/day for adolescents and adults)
    - Foods found in this category include pork, beef, chicken, turkey, and fish, along with eggs and nuts. Beans and peas are also considered protein and are found in both the protein group and vegetable group.
- Dairy (2-3 cups/day)
    - Foods found in this category include cheese, milk, ice cream, and yogurt.

OTHER: Oils (Oils are NOT considered a food group but offer essential nutrients and therefore included; recommended allowance of 3-7 tsp/day depending on age and sex.)

- Foods found in this category include any fat that is liquid at room temperature.

Nutrients Required by the Human Body and Age-Related Concerns

Macronutrients:

Protein	Requirements for healthy elderly individuals is 1.0 g/kg body weight, and approximately 12-14% of total caloric intake.
Fat	Necessary for life because they transport and help absorb fat-soluble vitamins (A, D, K, E). Fats impart flavor to food and enhance satiety. Digestion of fat is inhibited in the elderly, and fats should comprise, at most, 30% of total caloric intake.
Carbohydrates	The recommended daily intake is 50-100 grams minimum. At least 50% of total caloric intake should be provided by complex carbohydrate sources. Fiber intake should be 20-35 grams per day.

The caloric content provided by proteins, carbohydrates, and fats is as follows: Protein has 4 calories per gram, Carbohydrate also has 4 calories per gram, Fat has 9 calories per gram. **Vitamin requirements change with age:**

- Vitamin A requirements: Decreases
- Vitamin D requirements: Increases; sources include increasing exposure to sunlight and including foods rich in vitamin D, such as fish and fortified skim milk and orange juice
- Vitamin B12 requirements: Increases; sources include foods such as chicken, lean red meat, and skim milk
- Folate requirement: Decreases; there are no recommended changes

Functions and Classifications of Nutrients

Classifying Nutrients: Nutrients are generally divided into six categories: carbohydrates, vitamins, proteins, minerals, lipids (fats), and water. Nutrients are further classified as either essential or nonessential, which refer to the body's ability to produce the needed nutrient. For example, essential nutrients are nutrients that must be obtained through diet. These essential nutrients are required by the body on a daily basis for growth and health maintenance. Nonessential nutrients are those nutrients the body is capable of producing on its own.

Functions of nutrients are as follows:

- Lipids (fats), Proteins, and Carbohydrates: provide energy for body functions, aid in tissue growth.
- Vitamins: perform in a catalytic role to promote the use of nutrients for energy.
- Water and Minerals: Tissue repair and function; body temperature regulation.

Water-Soluble Vitamins

Water-soluble vitamins are those vitamins that the body cannot store, and need to be replenished on a daily basis. Water-soluble vitamins include all the B vitamins and vitamin C. A key fact to remember about water-soluble vitamins is that because they are excreted easily by the body/not stored, they need to be consumed regularly in order for the body to have an adequate supply.

Sources include citrus, tomatoes, cantaloupe, potatoes, green leafy vegetables, pork, liver, and enriched breads and cereals.

Functions and Sources of Major Vitamins

Vitamin	Major Functions	Found in
A	eyes, skin, immune system	dark green or orange fruits and vegetables, milk
B6	producing RBCs, brain/nerve function	spinach, beans, nuts, eggs, red meat, fish
B12	producing RBCs, nerve function	eggs, milk, chicken, red meat, fish
C	teeth, bones, skin	spinach, tomatoes, berries, citrus fruits
D	bones, absorbing calcium	milk, egg yolk, sunlight
E	protects cells from damage, involved in function of RBCs	nuts, grains, oils, green vegetables
Folic Acid	protects against heart disease, essential for cell health, fetal CNS development	fruits, dark green vegetables

Potassium

The mineral **potassium** is involved in both electrical and cellular physiologic processes. (In the human body, it is considered an electrolyte).

Potassium has various functions in metabolism and other body processes including:

- Assisting acid-base and water balance regulation in the bloodstream and tissues.
- Assisting in synthesizing proteins from amino acids and metabolizing carbohydrates.
- Building muscle and helping with normal body growth.
- Proper functioning of neurons.

Fish like salmon, cod, sardines, and flounder are rich sources of potassium. Some other meats contain potassium as well. Potassium-rich vegetables include broccoli, peas, tomatoes, lima beans, potatoes, and leafy green vegetables like spinach, lettuce, and parsley. Fruits sources include citrus fruits, apples, apricots, and bananas.

Sodium

Sodium is naturally-occurring in most foods. Table salt, the most common form of sodium, is sodium chloride. Milk, celery, and beets also contain sodium naturally, as does drinking water, but the amount of sodium varies depending on the source. Added forms of sodium include monosodium glutamate, sodium nitrite, sodium bicarbonate (baking soda), sodium saccharin, and sodium benzoate.

These additives are ingredients in seasonings and condiments such as bouillon cubes, garlic salt, onion salt, soy sauce, and Worcestershire sauce. Processed meats, like bacon, ham, and sausage, and canned vegetables and soups are all good examples of foods with added sodium. Fast foods are usually quite high in sodium.

Additionally, sodium can cause fluid retention in individuals with congestive heart failure, cirrhosis or liver disease, kidney disease, or hypertension. Patients with these conditions should follow strict sodium-restricted diets as recommended or prescribed by their physician.

Changes and Potential Complications in Nutrition for Adolescents

Adolescence is a time of accelerated growth and development, and thus brings with it different nutritional needs. The following are some of the common nutritional issues seen in this population:

- **Undernourishment:** Puberty can as much as double an adolescent's need for iron, calcium, zinc, and protein. Particularly for females, iron and calcium are crucial. Girls are more susceptible to iron deficiency at menarche due to blood loss. Also, maximum bone mass is acquired during the teen years, so the amount of calcium deposited determines risk of osteoporosis later in life.
- **Obesity:** related to an excess intake of calories. BMI equal to or greater than the 95th percentile for age and gender is considered overweight and should be investigated further. Obesity is found in all income, racial, and ethnic groups and both genders.
- **Eating Disorders:** May effect as many as 1/3 of adolescents in the United States. Signs and symptoms include recurrent dieting when not overweight, distorted body image, BMI below the 5th percentile, use of laxatives, emesis after meals (may see stained teeth, throat irritation), starvation.

Health Screening

Health Screening and Targeted Health Screening

Health screening, testing to determine if a problem exists, includes blood pressure checks, Pap smears, colonoscopies to screen for colon cancer, prostate exams, scoliosis assessment, blood glucose assessment, cholesterol screening, BMI assessment, HIV/AIDS, and osteoporosis screening. Screening is essential as a preventative measure because identifying a problem early and beginning treatment can help to prevent further complications. While some screening is recommended for all individuals, **targeted health screening** involves a subgroup of the population. For example, screening an entire population of HIV/AIDS or sexually-transmitted diseases would be a waste of resources because many individuals have almost no risk factors. With targeted screening, only those with multiple sexual partners, IV drug users, and/or males having sex with males would be screened because they have the greatest risk of developing the disease. Groups that have high rates of diabetes, such as African Americans or Hispanics, may be targeted for screening in a community.

Health Risk Factors Related to Ethnicity

Health risk factors related to ethnicity include:

- **Hypertension**: African Americans have consistently been shown to have higher rates of hypertension than Caucasian Americans, and age of onset is younger. These higher rates result in stroke rates that are double those of Caucasians and end-stage renal disease rates that are 5 times higher. Additionally, African Americans tend to respond differently to medications to control hypertension and heart failure. For example, African Americans tend to respond well to calcium channel blockers but not to ACE inhibitors, beta-blockers, or angiotensin II receptor blockers (ARBs).
- **Diabetes**: Ethnic minorities in America are at much higher risk of developing diabetes than Caucasian Americans: African Americans have 77% higher risk; Hispanics/Latin Americans, 66%; Asian Americans/Native Hawaiians/Pacific Islanders, 22%. Additionally, Alaskan Natives and Native Americans have death rates from diabetes that was 300% that of the general population and rates of kidney failure related to diabetes 3.5 times higher.

Pap Smear

A **Pap smear** is an exam that checks for changes in the cells of a woman's cervix. It is performed by a gynecologist during an annual exam. It is important for all women to have an annual Pap smear if they are sexually active or older than 18 years. The test is key to catching cervical problems and cancers early, allowing prompt diagnosis and treatment.

Considerations

The woman should avoid sex, douching, tampons, and the use of vaginal suppositories 24-48 hours before the test. There are no firm contraindications for a Pap smear, but it may be avoided during pregnancy, menstruation, or in patients with existing cervicitis until treated.

Procedure

On the day of the exam, the woman is placed in the lithotomy position, with her legs in stirrups. The doctor will then insert a speculum without lubricant into the woman's vagina, and open it up. A small brushing of the cells of the cervix is then taken to send to the laboratory. There the cells are tested for infection, abnormalities, and/or cancer.

Vaginitis

Vaginitis is a condition in which there is inflammation of the vagina. This most often occurs after menopause, but hormonal changes, medications (antibiotics, steroids, OCPs), STIs, IUDs, and douches/bubble baths can increase risk.

Signs and symptoms: pain with intercourse, vaginal itching/pain/discharge, vaginal irritation after intercourse.

Diagnosis: Pelvic examination, blood work (hormones), lab evaluation of vaginal secretions.

Treatment includes the following:

- Treat underlying cause: antibiotics for infections, removal of IUD, cease use of allergens, etc.
- Atrophic vaginitis: caused by low estrogen levels; hormone therapy and use of vaginal lubricant.
- Lifestyle modification: do not use douches/sprays, practice safe sex, use sufficient lubricant for comfort.

Bacterial Vaginosis

Bacterial vaginosis (BV) is a bacterial infection of the vagina, which can be caused by several different types of organisms. BV occurs when hydrogen peroxide–producing lactobacilli of the normal flora of the vagina are replaced by anaerobic bacteria, causing an increase in the pH of the vaginal secretions. Common causes of bacterial vaginosis include multiple sexual partners, frequent sex, douching, and the use of intra-uterine devices to avoid pregnancy.

Symptoms: white/gray vaginal discharge, "fishy"/foul smelling discharge, pain with intercourse, vaginal itching/irritation.

Diagnosis: gynecological exam, microscopic examination of vaginal secretions.

Treatment includes:

- Metronidazole (Flagyl) or other antibiotics: oral.
- Clindamycin 2% cream: vaginal suppository.
- Lifestyle modification: stop douching, condoms during sex, feminine hygiene education.

Trichomoniasis

Trichomoniasis is one of the most common sexually transmitted infections (STIs), caused by a species of the genus *Trichomonas*. Trichomoniasis can be found in both women and men. Those at highest risk of trichomoniasis are those with multiple sexual partners and those who have unprotected sexual intercourse with infected individuals.

Signs and symptoms: excessive vaginal discharge, genital irritation, difficult urination (dysuria), odor, painful sexual intercourse, suprapubic pain and discomfort.

Diagnosis: genital exam, microscopic examination of secretions

Treatment includes:

- Metronidazole (Flagyl): treat all sexual partners.
- Abstinence from sex to deter transmission until treatment is complete and patient is symptom free.
- Sex education.

Toxic Shock Syndrome

Toxic shock syndrome (TSS) is an infection of *Staphylococcus aureus* or another organism that ultimately causes shock and organ failure. It is generally associated with super-absorbent tampons, contraceptive sponges and diaphragms, but can also be related to recent surgery, infected wounds, or a viral infection. While more common in woman, TSS can affect both genders and all ages.

Signs and symptoms: seizures, headaches, hypotension, fatigue, multiple organ involvement, fever, nausea, vomiting; progress to shock and kidney failure.

Diagnosis: vital signs, urinalysis, blood work, CT scans, x-ray, depends on organ involvement.

Treatment includes:

- IV antibiotics.
- Vassopressors if hypotensive and fluid resuscitation.
- Dialysis if renal failure develops.
- Surgery to remove necrotic tissue.
- Teaching: change tampons frequently, and use lowest absorbancy.
- Wear pads at night. If had TSS, patient cannot use tampons or internal devices because TSS can occur again.

PID

Pelvic inflammatory disease (PID) is an infection of the fallopian tubes, uterus, or ovaries. It is commonly caused by an STI (generally chlamydia or gonorrhea), though it can be caused by intrauterine devices, childbirth/miscarriage, or abortion. Often, PID is asymptomatic; it is usually not diagnosed until fertility or pain problems are seen. Those with multiple sexual partners, recent IUD insertion, or a history of PID/STI are at an increased risk.

Signs and symptoms: Pain in pelvic region or with intercourse, discharge, fever, nausea, painful urination, irregular menstruation; untreated can lead to ectopic pregnancies, infertility, and chronic pelvic pain.

Diagnosis: Pelvic exam, laparoscopy, ESR, endometrial biopsy

WBC count, pregnancy test, cultures for infection

Treatment includes:

- Antibiotics: oral, or IV if severe infection. Partner should come in for testing and be treated as well.
- Surgery: could require drainage of abscess, or hysterectomy if severe.
- Lifestyle modification: abstinence until cleared from infection, safe sex, regular STI testing, don't douche, wipe front-to-back.

Breast Self-Examination

Breast self-examination should begin when patients are in their 20s and should ideally be performed monthly after menses when breasts are less tender (on day 5 to 7 with day 1 the first day of menses) or at any time in the month for postmenopausal women. Patients should begin by examining the breasts in a mirror to note any changes, such as skin dimpling, contour changes, discolorations, skin retractions, or nipple discharge. They should note any venous prominence, nipple inversion, or peau d'orange (orange peel appearance of tissue). Any abnormalities should be reported to their physician. The patient should palpate the breast when in supine position with the arm on the side examined extended above the head. The patient may use a circular, wedge, or vertical strip palpation pattern. If patients have had previous breast surgery, they should be advised to examine remaining breast tissue and the chest wall for any nodules or changes. Males who are at risk of breast cancer should also be advised to do monthly breast examinations.

Testicular Self-Examination

Testicular self-examination should begin during adolescence and should be carried out monthly, usually after a warm shower or bath because the scrotal tissue is more relaxed. The patient should hold the penis to the opposite side of the testes being examined. Steps include:

- Palpating the testicles with both hands to determine if they are smooth and uniform in size, shape, and consistency. It is not uncommon for one testis to be longer or larger than the other, but changes should be noted.
- Rolling the testes gently horizontally back and forth (thumb on top and fingers below) to feel for any abnormalities, such as lumps.
- Rolling the testes gently vertically in the same procedure as above.
- Using the index finger, palpate the epididymis, which is a cordlike structure superior and posterior to each testicle, and the spermatic cord on both testes.

Patients should be advised to report any changes, swelling, or lumps.

High Risk Behaviors

Educating Clients on High Risk Behaviors

High-risk behaviors and associated increased risks:

Multiple sex partners	STDs, including HIV/AIDS and HPV (which may result in cervical cancer).
Males-having-sex-with males	Hepatitis, STDs (including HPV), and HIV/AIDS infection.
Unprotected sex	STDs and pregnancy.
Alcohol abuse	Cirrhosis, liver cancer, oral cancer, colon cancer, breast cancer, heart disease, accidental injury, dementia, hypertension, fetal alcohol syndrome.
Drug abuse	Infection, accidental injury, seizures, coma, cardiac arrest, cognitive impairment, hallucinations, delusions, organ damage.
Unhealthy diet	Obesity, hypertension, diabetes mellitus, high cholesterol, breast cancer, colon cancer, osteoporosis.
Marijuana use	Impaired cognition (especially with use during adolescence), accidental injury.
Lack of physical activity	Obesity, heart disease, hypertension, osteoporosis.

Infectious Mononucleosis

Infectious mononucleosis ("mono"), sometimes called "the kissing disease," is a viral infection caused by the Epstein-Barr virus. Infectious mononucleosis characteristically occurs in young adults and most often is transmitted via saliva. Those at increased risk of infectious mononucleosis include students (both high school and college) and those with impaired immunity.

Signs and symptoms: generalized lymphadenopathy, sore throat/pharyngitis, dysphagia, fever, chills, splenomegaly (enlarged spleen), headache, anorexia, nausea/vomiting, and generalized malaise/extreme fatigue.

Diagnosis: blood work (antibody test/WBC), physical exam

Treatment includes:

- Rest: avoid contact sports, strenuous lifting / any other rigorous activity due to splenomegaly (risk of rupture).
- Antipyretics/mild analgesics for fever/discomfort.
- Saltwater gargles/cool drinks and smoothies for sore throat/dysphagia.
- Steroids possibly prescribed depending on severity.
- Educate on prevention: do not share drinks; spread by oral contact, can be spread by person who is asymptomatic.

Adolescent Pregnancy

Adolescent/teen pregnancy is defined as pregnancy in which the woman gives birth before the age of 20. Teenage pregnancies are considered high risk, as they have an increased incidence of poor outcomes for mom and baby.

Common complications are as follows:

- *Bleeding*: Likely to signal spontaneous abortion. *If a woman presents with bleeding and abdominal pain, the provider MUST rule out ectopic pregnancy.
- *Ectopic pregnancy*: Highest rate of mortality in teens; increased risk with history of intrauterine device, pelvic inflammatory disease/surgery or previous ectopic pregnancy.
- *Prolonged labor*: Labor may be prolonged in younger teens due to *fetopelvic incompatibility*, meaning the head of the fetus is too large to pass through the mother's pelvis. This is especially prevalent in pregnant mothers aged 12-16, due to their smaller stature and incomplete growth. This age group is at a greatly increased risk of cesarean delivery.

Prevention is as follows:

- Teaching abstinence as ideal.
- Educate on methods of birth control: condoms for younger teens, oral contraceptives for older adolescents.

Drug Use During Pregnancy

The use of **drugs during pregnancy** is extremely detrimental to mother and fetus. This is because the use of cocaine and other stimulant drugs causes systemic release of epinephrine and norepinephrine, resulting in vasoconstriction. This includes the arteries and veins in the umbilical cord. A decreased blood supply means a decrease in the amount of nutrients and oxygen to the fetus, causing impaired growth and intellectual disability. Women who continue to abuse drugs during pregnancy have an increased risk of abruptio placenta, abortion in the first trimester, growth limitations, premature, and non-living births. Babies who are born to mothers who ingest drugs have a tendency to have lower Apgar scores/neurological problems (often evidenced by a shrill, piercing cry), irritability, increased startle reflexes, and an increased risk of sudden infant death syndrome (SIDS).

Contraindications to Contraceptive Methods

The following are **contraindications to contraceptive methods** that must be communicated when family planning methods are discussed:

- **Oral contraceptives**: Contraindications include history of stroke or cerebrovascular disease, DVT, pulmonary embolism of CHF; hypertension, diabetes associated with vascular conditions; breast cancer, estrogen-dependent cancerous lesions; breast cancer; liver disease; cigarette smoking; age >35; possible pregnancy; and vaginal bleeding.
- **Barrier contraceptives** (condoms, diaphragms, cervical cap, contraceptive sponge): Some may develop or have an allergy to latex. Few contraindications unless the person is unable to apply correctly. Diaphragms may increase incidence of urinary tract infections and should be avoided with history of toxic shock syndrome. They should not be left in place for more than 24 hours. Contraceptive sponges contain nonoxynol, so they are contraindicated with allergy to the drug.
- **Intrauterine devices**: Contraindications include uterine anomaly, recent history of pelvic inflammatory disease, vaginitis, multiple sexual partners and high risk for STIs, and immunosuppression.
- **Injectable contraceptive (Depo-Provera®)**: Increases bone loss so should not be taken for longer than 2 years. Contraindications include history or current blood clots, breast cancer, or stroke; possible pregnancy; vaginal bleeding; liver disease, and allergy to ingredients.

Evaluating Massage Therapy and Acupuncture

Alternative or homeopathic health care practices include:

- **Massage therapy**: The reasons for the therapy may provide information about pain or other condition. While generally safe, massage should be avoided in areas with blood clots, infections, recent surgical procedures, fractures, wounds, or osteoporosis. Vigorous massage of the calves may dislodge clots or may cause bleeding in clients with bleeding disorders, anticoagulant therapy, or thrombocytopenia. Vigorous massage should also be avoided over areas of tumor because of risk of dislodging malignant cells and because tissue may be more friable.
- **Acupuncture**: It's important to ascertain the reason for the acupuncture in order to understand the client's needs. While generally safe, the needles may cause bleeding for those with bleeding disorders or anticoagulant therapy. Acupuncture with electrical stimulation should be avoided in clients with a pacemaker. Because acupuncture may stimulate labor, it should generally be avoided during pregnancy, especially in the abdominal area.

Uses and Possible Undesired Effects of Herbal Preparations

Herbal Preparation	Uses	Possible Undesired Effects
St. John's wort	Depression and anxiety	Nausea, dry mouth, headache, dizziness; may interact with antibiotics, birth control pills, antidepressants, warfarin, anticonvulsants, MAO inhibitors, antivirals, immunosuppressants and migraine drugs
Melatonin	Insomnia, Alzheimer's, cancer, ADHD, sexual disorders	Depression, lethargy, headache; may interact with NSAIDS, antihypertensives, steroids, and anti-anxiety medications
Ginseng	Stress, cancer, high cholesterol, diabetes, and to increase immunity and strength	Headache, anxiety, insomnia, rash, breast tenderness, hypertension or hypotension, and vaginal bleeding; may interact with cardiac drugs, anticoagulants, aspirin, anti-diabetic medications, diuretics, and NSAIDs
Ginkgo biloba	Alzheimer's, erectile dysfunction, mood elevation	GI disturbance, diarrhea, headache, muscle cramps, dizziness, seizures, increased bleeding, and skin irritation; may interact with aspirin, anticoagulants, diuretics, and NSAIDs
Echinacea	Viral infections, UTIs, allergic rhinitis, and fungal infections	GI disturbance, constipation, diarrhea, dizziness, and rash; may interact with immunosuppressants and steroids

Gram-Positive Neisseria Gonorrhoeae

Sexually transmitted **Neisseria gonorrhoeae** is a disease with horrific side effects if left untreated. While the organism is unable to survive dehydration or cool conditions, it is easily passed by sexual transmission from infected individuals and from mother to infant.

Signs and symptoms: asymptomatic during early infection.

- Males: urethritis with dysuria and purulent discharge.
- Female: purulent vaginal discharge and bleeding, pelvic inflammatory disease—this can lead to sterility, chronic pelvic pain, and ectopic pregnancy.

Diagnosis: laboratory examination of vaginal/seminal fluids.

Treatment is as follows:

- Antibiotics: ceftriaxone, ciprofloxacin, etc (penicillin [PCN] resistant).
- Chlamydia should be treated concurrently with gonorrhea using tetracycline or erythromycin.
- Monitor for: endocarditis, meningitis, septic arthritis.

Prevention: sex education/condoms, antibiotic eye drops prevent mother-baby transmission.

Positive and Negative Lifestyle Choices

Lifestyle choices are the choices that a person makes regarding how they live their life. While many of these choices do not affect one's health, some have a profound impact on a person's state of being throughout their lives. The following are considered basic examples of positive and negative lifestyle choices in regards to health:

The following are **positive lifestyle choices:**

- **Exercise** – increases bone-density, decreases chances of obesity, heart disease, diabetes.
- **A diet rich in fruits and vegetables** – increases overall health, decreases risk of cancers and numerous diseases.
- **Preventative care** – yearly physicals, follow-up with primary care physician; can help detect problems early and prevent complications.

The following are **negative/harmful lifestyle choices:**

- **Use of illicit drugs/excessive drinking** – increases risk of multiple diseases and complications; many drugs are addictive, even from first use. Can harm unborn children and others.
- **Smoking** – known to cause cancers and other diseases, including Buerger's and COPD.
- **Exposure to high-stress environments** – increases risk of heart attack and stroke; while unavoidable in some scenarios, patients should be referred to stress management techniques and counseling as needed.

Sexuality Issues Associated with Lifestyle Choices

Sexuality issues associated with lifestyle choices include:

- **Family planning**: When discussing family planning, the nurse should first ask clients their feelings about the issue as some clients, for religious or ethical reasons, may reject all or some family planning methods, such as contraception. Many have inadequate knowledge and may benefit from discussion of different options and associated contraindications and complications.

- **Menopause**: Clients are often concerned about body changes associated with menopause and may need information about dealing with the effects, such as mood swings and hot flashes. Some may be unaware that they may become pregnant during early stages when hormone levels fluctuate.
- **Impotence**: Clients are often reluctant to discuss impotence because of embarrassment or shame, so the nurse should address the issue matter-of-factly, providing information about possible causes (drugs, chronic health condition, alcohol use) and options available to the client, such as examination by a urologist, erectile dysfunction medications, alternative methods of sexual contact, and counseling.

Techniques of Physical Assessment

Assessing Vital Signs

Age-appropriate equipment and techniques for assessing vital signs include the following:

- **Blood pressure**: Use correct blood pressure cuff size for accuracy. The length of the cuff bladder should be equal to 80% of the arm's circumference, and the lower edge of the cuff when positioned should end about one inch above the antecubital fossa. For adults, inflate the cuff to 160 to 180 initially and increase pressure if pulse sounds are heard at that level. Usually, inflating the cuff to 100 to 120 initially is adequate for children. Extra-large cuffs are available for obese clients and pediatric cuffs for children. The BP is not usually assessed for infants.
- **Pulse**: Pulse should be assessed with the 3rd and 4th fingers for one minute with light pressure to count the rate and determine if the pulse is regular or irregular. The most commonly used site is the radial artery, but other sites include the temporal, carotid, apical (used commonly for infants and children), brachial, femoral, popliteal, and dorsalis pedis.
- **Respirations**: Includes assessment of the rhythm, breathing effort (dyspnea, wheezes), rate per minute (normal 12-20 for adults, 20-30 for children, and 40-60 for neonates), and comparison of inspiration/expirations (should be equal duration). Measure for at least 30 seconds.

Comprehensive Health Assessment

A **comprehensive system-based physical examination** is carried out methodically, moving from one system to another to ensure that all body systems are reviewed. The examination begins with a client and family history and then a general survey that includes assessment of psychosocial status, substance abuse, and domestic partner violence, and measurements (height, weight), vital signs as well as assessment of pain level and nutritional assessment. System-based physical examination utilizes inspection, palpation, percussion, and auscultation, While the order may vary somewhat, the usually order of examination is:

- Skin, nails, and hair.
- Head, face, and neck.
- Eyes, ears, nose, mouth, and throat.
- Breasts and regional lymph nodes.
- Thorax and lungs.
- Heart and neck vessels.
- Peripheral vascular/lymphatic system.
- Abdomen.
- Musculoskeletal system (may include functional assessment).

- Genitourinary system.
- Anus, rectum, and prostate.

Focused Health Assessment

A comprehensive health assessment is used to identify problems that a client may have and to determine baseline measurements while a **focused (problem-based) health assessment** focuses on an already identified problem. Often clients present with many health problems, so a focused (problem-base) assessment can be effective. Focused health assessments require a thorough history, including questioning family and caregivers when appropriate, to create a problem list. This approach does not preclude a complete exam, which might identify problems that the client has neglected, but the focus remains on the problem list generated. The list should be prioritized to ensure that the most critical issues (blood in the stool) are thoroughly assessed before less critical issues (occasional insomnia). Once a problem is identified, then differential diagnoses are determined. There may be a combination of physical and psychosocial elements to a problem. For example, urinary problems may relate to dehydration, lack of mobility, poor hygiene, medications, or disease. Appropriate diagnostic tests, further assessments, and interventions are completed as needed to diagnose and resolve problems.

Techniques When Conducting a Physical Assessment

A thorough and accurate **physical assessment** is the most important skill that a nurse performs, as it will determine the plan of care and help diagnose issues or complications that the patient may be having. There are four basic parts of physical assessment:

- **Inspection***:* Looking at the body area, assessing for symmetry and the presence or absence of normal features. Assess features bilaterally, noting size, color, odor, sounds, or any deviations from expected findings.
- **Palpation**: Placing your hands on the patient, palpating to determine softness, irregularities in texture, abdominal masses, edema, or other abnormalities. Palpation ranges from light (1-2cm) to deep (4-6cm), depending on what area of the body is being assessed. Remember to wear gloves when palpating mucous membranes.
- **Percussion***:* While not normally required in a nurses' daily assessment, percussion involves tapping one's fingers against a body part and listening to the sound. This can determine fluid build-up or thickness of underlying tissue. Percussion may also be used to determine tenderness.
- **Auscultation***:* This is listening to the patient's heart, lung or bowel sounds using your stethoscope. Ensure the environment is quiet, and the stethoscope is clean and fits into your ears. Expose the area you are listening to, and use firm pressure with the diaphragm for high-pitched noises and light-pressure with the bell for low-pitched sounds.

*Note: For an abdominal assessment, auscultate before palpation and percussion, as these can alter the presence of bowel sounds in the patient.

Assessment of Functional Abilities of Both Client and Primary Caregiver

Assessment of the **functional ability** (the ability of the client to carry out self-care activities of daily living with or without assistance) or the ability of a caregiver to assist should include both questioning and observation:

- **Feeding**: Assess the client's ability to hold utensils, cut food, eat and drink (including swallowing ability).
- **Preparing food**: Assess the ability to use stove, carry food, use refrigerator, and clean dishes. Consider the need for homemaking assistance and/or meals-on-wheels.
- **Grooming**: Assess the client's ability to wash hands and face, comb/brush hair, care for teeth, dress and undress. Ask about bathing facilities and need for assistance or assistive devices, such as grab bars and shower chairs.
- **Toileting**: Observe client getting on and off of toilet.
- **Continence**: Assess client's urinary and fecal continence and the need for incontinence supplies or bladder/bowel training.
- **Mobility**: Utilize the timed-up-and-go (TUG) test--Client stands from chair with armrests, walks 3 meters, and turns and sits back down. Those requiring ≥14 seconds are at risk for falls (Normal:7-10 seconds). If the client's gait speed in 5 meters is slow (<0.6 m/second), this is predictive of limitations. Age-Appropriate Equipment and Techniques for Assessment of Vital Signs.

Psychosocial Integrity

Abuse

Child Abuse

Child abuse is the intentional harm, either psychological or physical, of a child. The nurse's role is to identify, assist with treatment, and aid in the prevention of abuse and neglect. It is the nurse's duty to report suspected neglect/abuse to appropriate authorities; however, do not approach the abuser directly. Private interviews and asking, "Do you feel safe?" are common diagnostic tools for abuse; also, a thorough physical exam.

The **most common Signs and symptoms**:

- Bruises, especially those in multiple stages of healing or on the central part of the body.
- Burns with clear borders, such as immersion or cigarette burns.
- Fractures, especially spiral or rib fractures.
- Lacerations and abrasions may appear on the mouth, gums, around the eye area, and in the genital region.
- Bite marks, fingernail scratches, and puncture wounds.
- Head trauma may present with bulging fontanelle, cranial suture separation, hematomas and broken vessels in the eyes, bleeding from the ears, and decreased or impaired hearing.

Psychological signs include:

- Aggression and/or pulling back.
- Express fear with the home environment and/or the individual who is abusing them.
- Display no emotion/attachment with parents.
- Avoid eye contact, show signs of rigidity when they are approached, inappropriate responses to painful procedures.

Spousal/Partner Abuse

The following are characteristics of victims of spousal/partner abuse:

- Feelings of failure as a mother, wife, or caregiver; feel as if they deserve abuse.
- Accept the abuse as a normal healthy relationship; denial.
- Do not have close family relationships or friendships; social isolation.
- Low self-esteem; show lack of independence in decision-making skills.
- Express fear or anxiety related to confronting or upsetting the abuser.
- Have conflicting stories related to injuries; the spouse dominates the questioning and unexplained injuries present.

Note: It is very appropriate for the nurse to first interview a couple, and then do a single interview with the individual they feel is being abused. Also, remember that victims of abuse often are in denial. Best thing to say to an abused woman: "You don't deserve to be treated in this manner."

Sexual Assault/Abuse

The following are **warning signs of sexual abuse/assault:**

- Detailed and overly sophisticated understanding of sexual behavior in young children
- Regressive behavior (e.g., excessive clinginess in preschool children or the sudden onset of soiling and wetting)
- A child may appear disconnected or focused on fantasy worlds
- Sleep disturbances and nightmares
- Marked changes in appetite
- Fear states (e.g., anxiety, depression, phobias, obsession)
- Overly compliant behavior such as extensive grooming behaviors
- Parentified/adultified behavior (e.g., acting like a parent/spouse)
- Delinquent or aggressive behavior
- Poor or deteriorating relationships with peers
- Sudden inability to concentrate in school/deterioration in school performance
- Unwillingness to participate in physical/recreational activities, especially if this is due to symptoms of physical discomfort
- Truancy/running away from home
- Drug/alcohol abuse

Note: These signs are not diagnostic; must look at overall clinical picture before making a judgment.

Forensic Nursing

Treatment of Victims of Crime

Victims of crimes vary widely, from those with emotional distress to those with life-threatening injuries, so it is especially important to follow protocols for care. A complete detailed history of the injury sustained and any trauma should be taken, documenting carefully with direct quotations and objective observations, avoiding subjective observations that might not hold up in court. Clothing, which may contain evidence, should be carefully removed and placed in separate bags. A head-to-toe physical examination should be carried out, and injuries should be carefully noted and photodocumentation taken if possible, with the patient's consent. If the police have not been notified prior to the patient's admission for care, then a report may need to be filed, depending on the state laws and the type of injuries. For example, gunshot wounds generally must be reported to the police, while physical assaults, such as with domestic violence, may or may not require reporting.

Treatment of Rape Victims

Rape victims need to sign a consent before examination with a rape kit and can refuse any part of the examination. Patients should remove clothing while standing on a clean sheet or drape, placing each item of clothing into a separate paper bag. Female patients should receive a baseline pregnancy test and be offered emergency contraceptive prophylaxis (for up to 120 hours). Patients should be offered antibiotic prophylaxis for sexually transmitted infections and counseled about HIV prophylaxis. Drugs used to facilitate rape may be detected for up to 96 hours. Blood tests are done for the first 36 hours after a drug-facilitated rape and urine tests after that time. The assault should be carefully documented, using direct quotations. Patients often want to shower and should be advised when they will be allowed to do so. Toluidine dye may be applied to the labia and perineal/perianal areas to help identify superficial lacerations before a vaginal examination. Photo documentation should be completed following protocols.

Behavioral Interventions

Behavioral interventions may include:

- **Utilizing behavior modification**: Intended to change a client's behavior, include providing positive and negative reinforcement to promote desired behavior and utilizing cognitive behavioral therapy techniques to help the client control behavior by altering patterns of thinking and behavior.
- **Decreasing anxiety**: May include deep breathing and relaxation exercises, visualization and imagery, self-hypnosis, and meditation to help the client focus energy away from those things causing anxiety.
- **Orienting client to reality**: May include a memory board with pictures and important information, such as the date and names of family and staff; verbally reminding the client of important information; placing familiar items in the client's room; serving favorite foods; and playing the client's favorite music.
- **Minimizing environmental distractions**: May include reducing clutter, removing pictures from the wall, quieting alarms, keeping lights low, and lowering voices. Interventions may vary depending on what the client finds most distracting.

Behavioral interventions should be based on client assessment:

- **Appearance**: The client's appearance can give clues the person's mental status as well as physical ability to provide self-care. The nurse should note grooming and dress, hygiene, height, weight, and any piercings, scars, or tattoo as well as whether the person's age and mode of dress seem to correspond.
- **Mood**: Mood may be described as sad, labile, or euphoric. Affect may be blunted (shows little facial expression or is very slow to show expressions) flat (shows no facial expression), broad (shows a wide range of facial/emotional expressions), inappropriate (shows a range of expressions but they are inconsistent with mood or situation, especially exhibiting inappropriate laughter or crying) and restricted (shows one type of expression regardless of circumstances).
- **Psychomotor behavior**: The client may exhibit excessive or reduced movements or abnormal/peculiar movements (such as repetitive movements or tremors). Eye contact may vary. If a client avoids eye contact, this may indicate fear, dishonesty, or cultural difference.

Counselor Contracts with Clients

A **contract** is a type of agreement drawn up between people that is done to promote action and possible reward. A counselor may use a contract with a client who wants to change a behavior; for example, a client may express frustration about making rash decisions that significantly affect his personal life. As part of a contract, a counselor may require that the client agree to consult with a family member or professional before making any decisions that will affect his finances, family life, or health. The contract is drawn up with specific terms and signed by the client. The three characteristics of a good contract are:

1. *Feasible* - the contract should be written in such a way that the client can actually perform the terms.
2. *Specific* - leaving little room for interpretation.
3. *Retractable* - in that the client can decide that he/she does not want to meet the terms.

Learner Readiness

Learner readiness is the term used to describe whether the person being educated is willing to receive and implement the information given. The client, family, or support person will not learn, retain, or be able to repeat the material if they are not at a point in the care in which they are ready to learn. It is important to document the level of learner readiness in the chart to prevent the nurse from being liable if the patient is readmitted or noncompliant with care. The nurse may also assist in identifying barriers to learning and addressing those barriers to enhance the learning process.

Barriers to Learning: terminal diagnosis, cognitive disability/injury, denial of health problems, low educational/reading level.

The following are **methods to increase learning**:

- Use visual aids, videotapes, and clearly written handouts.
- Ensure material is appropriate to patient learning level.
- Encourage family participation.
- Limit what is taught during each session.
- Put special emphasis on the needs of the patient after the patient goes home, rather than just focusing on the here and now.
- Allow time for questions and answers.

Supporting Clients with Unexpected Altered Body Image

With any **altered body image**, the nurse should recognize that the client is likely to experience a period of grieving with emotions ranging from anger to sadness. The client needs support, patience, and understanding, especially if also dealing with pain and altered physical abilities:

- **Alopecia**: Hair loss may be partial or total, temporary or permanent, but the client may feel very self-conscious and depressed. Information about hair coverings and wigs may be particularly helpful to females; but males, who may be considered stylish with a shaved head, may still be as distressed as females.
- **Amputations**: Clients may benefit from focusing on areas of strength and helping them to be as independent as possible while recognizing that some may overcompensate by refusing needed assistance. Managing pain, preventing complications, and reinforcing positive coping skills are important.
- **Burns**: Pain control is especially important for burn clients. Clients may be very concerned about their appearance (especially if burns involve visible areas of the body) and their ability to function, so acceptance and reassurance are essential. Clients should be helped to be as independent as possible and encouraged to take an active role in wound care and recovery.

Coping Mechanisms

Coping mechanisms (also known as *defense mechanisms)* are ways that an individual responds to increased stress or a crisis in order to process the event and maintain their psychological integrity. Coping mechanisms are considered a healthy response to stress; however, disproportionate or exclusive use of one coping mechanism over others is considered unhealthy. Coping mechanisms include:

- **Compensation:** Making up for a perceived weakness by exaggerating a different feature

  John is failing math, but becomes an all-star basketball player.

- **Conversion:** Changing psychological stress into a physical problem

  John gets nauseated before his midterm in math.

- **Denial:** refusing to accept an unpleasant reality

  John refused to study for his math test, thinking he will probably pass it.

- **Displacement:** directing anger at situation at another person/object

  John screams at his little sister after his parents chide him about his math test.

- **Dissociation:** Separating the emotions from an event/situation

  John jokes and laughs with his friends about failing his class and repeating the grade.

- **Fantasy:** a conscious creation of an alternate reality as an escape from unpleasant feelings

  John fantasizes about playing basketball during math class.

- **Identification:** Assimilating feelings/actions of a desired person

  John buys expensive shoes endorsed by his favorite basketball player.

- **Introjection:** Unconsciously assimilating behaviors external to one's self

  John swears at his opponents during an intense game, as he has heard his father do before.

- **Projection:** Ascribing undesirable feelings, motivation, and behaviors to another person

  John states that his teacher just hates him, and doesn't want him to pass the class.

- **Rationalization:** Deciding that undesirable feelings or actions are bearable and satisfactory

  John decides that math is not an important subject, and he doesn't need to pass it

- **Reaction Formation:** Feelings and motives are completely opposite of actions and behavior displayed

  John skips and whistles as his goes into math test, stating math is his favorite subject.

- **Regression:** A retreat back to an earlier stage of comfort

  John begins to hang out with younger kids and avoid his older friends.

- **Repression**: Unconscious amnesia regarding unpleasant circumstances and feelings

  John completely forgets to attend his math tutoring session at school.

- **Restitution:** Trying to alleviate subconscious guilt regarding an event

  John gives extra effort in English class to impress his parents.

- **Sublimation:** converting unacceptable behaviors into acceptable ones

  John uses his obsession with basketball to participate in an after-school program for troubled youth.

- **Substitution:** Decision to change a negative attitude into a more positive emotion

  John has decided that while math is not his favorite, he really likes English.

- **Suppression:** Choosing not to think or dwell on an unpleasant experience or emotion

  John refuses to talk about his failing math grade with his siblings.

- **Symbolization:** using a physical object to represent an internal emotion or idea

  John burns his math book at the end of the semester.

- **Undoing:** An attempt to alleviate conscious guilt regarding a negative event

  John apologizes to his parents for failing math and promises to try harder in the future.

Crisis Intervention

Assessment for Potential Client Violence

Assessing a client for potential violence includes:

- **Reviewing the client's history** for evidence of history of violent or aggressive behavior to determine the degree of risk.
- **Assessing the client's arousal state**: For example, does the client appear to be angry, anxious, or fearful because these states may lead to aggression.
- **Noting the client's choice and use of language**: Swearing and speaking loudly or yelling are indications that a client may become violent.
- **Assessing confusion, delusions, and hallucination** and avoiding challenging the client but remaining supportive to prevent the client from acting out or feeling humiliated.
- **Orienting the client** who appears disoriented by introducing self and providing and explanation of place and purpose of meeting with the client.
- **Reviewing the environment for safety** to make sure that security personnel are within sight (if necessary) and that the room allows easy and rapid exit if the client becomes violent.

Crisis Intervention Techniques

Crisis intervention techniques include:

- **Active listening**: Looking at the client, nodding the head, and responding with comments and questions as appropriate to help the client feel in control.
- **Distracting/Redirecting**: Directing the client's attention to another topic or thing, such as suggesting that the client take deep breaths and concentrate on breathing. In some cases, the client may be so overwhelmed that the nurse may need to assume direction to give the client time to control emotions.
- **Supporting self-direction**: Encouraging the client to take responsibility for dealing with the crisis, "What do you want to do now?" or "What will help you at this time?"
- **Collaborating**: Working together with the client to arrive at a plan to deal with the crisis.
- **Providing resources**: Providing self-help materials, such as books and pamphlets, as well as websites that may provide information that the client can use in mediating crises.

Resources for Recovery from Personal Crises

Resources for recovery include:

- **Loss of loved one**: Support groups, often available through hospitals or hospices; websites, such as Webhealing.com, which provides articles, forums for discussion, videos, and links to other sites; and books, such as *When God Doesn't Fix It* (Story), *You Can Heal Your Life* (Hay), and *Healing after Loss* (Hickman).
- **Smoking cessation**: Support groups, locally and online forums, such as *StopSmokingCenter.net,* and informational websites, such as *Smokefree.gov.*
- **Job loss**: Information about Unemployment Insurance (joint state-federal program to provide monetary benefits to those who have lost a job) and employment office services may be helpful. Some clients may experience depression and anxiety and may need counseling to help with coping.
- **Addiction recovery**: Rehabilitation programs (both inpatient and outpatient), 12-step programs (Narcotics Anonymous®, Alcoholics Anonymous®), support groups, and free clinics.

Suicide

Suicide is among the most frequent causes of death in the United States, and the third most common causes of death in 10-14-year olds, and second among 15-34-year olds. The risk of suicide is increased in men over 50 years, those with mental illness, gay/lesbian youth, and those of Native American or Alaskan descent. While males are more likely to commit suicide than females, the attempt rate is higher among females. Counselors should be aware of support groups, have a crisis plan, and involve the community when working with at-risk clients.

Warning signs include depression and anger, experiencing loss or rejection, talking about suicide, planning and securing the means to commit suicide, and giving away possessions.

A sudden, unexpected uplift in mood is considered a red flag, as it may indicate the person has finalized a plan; educate family and caregivers to look out for this.

Suicide precautions: locked windows and stairwells, breakproof glass and mirrors, break away shower heads/wall railing, plastic flatware, no cords of any kind, no belts, sharps, razors, matches or cigarettes, frequent observation or 1 to 1 care, communicate therapeutically, make a behavior contract, restraints if ordered, medications if ordered, monitor and restrict visitors.

Cultural Awareness

Cultural Views on Physical and Mental Illness

Many cultures have specific traditional beliefs regarding the **source and meaning** of illnesses. For instance, some cultures may believe that illness is the result of an imbalance between a person's body and spirit or that it is a punishment for actions taken earlier in life. **Mental illnesses** are particularly subject to these types of beliefs. Even in cultures where beliefs are not primarily based on superstition, mental illness frequently has a stigma attached to it. Many Eastern cultures value conformity to social norms and emotional control, and mental illness directly interferes with a person's ability to achieve these things. In Western cultures, mental illness is still often misunderstood and stigmatized, seen by many as a sign of a weak mind or simply a lack of willpower on the part of those affected.

The nurse should be aware that the client's **cultural background** may significantly impact how the client receives a diagnosis of mental illness and what information, support, and resources they will require. Beliefs held by the **client's family**, regardless of whether they are shared by the client, can directly affect the client. If the client has a strong negative reaction to a psychiatric diagnosis, the nurse should attempt to determine the source of the distress and address it appropriately, including offering reassurance that the client will not be forced to receive any treatment he or she does not wish to receive.

Caring for Clients with Language Barriers

Language barriers may relate to non-English speakers as well as client with aphasia or deafness. The nurse should first assess the type of barrier and how the client is able to communicate (in another language, sign language, gestures) to know best how to proceed. Family members or caregivers may be able to provide useful guidance. For example, an aphasic client may be able to understand but not speak. The nurse should always try to communicate what the nurse plans to do (give the client medication, take a blood pressure, change a dressing) and should address the client directly, even if using a translator. If a translator is needed, then having one present is ideal. If this is not possible, then the nurse should use gestures or pictures to try to communicate meaning. Google Translate® is a very helpful free application that provides translation of 100 languages and is available on smart phones and other devices and may be utilized for non-critical communication.

Cultural Health Considerations

The following are cultural health considerations:

- **Proxemics** (space considerations): Cultures vary in the amount of personal space they require, and people may feel uncomfortable if others stand too close or too far away. North Americans and Northern Europeans tend to want the most space and may feel uncomfortable if someone stands within arm's length. Latin Americans, Asians, Middle Easterners, and Southern Europeans often feel comfortable standing very close to others.
- **Eye contact**: While direct eye contact is a cultural norm in North America and many European countries, it may be considered aggressive by some cultures and disrespectful by others. African Americans, Native Americans, Asians, and Mexicans often avoid eye contact to show respect.
- **Time**: While punctuality is considered the norm in the United States, time is much more flexible in many cultures, so some people, such as Latin Americans and Mexicans, may consider time in relation to day and night or before or after meals rather than by the clock.

- **Complementary/Folk medicine**: People from other cultures may utilize alternative medical systems (such as Chinese herbal medications), healers, meditation, manipulative or body-based therapies, or practices such as coining and cupping (which may leave distinctive bruising).
- **Touch**: There may be restrictions in touch between males and females in some cultures (such as Middle Eastern), and some in Asian cultures may be upset if the head is touched without permission because they believe the spirit resides in the head.
- **Holiday/Religious observance**: Patients may want to continue to observe cultural holidays or religious practices, such as eating kosher meals and fasting during Ramadan. They may have restrictions as to what they are able to do during religious days, such as ultra-conservative Jews on the Sabbath.
- **Family hierarchy**: In some cultures (Mexican, Asian, and Middle Eastern) decisions are made by the males or the head of the family rather than by the individual, so a wife, for example, may expect her husband to make decisions about her care.

Religious and Spiritual Influences on Health

A person's **spiritual and religious beliefs** can often have a pronounced impact on their health. While it is not the nurses' duty to try to change those beliefs, the nurse should be aware of them in order to respect the patient's wishes and give safe and effective care. This will always start with an assessment of the patient's beliefs: the nurse should ask the patient if they have any religious or spiritual beliefs that they would like their health care team to be aware of, and then use open-ended questions to determine if there is anything that may potentially cause a spiritual conflict during the course of treatment. For example, if the patient is Jewish and wishes to abstain from pork, a note should be made to the dietitian. More commonly, a patient who is a Jehovah's Witness will often refuse blood products, so special planning will be necessary for these patients when they undergo surgery or other medical procedures. If a patient has religious/spiritual preferences, the nurse's responsibilities are to be respectful of the patient and to facilitate their preferences as much as possible while still providing excellent care.

Emotional Problems Related to Religious/Spiritual Beliefs

Emotional problems related to **religious/spiritual beliefs** include:

- **Spiritual distress**: Clients may experience spiritual distress if they feel that they have lived in a way inconsistent with their beliefs or may feel that they have been abandoned by their deity or deities. Some may lose faith or question their beliefs when confronted with illness or death and feel at a loss to fill the void and may react with anger or depression. Clients may have difficulty sleeping and eating. Actively listening to clients express their feeling and providing emotional support may help relieve the distress.
- **Conflict between beliefs and treatment**: Clients may have cultural or religious beliefs in conflict with treatment, and this can cause anxiety and distress and often feelings of guilt. For example, a Christian Scientist who takes chemotherapy or a Jehovah's Witness who accepts blood transfusions may be distressed by their failure to uphold their beliefs and may need much reassurance.

End-of-Life Care

End-of-Life Issues

End-of-life issues include:

- **Financial needs**: The costs of end-of-life care, especially if caregivers or nursing home care are needed, may be prohibitively high, requiring clients and family to liquidate assets and/or apply for Medicaid. Bills may go unpaid and clients and family members may do without essential items or services.
- **Fear**: Both client and family may be fearful of pain and/or physical changes associated with end-of-life, and the client may be fearful of death, especially if the client has issues that are unresolved.
- **Loss of control**: Clients experience increasing loss of control as their physical condition weakens and they are able to do less and less for themselves and must depend on others for their basic needs.
- **Role changes**: Children and spouses often become the caregivers of clients, reversing roles that are long established. This can lead to conflict, confusion, insecurity, and resentment at times.

Hospice Care

Hospice care is for the terminally ill, usually within the last 6 months of life (two 90-day periods) although this may be extended by physician authorization every 60 days. Medicare clients must be eligible for Medicare A, and a physician must certify that the client is terminal with life expectancy ≤6 months. The client (or responsible family member) must agree to receive Hospice care rather than regular Medicare, requiring that the client receive palliative rather than curative treatment. The goal of hospice care is to maintain the person in the home environment, so the client is provided home health aides and homemakers, durable goods (dressings, adult diapers, under pads), pain management, case management, counselling, and social worker assistance. Routine home care is intermittent. In-home continuous care is available only during crisis for short periods. In-client hospice (often beds assigned in a skilled nursing facility) may be used for 4-5 days for symptom management and/or a 5-day respite period for caregivers.

Nurse's Role in End of Life Care

The nurse often plays a crucial role in **end of life care**. End of life care (also known as *palliative* or "comfort care") is care centered on providing patient ease as they transition into the end of life. There are few things the nurse should keep in mind when providing palliative care:

- **Pain Control**: This is the #1 priority for palliative care patients. Adequate pain control in these patients often includes opioids and anxiolytics in high doses. For some nurses this may cause moral distress, as drugs at this level may shorten the life of the patient. However, the nurses' creed is to "first, do no harm"; thus, this practice is deemed ethical and compassionate for the patient.
- **EENT**: Dying patients will often require frequent suctioning due to increased secretions; the MD may even order a scopolamine patch to help dry up the excess saliva and mucous in the back of the throat that causes the characteristic "death rattle." These patients will also need the mouth swabbed frequently for comfort, and sometimes artificial tears to treat dry eyes.
- **Positioning**: Turn and support with pillows to increase comfort; it may help to elevate the head of the bed to facilitate breathing for the patient.

- **Psychological**: If the patient is still coherent and talking, allow them to verbalize their feelings about death and reminisce. Do not patronize or dismiss their concerns, but be honest regarding their condition and treatment options. Spiritual interventions are considered high priority during this time.

Phases of Grief Defined by Kübler-Ross

Kübler-Ross is famous for her five phases of grief, the process that people move through when losing something important to them, including the loss of a loved one, successful job, or even body image changes. It is important to realize that Kübler-Ross taught that a person does not necessarily move through the stages in exact order, and may skip or regress to different stages. Children especially move through the phases faster than adults. The five phases (DABDA) are:

1. **Denial**: does not really believe loss has happened, talks as if nothing has changed. Family/caregivers may fear delirium; educate that this might be a normal part of grieving process.
2. **Anger:** upset about loss, may act out, exhibit previously unfelt aggression at the lost individual; may blame caregivers or others for loss.
3. **Bargaining**: trying to change results of loss/avoid consequences of loss; may ask God to change what happened.
4. **Depression**: loss of interest, may feel life is not worth living/fatalistic, withdraw from friends/family. Offer support, and do not try to prematurely pull out of grief.
5. **Acceptance:** come to terms with loss and able to cope, accepted consequences; back into a pattern of daily living.

Impaired/complicated grieving*:* when debilitating feelings of grief and sadness remain ≥6 months after event; requires medical intervention.

Review Video: Patient Treatment and Grief
Visit mometrix.com/academy and enter code: 648794

Mental Health Concepts

Impaired Cognition

Signs and symptoms of **impaired cognition** include:

- Short-term memory loss, such as forgetting recent activities.
- Misplacing and/or losing items.
- Confusing people's names or relationships (such as thinking a daughter is a sister) or failing to recognize family members.
- Poor hygiene out of character with usual habits.
- Wearing mismatched clothing or the same clothing day after day.
- Missing appointments and/or social engagements.
- Exhibiting changes in personality, increasing episodes of anger or aggressive behavior.
- Losing track of ideas when conversing and forgetting words or using incorrect words.
- Having increasing difficulty making decisions, such as what food to order or what to do next.
- Losing track of finances and forgetting to pay bills, spending money excessively (sometimes without memory), or giving money away.
- Exhibiting apathy and/or depression, fearfulness and/or paranoia.

- Exhibiting impaired motor coordination.
- Overeating or forgetting to eat.
- Regressing to manner of dress or behavior more common in earlier years.

Assessing Adherence to Mental Health Treatment Plan

Assessing adherence to treatment plan includes:

- Discussing adherence directly with the client and family members (when appropriate).
- Checking prescriptions bottles for the dates and amounts of drugs.
- Observing client's behavior and noting any changes that may indicate non-adherence.
- Assessing client's motivation to follow the treatment plan.
- Recognizing reasons for non-adherence:
    - Adverse effects, such as tremors, erectile dysfunction, weight gain, lethargy, fatigue.
    - Costs: Many drugs require out-of-pocket costs even with insurance, and those with low income may not be able to afford the drugs or may not have the knowledge or ability to compare prices or to apply to drug companies for prescription assistance.
    - Polypharmacy may result in confusion when clients must deal with multiple prescriptions.
    - Inconvenience: Clients may lose patience or forget when drugs must be taken at different times, such as before meals or with food.
    - Reluctance to be confronted about non-adherence may cause clients to miss appointments, support groups, or other treatments.

Sensory/Perceptual Alterations Upon Appearance of Symptoms

Sensory/Perceptual alterations should be explored when assessing the appearance of symptoms:

- **Time**: Clients are often vague about when symptoms first began but can sometimes associate the symptoms with events in their lives to help pinpoint the time. For example, if a client took a vacation a few months earlier, the client may be able to remember whether the symptoms started before or after the vacation.
- **Place**: Identifying the place where symptoms began and/or continue may help to determine triggering factors. For example, if a client started having asthma attacks at home, then the home environment should be explored for allergens.
- **Stimuli**: The nurse should question sensory elements—sounds, smells, sights, taste, touch (cold, hot, pain, itch)— to determine exactly how the symptoms began because sensory elements that are associated with onset of symptoms may give a clue to an environmental cause. For example, if a client developed nausea after noting a foul smell, then the cause may be a toxic substance.

Dealing with Sensory and Thought Disturbances

Strategies for dealing with **sensory and thought disturbances** include identifying the cause of the disturbance, such as exploring whether it may be drug-induced (a common finding), caused by a physical disease, or associated with psychological problems. Sensory disturbances may vary widely; for example, some clients may complain of ringing in their ears, blurring of vision, difficulty smelling or odd smells, and/or changes in perception of touch or feeling. Listening carefully and exploring how and when the disturbance occurs is essential as well as helping the client compensate. For example, white noise may help client's tolerate ringing in the ears. Clients may be less self-aware of thought disturbances, disorders in thinking often associated with disorders in verbal expression (poverty of speech, perseveration echolalia, blocking, stilted speech, neologisms).

Strategies include orienting client to reality, teaching the client relaxation techniques, ensuring client safety, monitoring medications, and encouraging family to be supportive of client.

Levels of Intellectual Disability

There are four levels of **intellectual disability** (formerly known as *mental retardation*):

1. Mild intellectual disability: IQ of 52 to 69; This individual will achieve a mental age of 8 to 12 years, can learn daily living activities, elementary-level communication skills, and be able to function with minimal vocational skills to provide self-care and maintenance.
2. Moderate intellectual disability: IQ of 36 to 51; This individual will achieve a mental age between 3 and 7 years, has noted developmental delays, shows simple communication skills, and can learn self-help skills.
3. Severe intellectual disability: IQ of 20 to 35; This individual will have the mental age of a toddler, marked developmental delay, and little or no communication ability. They can learn repetition related to activities. This individual must be supervised continuously with self-protective mechanisms in place.
4. Profound intellectual disability: IQ ≤19; This individual will have the mental age of an infant, obvious developmental delays in all aspects of life, and require total care.

Bipolar Disorder

Bipolar disorder or **manic-depressive disorder** is a psychological condition in which the patient swings between depressive and manic episodes. These swings can be sudden or the phases can last for long periods of time:

- **Depressive symptoms**: chronic pain, decreased energy, loss of interest in activities, weight/appetite changes, excessive crying, suicidal thoughts and/or attempts, feelings of helplessness, changes in sleep patterns, social withdrawal.
- **Manic symptoms**: overly inflated self-esteem, decreased need for rest and sleep, irritability, distractedness, physical agitation/aggression, provocative or destructive behavior, increased talkativeness, excessive "high" or euphoric feelings, increased sex drive/energy level, denial, uncharacteristically poor judgment.

Treatment includes:

- Medication: Mood stabilizers (lithium), antipsychotics, anticonvulsants, antidepressants.
- Psychotherapy.
- Teaching: stress medication compliance, increased risk of self-harm/suicide, feed finger foods and engage in nonviolent activities during manic phase.

Schizophrenia

Such dysfunctions as delusions, hallucinations, inappropriate emotions, disorganized speech, and inappropriate behavior make up the category of mental illness called **schizophrenia**. A person with schizophrenia may not have any outward appearance of being ill. In other cases, the illness may be more apparent, causing bizarre behaviors. Advanced paternal age, illegal drug use, family history, and autoimmune diseases increase a person's risk of developing schizophrenia. Signs and symptoms include social withdrawal; depersonalization (intense anxiety and a feeling of being unreal); loss of appetite; poor hygiene; delusions; hallucinations; paranoia; and disrupted or disturbed thought processes, perceptions, speech, and movement ("negative symptoms").

Treatment includes:

- Medications: antipsychotics (atypical preferred)
- Psychotherapy: individual and family therapy, social skills training, vocational rehabilitation.
- Teaching: stress medication compliance, support groups, increased suicide/self-harm risk.

Note: Schizophrenia is NOT multiple personality disorder.

Additional Mental Health Disorders

Anxiety Disorders

Anxiety is a state of uneasiness or apprehension, which can cause physical tension. Severe anxieties or multiple anxieties, especially when they have comorbidity with another disorder, are abnormal behavior. Panic disorder, phobias, posttraumatic stress, and obsessive-compulsive disorder are examples of anxiety disorders.

Medication, relaxation techniques, cognitive behavioral therapy, and exposure exercises are acceptable treatments for anxiety disorders.

Somatoform Disorder

Somatoform disorders involve physical symptoms for which no specific physical cause is present. The disorders include hypochondria, somatization disorder, conversion, and pain disorder.

Treatment is more management than cure and may or may not include medication.

Dissociative Disorders

Dissociative disorders involve the breakdown of a person's perceptions of his environment, memory, or identity. Dissociative disorders include dissociative amnesia, dissociative fugue (flight), dissociative identity disorder (multiple personality) and depersonalization disorder.

Psychotherapy and sometimes hypnosis are among the treatments for dissociative disorders.

Mood Disorders

Mood disorders are conditions in which the person's prevailing mood is disturbed or inappropriate. The disorders include depression, anxiety, and bipolar syndrome. The mood disorders are the most common psychological illnesses.

Treatment includes medication and counseling and is disorder-specific.

Substance Abuse

Substance abuse, which includes the abuse of alcohol, prescription drugs, and illegal drugs, is a major problem in the United States. Of the 14% of adults who admit to dependence at some time in their life, half have experienced the problem during the last year. More than 3 million teenagers have a problem with alcohol. There is a strong connection between drinking and teenage problems such as suicide, early sexual activity, and driving accidents. Abuse of alcohol and drugs affects not just the addict, but family members, friends, and coworkers as well.

Characteristics include low self-esteem, anxiety, sexual problems, suicidal impulses, fear of failure, and social isolation. The Substance Abuse Subtle Screening Inventory (SASSI) can be used to detect indications of addiction.

Since addictions are both physical and mental, successful **treatment** must involve both. With certain substances, hospitalization and medications will be required to treat acute withdrawal symptoms. For long-term recovery, one effective treatment method is a 12-step program coupled with individual, group, and family counseling. It is especially important that counseling involve the family. Behavior modification and social learning theory can be used effectively in a residential program.

DT

Delirium tremens (DT) is a potentially fatal form of ethanol (alcohol) withdrawal. Symptoms may begin a few hours after the cessation of ethanol, but may not peak until 48-72 hours. Physicians and nurses must recognize that the presenting symptoms may not be severe and identify those at risk of developing DT.

Signs and symptoms: tremors, agitation/irritability, insomnia, nausea/vomiting, hallucinations, confusion, seizures

Diagnosis: based on patient history and symptoms, blood alcohol levels

Treatment includes:

- IV sedation; IV midazolam or lorazepam.
- Close monitoring; generally in ICU during acute withdrawal; may require restraints if they become violent with hallucinations.
- Teaching: Drinking cessation- join support group such as Alcoholics Anonymous.

Must ask patient the time of last drink, and realize symptoms may not manifest for 6-48 hours.

Non-Substance-Related Dependencies

Non-substance-related (behavioral) dependencies can be as disruptive to life as drug and alcohol addiction. Non-substance-related dependencies include the inability to resist the activity, a recurrent pattern of behavior, and interference with functioning in other aspects of life. Clients may feel anxiety prior to engaging in the behavior (akin to cravings) and relief (high) afterwards. Some clients also engage in substance-abuse. Non-substance-related dependencies include:

- **Pathological gambling**: The client may engage in all types of gambling or focus on one type (blackjack), but continues to gamble despite major losses and tends to gamble more and more as losses pile up.
- **Sexual addiction**: The client gains a feeling of self-worth through conquest and often ignores risks, such as HIV/AIDS infection and STDs, even when putting a partner at risk as well.
- **Kleptomania**: The client cannot control the urge to steal, even things that are of little or no value to the client.
- **Compulsive shopping**: The client may have closets and drawers full of unused clothing and items and may buy multiple units, often hiding receipts and lying about purchases.
- **Internet/Video game addiction**: The client may forego personal associations and interactions in favor of hours spent on the computer or playing video games.

Stress Management

External Factors That Can Interfere with Recovery

External factors that can interfere with recovery include:

- **Stressors**: Clients may experience multiple stressors, including physical stress (pain, weakness, fatigue, disability) and psychological stress (anger, depression, anxiety, fear) during recovery, and these stressors may overwhelm the clients' abilities to cope, thus interfering with recovery. See below for the assessment of these stressors.
- **Family dynamics**: Clients may be concerned about the need for others, such as a spouse, to take over the role of primary breadwinner; and may be worried about their ability to care for their families or for their families to accept changes. Family members may become resentful of the clients' needs and limitations, and conflicts may arise.
- **Socioeconomics**: Clients may be concerned about the costs associated with illness/injury and recovery, especially if they lack insurance, and may be faced with loss of employment or prolonged periods of unemployment as well as loss of savings. Clients may feel shame if forced to accept Medicaid or assistance from others and may be concerned about the possibility of losing a home and belongings and becoming homeless.

Assessment of Environmental Stressors

When assessing **environmental stressors,** the nurse should observe for the client for both verbal and non-verbal indicators of stress. Non-verbal indicators of stress may include rapid speech, self-comforting measures (rubbing hands together, wrapping arms around torso, folding arms tightly), physical complaints (headache, nausea, diarrhea), covering the mouth (may indicate discomfort with a subject), and wrapping feet around chair legs. Environmental stressors may include:

- **Noise**: Machines, heavy equipment, conversation, repeated alarms, and other noises in the home or working environment may interfere with the client's ability to think and focus, increase anxiety, and decrease the perception of other stimuli.
- **Fear**: The nurse should help the client identify fears and find strategies for alleviating fear (more lighting, better locks, reality orientation).
- **Uncertainty**: Clients are often unsure of what action to take or what to believe, and this uncertainty can lead to ongoing stress because of inability to make decisions.
- **Change**: Some clients do not react well to change of any kind because the change threatens their sense of control.
- **Lack of knowledge**: Clients may feel inferior or anxious if they recognize that they lack sufficient knowledge and may withdraw or seek to gain more knowledge.

Stress Management Techniques

Stress management techniques include:

- **Reducing environmental stressors**: Reducing ambient noise with sound barriers, sound reduction, and/or sound-proofing; reducing clutter; eliminating unpleasant or cloying odors; adjusting lighting; and changing color schemes.
- **Taking a break from the environment**: Urging the client to take a break for a short period may help the person feel less overwhelmed.
- **Practicing relaxation/visualization**: Can help the client control responses to stress.
- **Meditating**: May help the client to be more accepting and less bothered by distracting elements.

- **Utilizing social support**: Trusted friends and family members may serve as listening boards and provide emotional support.
- **Exercising**: May improve the client's sense of well-being and control, allowing the client to better tolerate stressors.
- **Setting limits**: Helping the client find ways to say "no" to those things (such as serving on yet another committee) that will likely increase stress.
- **Learning time management**: Help the client develop a realistic schedule that includes some free time.

Support and Therapeutic Communication

Support Systems for Patients

A large factor in a patient's recovery from illness is the patient's **support system** at home. This usually refers to the patient's friends and family members who are involved in the patient's life, and who will be largely involved in the patient's care. An adequate support system may require different levels of involvement depending on patient condition and situation; the nurse should assess:

- What are the patient's thoughts about their support at home? Is it adequate? Is the family in the home supportive and agreeable with the care that is going to be required?
- What support systems have worked for the patient in the past? What has changed this time that might necessitate a different level of involvement?
- Will the patient require outside help, such as a support group (e.g. AA, group therapy sessions, etc.)?

Once the nurse has answered these questions, he/she should work closely with the case manager to get the patient the help they need to have a successful recovery.

Family Types

Nuclear

This husband-wife-children model was once the most common family type but is no longer the norm. In this model, the husband is the provider, and the mother stays home to care for the children, but this makes up only about 7% of current American families.

Single-Parent/Divorced

Usually the mother is the single parent, but it may be the father. The single parent may be widowed, divorced, or separated, but more commonly the person has never married. In cases of divorce or abandonment, the child may have minimal or no contact with one parent, often the father. Single parents often face difficulties in trying to support and care for a child and may suffer economic hardship.

Blended

Because of the high rate of divorce, stepparent families are common, and this can result in stress and conflict when a new child enters the picture. There may be jealousy and resentment on the part of siblings and estranged family members.

Adoptive

Adoptive families may consist of a child or children and one parent, two traditional parents, and/or two parents of the same gender. In some cases, one parent is a natural parent and the other an adoptive.

Parenting Styles

Parenting has an essential role in the social and behavioral development of the child. The degree of **warmth** the parents exhibit and the type of **control** have a profound effect on the child.

Style	Parental behavior	Effects on child
Indifferent	Shows little warmth and rarely imposes limits, may neglect or dislike child.	Child feels unloved and lacks direction or a positive sense of self, resulting in destructive or delinquent behavior.
Permissive	Shows much warmth and affection for the child but imposes few limits and little guidance although communication remains good.	Child may be creative and extroverted but doesn't negotiate or cooperate well with others, making acceptance by peers difficult. The child may become very self-centered and impulsive with impaired social functioning. The child may bully others or become aggressive and rebellious.
Authoritarian	Shows little warmth or affection for the child and communicates little. Is often inflexible and sets very restrictive limits that allow little independent thought or activity.	Child does not learn to negotiate or direct own behavior and has difficulty learning autonomy. Child may be fearful, passive, withdrawn. During adolescence, girls tend to be more passive and needy while boys tend to become aggressive.
Authoritative	Shows much warmth and affection for the child and provides guidance with minimal restraints. Maintains flexibility and communicates freely with the child, encouraging autonomy.	Child often has a positive self-image and is able to act independently and gets along well with others. The child is accepting of restrictions and often does well in school.

Caregiver Strain

Signs and symptoms of **caregiver strain** are as follows:

- Caregiver appears anxious or depressed and easily irritated.
- Caregiver complains of fatigue and difficulty sleeping.
- Caregiver gets upset or lashes out excessively in response to irritating or stressful events.
- Caregiver complains of new ailments or of worsening health.
- Caregiver is forgetful and has difficulty concentrating or carrying through with activities.
- Caregiver is increasingly angry and resentful toward the patient.
- Caregiver no longer engages in leisure activities.
- Caregiver increasingly withdraws from outside relationships and social activities.
- Caregiver begins to neglect the patient and other responsibilities.
- Caregiver shows signs of compensatory behavior, such as excessive drinking, eating, or smoking.

- Caregiver neglects personal care and needs.
- Caregiver complains of feeling hopeless about future.
- Caregiver increasingly blames patient for things beyond patient's control.

Treatment consists of the following:

- Offer support/therapeutic listening; community support groups/social services for relief care.
- Notify social services if abuse is suspected.

Elements of Therapeutic Communication

Therapeutic communication begins with respect for the patient/family and the assumption that all communication, verbal and non-verbal, has meaning. Listening must be done empathetically. Techniques that facilitate communication include the following:

- *Introduction*: Make a personal introduction and use the patient's name: "Mrs. Brown, I am Susan Williams, your nurse."
- *Encouragement*: Use an open-ended opening statement: "Is there anything you'd like to discuss?"
- *Acknowledge comments*: "Yes," and "I understand."
- Allow silence and observe non-verbal behavior rather than trying to force conversation. Ask for clarification if statements are unclear.
- Reflect statements back (use sparingly):
    - Patient: "I hate this hospital."
    - Nurse: "You hate this hospital?"
- *Empathy*: Make observations: "You are shaking," and "You seem worried."
- Recognize feelings:
    - Patient: "I want to go home."
    - Nurse: "It must be hard to be away from your home and family."
- Provide information as honestly and completely as possible about condition, treatment, and procedures and respond to the patient's questions and concerns.

Methods to promote a caring and supportive environment with **therapeutic communication** include:

Exploration	Verbally express implied messages: Patient: "This treatment is too much trouble." Nurse: "You think the treatment isn't helping you?" Explore a topic but allow the patient to terminate the discussion without further probing: "I'd like to hear how you feel about that."
Orientation	Indicate reality: Patient: "Someone is screaming." Nurse: "That sound was an ambulance siren." Comment on distortions without directly agreeing or disagreeing: Patient: "That nurse promised I didn't have to walk again." Nurse: "Really? That's surprising because the doctor ordered physical therapy twice a day."
Collaboration	Work together to achieve better results: "Maybe if we talk about this, we can figure out a way to make the treatment easier for you."
Validation	Seek validation: "Do you feel better now?" or "Did the medication help you breathe better."

THERAPEUTIC MILIEU

The **therapeutic milieu** (AKA therapeutic community) is a method of structuring inpatient and outpatient rehabilitation programs so that all aspects of the environment are therapeutic in order that the client learn coping and relationship skills that the client can utilize in all aspects of life. The environment usually includes both areas for group activities as well as private areas and may include, for example, recreational facilities (swimming pool, gym). Clients typically receive a rule book that includes the schedule of activities and that outlines boundaries and limits so that the clients can feel safe and secure and understand expectations. Staff is available to provide emotional support. Clients are monitored and interventions carried out for inappropriate behavior as well as consistent positive feedback provided for constructive efforts to help build self-esteem. The focus of therapy is on the clients' emotions, behavior, and cognitive thought processes.

EMPATHY

Empathy is the process of understanding another person by identifying with his/her situation, rather than seeing it from an outside perspective. It involves putting oneself into another's shoes and seeing the situation as the affected person does. When used in a helping relationship, the counselor can utilize empathy by trying to see the client's viewpoint and consider the situation from the client's perspective, rather than the counselor's. Empathy comprises **two stages**:

1. The first stage is *experiencing the same emotions as the affected person.* An example of this might be when a counselor cries with a client who is experiencing significant emotional pain.
2. Stage two of empathy involves *realistically looking at the situation from the other person's point of view.* An example of this situation might be when a counselor listens to the client and examines his own reaction by considering how he might feel in the same situation.

Active Listening

Attributes of **active listeners** include conveying warmth and respect, and offering acceptance of the client. The nurse must:

- Acknowledge all behavior of the client and realize it has meaning.
- Set boundaries and abide by them when taking part in a conversation.
- Do not lead the client in a direction; allow client to direct conversation as appropriate.
- Give ample time for expression.
- Ask questions related to the topic of discussion.
- Body language: maintain eye contact, and face the client, lean in as listening intently, nod, smile, and frown to show agreement or disagreement.

The nurse must be aware of his or her own experiences and how they can alter the relationship with the client. If a nurse feels she is unable to adequately care for a client related to the nurse's past experience, she must relay this information to her superiors.

Barriers to Effective Communication

Barriers to communication exist when the nurse is unable to effectively communicate the wants, needs, and desires of the patient, as well as to effectively discuss and explain the care and rational for the care needed. Barriers to communication may include:

- Minimization of concerns/belittling the patient or concerns.
- Offering false reassurance/approval to the patient.
- Rejecting individuals.
- Choosing sides: the patient, the family, or the physician.
- Placing blame on external factors or patient /family.
- Conflicting opinions from the patient or family, giving advice.
- Minimal feedback to questions – one-word answers, cutting off.
- Shifting the focus of concern.
- Using medical terminology/jargon.
- Offering unrealistic ideation or ignoring patient's concerns.

To fix these common barriers, the nurse needs to speak honestly and openly with the client about health concerns and treatments. The nurse should use language that is easy to understand, and take time to listen to all the patient's concerns and questions. Open-ended questions and open body language reinforce the nurses' concern for the patient. Never offer opinions and false reassurances to patients, and always speak positively of others.

Basic Care and Comfort

Elimination

Types of Incontinence

Urge	An urgency to urinate as soon as the bladder feels full, so person may urinate on the way to the toilet or in bed during the night. Diuretics may exacerbate urge incontinence.
Overflow	An overfull bladder causes dribbling of urine, usually in small amounts but the leakage can be almost constant.
Functional	Incontinence caused by physical or mental impairment, such as dementia. May also be related to environmental barriers to urination, such as no accessible bathroom.
Reflex	Loss of urine takes place without awareness of person because of fistula or bladder leak.
Mixed	There may be more than one type of incontinence, so symptoms may vary.
Induced	Some surgical procedures (hysterectomy, prostatectomy, rectal surgery) can damage nerves or muscles that control urination.

Stress Incontinence

Stress incontinence is an involuntary leakage of urine due to a laugh, sneeze, urge to urinate, or activity that causes increased pressure on the bladder. It is generally due to urethral sphincter dysfunction. Increased age, childbirth, trauma, certain medications, and other factors may increase the risk of stress incontinence.

Diagnosis: Rectal exam, x-rays, pad test, urine analysis, PVR test, cystoscopy, pelvic exam, prostate exam (men).

Treatment includes:

- Medications - pseudoephedrine/phenylpropanolamine, estrogen, and other medications may help treat underlying cause.
- Physical therapy - Pelvic floor re-training; biofeedback training.
- Lifestyle modification: fluid restrictions, can wear pads/briefs, teach Kegel exercises for strengthening.

Bladder Irrigations

Bladder irrigations are carried out to flush residue (clots, mucous) out of the bladder and to maintain patency of indwelling catheters. Procedure:

1. Gather supplies (catheterization set if needed, sterile irrigation tray with 60 mL catheter-tipped syringe, alcohol swabs,) container of sterile water/NS, and container for urine collection) and verify the maximum volume that should be used (especially important for neobladders).
2. Wash hands.
3. Insert straight catheter using sterile technique if an indwelling catheter is not already in place.
4. Place sterile drape under the perineal area and catheter. Wipe catheter/tubing connection with alcohol and let dry.

5. Draw up 30 to 50 mL of sterile water/NS into the catheter-tipped syringe and insert syringe into the end of the catheter.
6. Place the urine collection container between client's legs.
7. Disconnect catheter/tubing and swab end of catheter with alcohol swab and place sterile cap from syringe on tubing.
8. Gently inject 30 to 50 mL of water through the catheter.
9. Aspirate the fluid but avoid excessive pulling on the plunger because the negative pressure created may damage tissue. Empty syringe into urine collection container.
10. Repeat until urine is clear and allow any remaining liquid to drain into the urine collection container.
11. Reconnect catheter and tubing.
12. If straight catheter was inserted for irrigation, remove.

Types of Enemas

Medicated retention	May contain antibiotics, nutritives, or anthelmintics.
Oil retention	Prepackaged in 3-8-ounce bulb-type devices. Use mineral oil to coat, lubricate, and soften stool in the rectum. Often used for children and as first step in removal of fecal impaction.
Tap water (hypotonic)	Used for mechanical flushing of the rectum, but tap water if used consistently can deplete electrolytes as well as causing acute water intoxication, especially in children and the elderly, if water is retained. However, the risk if very slight if small volumes (500 to 1000 mL) of water are used. Effective in 15-20 minutes.
Phosphate	Come prepackaged for one-time use with about 120 ml of solution. They stimulate contractions, and, because they are hypertonic, they draw fluid back into the intestines. Frequent use can result in hyperphosphatemia and hypocalcemia.
Soapsuds	Use Castile soap as an irritant to promote contraction and defecation. Usually about 5 ml of soap is added to 1000 ml of tap water. The enema is effective in about 10-15 minutes, but the soap can cause mucosal irritation.

Skin Care to Prevent Irritation from Fecal or Urinary Incontinence

Skin care for fecal or urinary incontinence includes:

- **Cleanse skin** with water after each episode of incontinence. Soap tends to be drying and can cause irritation, but if soap is needed, people can use baby wash, which is quite mild, or disposable pre-moistened alcohol-free, perfume-free wipes. After cleansing, the area should be dried thoroughly, patting dry or using a hair dryer on low heat.
- **Apply cream or powder** if there is any sign of skin irritation. Moisture-barrier creams, such as Desitin® and A & D ointment can prevent urine or feces from directly contacting skin. Non-medicated, non-perfumed talcum powder or cornstarch may help to keep perineal area dry.
- **Wear loose clothing** to allow for airflow as tight clothes can make skin irritation worse. Many synthetic fibers, such as polyester, constrict air and should be avoided. Underwear should be 100% cotton.
- **Use incontinence pads**, which should contain an absorbent wicking layer to keep moisture away from the skin and should be changed promptly when soiled.

Promoting Voiding

Methods for **promoting voiding** include:

- **Stimuli**: Pouring warm water over perineal area, having the person blow bubbles through a straw to relax the sphincter, or turning on the faucet so the person hears the sound of running water may promote voiding.
- **Bladder training**: Usually requires the person to keep a toileting diary for at least 3 days so patterns can be assessed. There are a number of different approaches:
- **Scheduled toileting**: Toileting or a regular schedule, usually every 2 to 4 hours during the daytime.
- **Habit training**: Involves an attempt to match the scheduled toileting to a person's individual voiding habits, based on the toileting diary. This is useful for people who have a natural and fairly consistent voiding pattern. Toileting is done every 2-4 hours.
- **Prompted voiding**: Often used in nursing homes and attempts to teach people to assess their own incontinence status and prompts them to ask for toileting.
- **Bladder retraining**: Behavioral modification program that teaches people to inhibit the urge to urinate and to urinate according to an established schedule, restoring normal bladder function as much as possible. Bladder training can improve incontinence in 80% of cases.

Ostomy

An **ostomy** is either a permanent or temporary artificial opening created to allow stool or other substances out of the body. An *ileostomy* occurs as the result of total removal of the colon and the rectum; the anus is sutured closed and an opening in the lower abdominal wall in the area of the ileum is formed to allow for fecal evacuation. A *colostomy,* however, is formed when the colon is routed to an opening in the abdominal wall forming an artificial opening for feces to be removed and collected. The anus is also sutured with a colostomy. A *urostomy* is the diversion of one or both ureters to an opening in the abdominal wall.

Teaching:

- Avoid gas-producing foods, can use deodorizers.
- Stool from ostomy more formed than ileostomy (pure liquid).
- Ostomy should be healthy, pink, beefy color. Report pale color (could mean loss of blood flow to tissue) or dark red with irritation or drainage (infection).
- Change as directed; teach patient to cut wafer to correct size to prevent skin irritation.
- Body image disturbance is problem for these patients. Educate to alleviate fears and embarrassment.

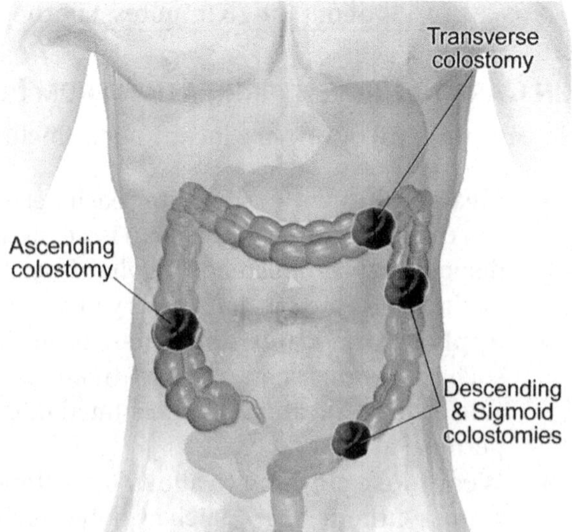

Colostomy Types

Mobility/Immobility

Assessing Mobility

About 20% of noninstitutionalized older adults and 54% of institutionalized older adults (≥85) have **gait and mobility issues** that limit their independence and predispose them to depression and falls. Risk factors include arthritis, peripheral neuropathy, hypothyroidism, Parkinson's disease, orthostatic hypotension, deformities, stroke and heart attack, medication effects, and orthopedic problems/surgery. Weakness, loss of muscle mass, and confusion may contribute to gait disorders. During assessment, the client should be carefully observed for gait abnormalities, include unsteadiness, uneven weight distribution, abnormal position of limbs, and type of gait. Gait assessment includes:

- Gait speed in 5 meters with slow gait (<0.6 m/second) predictive of limitations.
- Timed up and go (TUG): Client stands from chair with armrests, walks 3 meters, and turns and sits back down. Those requiring ≥14 seconds are at risk for falls (Normal:7-10 seconds).
- Performance oriented mobility assessment (POMA) tests mobility and gait under different conditions.

Treatment includes identifying and treating underlying cause, gait and strength training, environmental modifications, assistive devices, and orthotics.

Complications of Immobility

Complications of immobility include:

- **Skin breakdown**: Irritation of the skin and pressure sores may develop because of pressure on bony prominences or friction and shearing from the client sliding against the bedding, especially if the client is not repositioned correctly at least every 2 hours. Additionally, skin about the perineal area and in folds of skin (under abdominal fold, breasts, scrotum) may break down if skin care is inadequate. Risk increases for those who are underweight or overweight and those with decreased sensation.
- **Contractures**: A contracture results from lack of joint mobility because of changes in non-bone structures (muscles, tendons, ligaments). With immobility, joints tend to become stiff and over time muscles begin to atrophy, tighten, and shorten, resulting in flexion at the elbows, hips, and knees. Fingers may curl inward, and ankles and toes may go into foot drop (weakness in muscles of dorsiflexion) because of damage to the nerves or muscle paralysis.

Methods of Fixation/Traction

External fixation	Used to stabilize fractures without further damaging soft tissue. In the US, used primarily when extensive soft tissue damage precludes cast application. Types of external fixation devices includes simple pin fixations, clamp fixators, and ring fixators. Fixation pins are applied into the bones and attached to external devices, such as rods, to keep bones in alignment.
Halo traction	Comprises a halo ring about the head secured by in place in the frontal and temporal bones. Rods connect from the halo ring to the rigid body jacket/brace in order to maintain traction or for immobilization. Halo traction may be utilized for cervical and upper-thoracic fractures, nerve damage, head and neck tumors, and rheumatoid arthritis.
Skeletal traction	Skins, screws, tongs, or wires are used to attach traction devices directly to the bones (such as the femur), allowing more traction and heavier weights than skin traction.

Methods to Promote Circulation

Methods to promote circulation include:

- **Active range of motion (AROM)**: The client moves the joint through the range of motion appropriate for each joint without assistance or support of surrounding muscles. With assisted active range of motion (AAROM), the nurse may provide some assistance or equipment to assist the client, such as using a strap to help provide lift.
- **Passive range of motion (PROM)**: The nurse moves the client's joint through the range of motion appropriate for each joint with no effort on the part of the client. This type of range of motion is appropriate for clients who have paralysis or are unable to assist because of coma or severe weakness.
- **Positioning**: The client should be repositioned at least every 2 hours to prevent stasis and pressure and encouraged to change positions independently if able to do so.
- **Mobilization**: Early mobilization to the client's ability may begin with simply sitting up or standing at bedside but should progress to full mobilization to tolerance as soon as possible in order to prevent muscle atrophy and contractures and to improve venous return.

Pressure Ulcers

Pressure ulcers are ulcers that appear in areas of prolonged pressure on the human body. They are often the end result of pressure on overlying skin of bony prominences in patients who are debilitated or immobilized for any reason. "Bed sores," "decubital gangrene," "pressure sores," and "hospital gangrene" are all alternate names given to pressure ulcers. The most frequent location of pressure ulcers is the base of the skull, sacrum, elbows, ischial tuberosities/hips, and heels. The staging of pressure ulcers indicates their severity and helps mark the progress or regression of the wounds. They can be prevented by frequent turning, protecting bony prominences, shear precautions, and good nutrition.

- **Stage One**: skin may be cool to touch, does not blanch, and may be accompanied by pruritus and tenderness; skin intact.
- **Stage Two**: partial loss of skin thickness; epidermal and dermal involvement; may appear as a blister or abrasion.
- **Stage Three**: subcutaneous tissue involvement; can see yellow tissue (fat) in wound; may involve necrosis.
- **Stage Four**: tissue loss into layers of muscle and/or bone; widespread loss of tissue and broad tissue necrosis.
- **Unstageable**: full tissue loss across all layers; base of wound is covered in necrotic tissue, may appear yellow, green, or black; unable to see underlying structure.

Amputations

Amputations are explained below:

- **Types**: Lower extremities—toe, metatarsal (mid-foot amputation), Syme (removal of foot at ankle), knee disarticulation (amputation through knee joint), below knee (BKA), and above knee (AKA). Upper extremities—digit, wrist articulation, below elbow (BEA), above elbow (AEA), elbow disarticulation, shoulder disarticulation, and forequarter amputation (removes a large portion of shoulder and the arm). Others include hemipelvectomy (removal of half of pelvis and all of legs), hemicorporectomy (removal of lower half of body with resultant colostomy and urinary diversion).

- **Postoperative care**: Patients must be carefully monitored for signs of shock or bleeding. Focus is on stump care to provide correct molding and prevent infection, pain control, emotional support, acceptance of change in body image, and mobility. Place patient in prone position several times a day to improve oxygenation and prevent contractures.
- **Patient teaching**: Patients should have a clear understanding of prognosis and rehabilitation efforts needed. Patients may need to learn how to provide stump care and many need to be taught to use assistive devices and prostheses. Patients should understand pain control and be taught about phantom pain.

Non-Pharmacological Comfort Interventions

Non-Pharmacological Interventions for Pain

Non-pharmacological interventions are nursing interventions that decrease pain and discomfort in patients without the use of drugs. Listed below are some common interventions that may be seen:

- **Heat/Cold**: Usually requires a physician order; can be moist or dry. Be cautious as intense temperatures may cause burns or damage the skin. Always use a barrier between the source and the patient's skin, and instruct patients to never lay heating devices or sleep with them in use. Always maintain the prescribed temperature, and check the skin every 15 minutes. Heat/cold is contraindicated with sensory loss or cognitive impairment (diabetics, altered mental status, stroke patients, etc.)
- **Music/Distraction**: Multiple studies have shown that calming music or other forms of distraction can help to relieve mild pain and discomfort. Always remember to ask the patient's preferences, and keep the volume low so as not to disturb others. Remember that pain relieved by distraction does not indicate that the pain is not "real."
- **Mobility/Positioning**: Early ambulation and increased activity as tolerated (e.g. up in the chair for meals) are interventions which can greatly increase patient comfort/decrease risk for complications during the hospital stay. For bedridden patients, active and passive ROM and frequent turning (every two hours) can increase comfort and decrease risk of bedsores.

Complementary and Alternative Therapies for Pain Management

Reiki	This is a form of light therapeutic touch, primarily involving the head and torso but can also involve the extremities. The practitioner's hands may be held above an area that is painful or has an open wound rather than touching. Reiki is useful to help patients relax and relieve anxiety.
Hypnosis	Hypnosis increases susceptibility to suggestions, and some patients respond better than others, but it can help to relax patients and to reduce the perception of pain, both acute and chronic as well as nausea and vomiting. Some patients are able to utilize progressive relaxation and self-hypnosis techniques to help to control pain.
Acupressure	Similar to acupuncture, pressure instead of needles is applied to pressure points (meridians). Acupressure may relieve muscle tension, bring about relaxation, and help to reduce pain as well as nausea. Different methods (finger pressure, energy roller, electrical stimulation) may be used to stimulate the acupressure points.
Pet therapy	The most common animal used for pet therapy is the dog, although cats and other animals may be used as well. Petting an animal can relieve pain by providing distraction and releasing endorphins that help to increase a feeling of well-being. Patients may feel less fear and depression as well when interacting with animals. Caring for an animal may motivate patients to be more active.
Music therapy	Music can help to improve a patient's mood, resulting in relaxation and reduced anxiety, which in turn helps to reduce pain. Listening attentively to music, especially through a headset to block out other environmental noises, also can distract patients from perceptions of pain. There is no one type of music that is ideal, so the music selected should be that preferred by the patient. However, for relaxation, soft or classical music is often preferred.
Massage	Manual massage may improve circulation, relax muscles, reduce anxiety, and reduce pain although it should be avoided with low platelet counts (risk of bleeding), over cancerous bone lesions (fracture risks), and over areas of blood clots (risk of emboli).

Contraindications to Aromatherapy, Acupressure, and Supplements

Contraindications to complementary therapies include:

- **Aromatherapy**: Because some essential oils can be toxic, clients should avoid applying most of them to skin and should limit diffusion of oils to no more than 60 minutes (three times daily for 30 minutes is recommended) to avoid overexposure. The area with the diffuser should be well-ventilated and animals (such as cats) should be left outside the area as they may be sensitive to the odors. Clients should use care to dilute the essential oil as recommended.
- **Acupressure**: Pressure should not be applied over the abdominal area (especially if the client has a disease affecting the abdominal organs, such as cancer, or is pregnant) or areas of burns, infections, injuries, or scars. Acupressure should never be used as a sole treatment for a disease.
- **Supplements**: Some supplements may interfere with medications (such as coenzyme Q10 interfering with the effectiveness of warfarin) and others may be toxic if taken in high doses (such as vitamin A). Some clients may take supplements rather than medical treatment for disease even though studies do not support their use.

Nutrition, Hydration, Hygiene, and Rest

BMI

The **Body Mass Index (BMI)** formula is a measurement that uses height and weight as an indicator of obesity/malnutrition. This cannot be used alone to diagnose obesity because body types differ. Women often have more body fat than men. Tables are available to make calculations simple, but the BMI can be calculated manually using either metric or English units:

$$BMI = \frac{Weight\ in\ kilograms}{(Height\ in\ meters)^2} = \frac{(Weight\ in\ pounds) \times 703}{(Height\ in\ inches)^2}$$

Resulting scores for adults age 20 and over are interpreted according to this chart:

- Below 18.5: Underweight.
- 18.5-24.9: Normal weight.
- 25.0-29.9: Overweight.
- 30 and above: Obese.

The BMI for those under age 20 uses age-sex specific charts provided by the CDC, containing a curved line that indicates percentiles. Criteria for obesity based on these charts and BMI for age <20 follow:

- <5th percentile: Underweight.
- 85th-<95 percentile: At risk for overweight.
- ≥95th percentile: Overweight.

Monitoring of the Ability to Eat

Monitoring the ability to eat (chew, swallow) is an important responsibility of the practical nurse. This should first be assessed by a registered nurse or speech therapist, which begins with a history to determine if the client/caregiver is aware of problems and whether the client has dental problems that may interfere with chewing or wears/needs dentures. Additionally, any recent weight loss should be noted as this may indicate a problem with intake. If problems with chewing and swallowing (such as dysphagia after a stroke) are evident, then assessment should be carried out by a speech therapist with a videofluoroscopic or videoendoscopic exam. For routine assessment, the client should sit upright and first be asked to swallow normal secretions. If the client can do that without problem, then the client can be asked to swallow small amounts (about 5 mL) of liquids and foods of various consistencies. It's important to note whether the client can sense liquids and solids in the mouth. If tolerating solids, the client should be observed carefully while chewing to ensure that the chewing is adequate for the solid and then observed while swallowing, which should require less than 10 seconds. If the client needs to lower the chin to swallow or requires a longer time, this can indicate some impairment. The nurse should notice any coughing, choking, gagging, or spitting during the assessment. The practical nurse should monitor for these symptoms during patient feeding/meals and report any irregularities to the appropriate health care provider.

Common Food-Drug Interactions

Food and drug interactions can impact the drug's effect on the body:

Drug	Caution
ACE inhibitors	Avoid potassium supplements or foods high in potassium.
Antibiotics	Avoid milk products. Avoid vitamins and minerals containing iron and avoid caffeine.
Anticoagulants	Avoid foods high in vitamin K. Avoid vitamin E supplements.
Antifungals	Avoid milk products and alcohol.
Antihistamines, antidepressants, anti-anxieties	Avoid alcohol. Avoid grapefruit juice.
Beta blockers, nitrates, narcotics, NSAIDs	Avoid alcohol.
Bronchodilators, histamine blockers	Avoid caffeine and alcohol.
Carbamazepine, cyclosporine and tacrolimus, HIV medications, statins	Avoid grapefruit juice
Diuretics, potassium sparing	Avoid food high in potassium.
MAO inhibitors	Avoid alcohol and non-alcoholic substitute for beer or wine, foods high in tyramine, and products containing caffeine.

Indications for Special Diets

Indications for the following **special diets** include:

- **Low sodium**: Utilized to help control hypertension and to reduce edema. Diet used to prevent fluid overload for clients with renal failure and heart failure.
- **High protein**: Utilized primarily for weight loss. Some controversy remains regarding the long-term safety of a high protein diet because the diet is generally high in saturated fats.
- **Calorie restrictions**: Limiting calorie intake to that below the amount that maintains weight is primarily utilized for weight reduction. Some studies indicate that calorie restriction may prolong life, but those who restrict calories too much may have health risks.
- **Nutritional supplements**: May be utilized to compensate for deficits (such as a low vitamin D level) but often taken for no specific reason out of a belief that more is better, although this is not always the case as some nutritional supplements may be toxic if taken in large doses.

Progression of Diet Types

For patients who are having severe nausea/vomiting, prolonged fasting, or other digestive difficulties, the doctor will often give a restricted diet order. Additionally, they will often include "**Advance as Tolerated**" order, which will allow the patient to progress through the types until their normal digestion is restored.

1. **Nothing by Mouth (NPO)**: No food or liquids (including water or ice chips). Often before procedures; may be exception such as "sips and chips"), or "may give medications with small sips of water."
2. **Clear Liquid Diet**: Liquids that are clear and in liquid form at body temperature. This may include coffee (no creamer), gelatin, and broth.

3. **Full Liquid Diet**: Similar to clear liquid diet, with the addition of milk, soups, and other opaque liquids.
4. **Pureed Diets**: Foods that are smooth in consistency; often normal food items that have been blended. This diet is often seen in patients with chewing/swallowing difficulties.
5. **Mechanical Soft Diet**: A mechanical soft diet provides nutrition in the form of foods that require only a nominal amount of chewing.
6. **Soft Diet**: Foods that are easily digestible for the patient, such as bland food, white breads, or cooked vegetables. Soft diets are used when a patient is progressing from a clear to a regular diet.
7. **Regular Diet**: The term regular diet is for a diet that has no limits or needed modifications.

Impact of Disease on Nutritional Status

The impact of disease on **nutritional status** may vary widely, depending on the condition and the age and general health of the client. For example, a client with limited mobility may burn fewer calories but eat the same amount and may begin to gain weight. Some medications, such as steroids, may increase the appetite and cause the client to retain fluid and store fat. Clients with severe diseases, such as cancer, may find they lose their appetite or cannot tolerate some foods, so they may begin to eat less and lose weight, eventually suffering from malnutrition. With infection, intake of nutrients decreases while losses increase. Some metabolic disorders, such as diabetes (carbohydrates) and celiac disease (gluten), may impair the bodies' ability to digest certain foods or food constituents. Diseases with diarrhea, such as inflammatory bowel diseases, may result in excess loss of nutrients and inability to absorb nutrients, and the chronic blood loss that may occur may result in anemia. In many cases, the client's diet may need to be adjusted to compensate for disease.

NG Tubes and NJ Tubes

NG/NJ tubes are long, thin tubes that inserted through the nose of the patient and then down the throat and esophagus and into the stomach or intestine for either feeding or suctioning. The tube length is determined by measuring the patient from the tip of their nose across to one earlobe and down to the tip of the xiphoid process; in children, this measurement is extending to the umbilicus. It is crucial to remember to verify correct placement before feeding or administering medications through the tube. This can be done by either aspiration or checking gastric content pH. The initial placement is typically verified with x-ray.

- **NG tube (nasogastric)** – This tube ends in the stomach. Food could be supplied through the tube using a pump or gravity. Feeds may be provided in either a bolus or more continuous amounts. Bolus supply is large volume supplied over a short time. For instance, mealtimes can be modeled by providing three large meals (boluses) a day through the tube. For patients needing extra calories, or for those who do not tolerate bolus feeds, continuous or overnight feeds may be used. Patients with intestinal blockage, severe vomiting, or a high risk of aspiration may benefit from suction via an NG/NJ tube.
- **NJ tube (nasojejunal)** – Similar to an NG tube, the NJ tube passes through the patient's stomach and into the jejunum where it ends. Ending in the jejunum instead of the stomach helps reduce acid reflux-associated vomiting. Therefore, an NJ tube is used when bypassing the stomach is desirable.

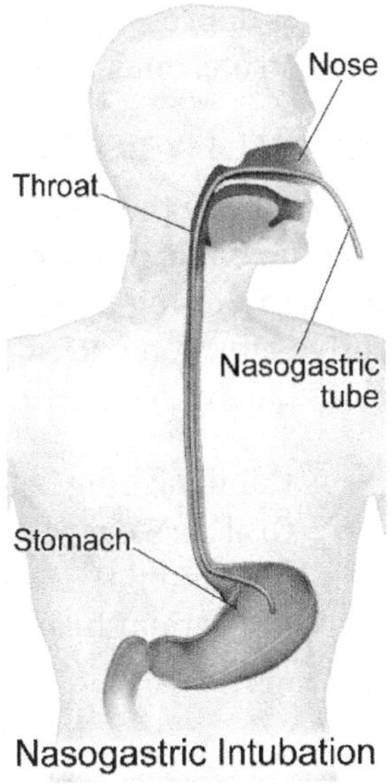

Nasogastric Intubation

Common Side Effects from Tube Feeding

Feeding tubes may be place nasally, orally, or percutaneously to provide feedings for those unable to take foods/fluids orally, such as with dysphagia after a stroke or with head and neck cancer. Nasogastric and orogastric tubes are usually used for short durations only. If prolonged feeding is needed, then a percutaneous endoscopic gastrostomy (PEG) tube or jejunostomy (J) tube is generally placed. Older adults, especially those with comorbid conditions, are more likely to encounter problems than others. Common side effects from tube feedings include:

- Nausea and vomiting, especially if feedings are given too quickly or if volume is too large.
- Dehydration if fluid intake is inadequate for needs.
- Constipation and/or diarrhea, depending on the formula utilized.
- Skin irritation about insertion site of tube.
- Intestinal perforation.
- Abdominal infection (peritonitis).
- Aspiration (with displacement, regurgitation).
- Generalized infection, sepsis, generally as a progression of peritonitis.
- Clogged tube preventing feedings, usually because of inadequate flushing of tube before and after feedings.

Hydration Status

Monitoring hydration status includes not only measuring/estimating intake and output and ensuring intake is adequate but also assessing the client for signs of fluid deficit. Fluid intake recommended for infant and children includes:

Weight in kg	24-hour fluid requirement
<10 kg	100 mL/kg
10-20 kg	1000 mL and 50 mL/kg for each kg >10 kg.
>20 kg	1500 mL and 20 mL/kg for each kg >20 kg.

Urinary output increases over the first 6 days of life from one time to 6 to 8 diapers in24 hours (average l-2 ML/kg/hr for infants). For older children and adults, the normal output varies from 800 mL to 2000 mL per day with intake of 2000 mL. Signs of fluid deficit include: dry mucous membranes, tachycardia, decreased urinary output, normal BP progressing to hypotension, fontanels depressed (infants), and 3-10% decrease in body weight. Intake and output should include urine, emesis, liquid stools and any other measurable drainage, such as from an NG tube.

Personal Hygiene for Hospitalized Patients

In the midst of the chaos of special tests, doctor's rounds, and medication passes, it can be easy to forget the **basic personal hygiene needs of the patient.** While they may not seem to be a top priority, adhering to basic hygiene during patient care can reduce the risk of infection and have a positive effect on patient outcomes. The following practices should be followed for every patient, as well as taught to those in an outpatient setting:

- Handwashing before meals/after using the bathroom (minimum).
- Oral care every day; every two hours if the patient is NPO/ventilated (prevents pneumonia); if the patient has dentures, these should be cleaned every night and given to the patient before meals.

- The patient should receive a full bath and linen change every day and when they are soiled; offer the patient lotion and deodorant at this time, as well as a clean gown.
- Toilet frequently and change incontinent patients every time they are soiled (check hourly and as needed). Educate female patients to wipe "front to back" to prevent UTIs.

**Note: If the patient refuses any part of personal hygiene, be sure to document that it was offered and the patient was educated about its importance.*

Rest and Sleep During Illness Recovery

Good quality sleep is hard to come by for the hospitalized patient. While it may not be a high priority to the nurses, **sleep and rest** are key components to recovery in patients. Lack of sleep may lead to agitation, delirium, falls, and many other adverse events. The following are interventions which the nurse may implement to promote rest and sleep in his/her patients:

- Turn down lights in the evening hours and offer personal hygiene before rest.
- Ensure the patient is positioned comfortably and linens/gown are clean and straightened.
- Keep the area around the room quiet at night, and limit loud talking/noises from the nurse's station.
- "Cluster" care: minimize disturbances to the patient by doing multiple tasks during one visit into the room. Work quietly and as quickly as possible to help the patient fall back asleep when finished.
- Realize some medications that promote sleep actually shorten or eliminate the REM cycle, preventing the patient from feeling well rested and mentally alert.

**Note: While sleep is important, it must be noted that sleep and rest are not an valid excuse to avoid required nursing duties and checks. It may seem difficult to arouse a resting patient, but their safety comes first.*

Pharmacological Therapies

Principles of Pharmacology

Pharmacokinetics

Pharmacokinetics includes the absorption, distribution, metabolism, and elimination of drugs/medications. These processes must all take place during the course of drug therapy for the drug to be safe and effective. A helpful mnemonic for remember the four parts is "AD ME!":

- **Absorption** is the rate a drug leaves the site of administration and the extent of the drug's entrance into the cells. Absorption determines the *bioavailability* of the medication. This refers to the amount of drug available when it reaches its target destination or organ system.
- **Distribution** involves the mechanism of distribution of the drug throughout the body, sometimes involving carrier proteins.
- **Metabolism**: The breakdown of the drug, usually occurring in the liver. This results in metabolites, which can either be more or less potent than the parent drug, depending on mechanism of action.
- **Excretion** is the way drugs are eliminated from the body, generally taking place in the kidneys. This is an important concept, as impaired excretion can lead to increased serum levels and toxicity.

Eight Rights of Medication Administration

The **Eight Rights of Medication Administration** are as follows:

1. Right Patient
2. Right Medication
3. Right Dose
4. Right Route
5. Right Time
6. Right Documentation
7. Right to Education
8. Right to Refuse

Nurses' Role in Preventing Medication Errors

The following are nursing duties to prevent medication errors:

- Checking the first five rights before medication administration against the medication administration record (MAR). These should be checked a minimum of 3 times each.
- Ensure the right patient by using three patient identifiers—this generally means checking the name, DOB, and medical record number (MRN) on the patient's armband with the MAR, and have the patient state name and DOB.
- The nurse should inform the patient what they are giving them and how it works, as well as expected side effects before administration; allergies should also be checked at this time.
- Realize that the patient has the right to refuse any and all medications. NEVER force a medication on a patient unless it is a safety issue.
- Sign off on **all** medications **after** they are administered.

Injections

The different types of injections are described below:

- Intradermal injections (ID)
  - Dermal layer of the skin; shallow, causes "bleb"; given into skin of inner forearm, or back, rarely chest
  - Angle: 10-15°
  - 27-30 g; 1/4-3/8 inch length
  - ≤1 mL fluid: Mantoux test for TB exposure, allergy testing, etc.
- Subcutaneous injections (SQ)
  - Adipose (fat) tissue; upper, outer arm, the anterior thigh, and the abdomen
  - Angle: 45° (90° for insulin and heparin)
  - 25-28 g; 5/8 of an inch long
  - 0.5-1 mL of fluid; insulin, heparin, enoxaparin, etc.
- Intramuscular injections (IM)
  - Deep into muscle; ventrogluteal, dorsogluteal, vastus lateralis, or deltoid muscle
  - Angle: 90°
  - 23 g; 1-1½ inch length.
  - ≤3 mL of fluid; only 2 mL in deltoid
  - **MUST** aspirate for blood prior to giving an IM injection to ensure medication will not be delivered intravenously

Pharmacologic Prefixes and Suffixes

Drug Class	Prefix/Suffix
ACE Inhibitor	-pril
Alpha-1 Antagonist	-zosin
Angiotensin Blocker	-sartan
Antifungal	-azole
Barbiturates	-barbital
Benzodiazepine	-pam OR -lam
Beta-2 Agonist	-terol
Beta Antagonist	-olol
Calcium Channel Blocker	-dipine
Cephalosporin	Ceph- OR Cef-
Fluoroquinolone	-floxacin/-floxin
H2 Antagonist	-tidine
Methylxanthine	-phylline
Penicillin	-cillin
Phenothiazine	-azine
Pituitary Hormone	-trophin
Protease Inhibitor	-navir
Sulfonamides	Sulfa-
Tetracyclines	-cycline
Thrombolytics	-ase
Tricyclic Antidepressant	-ipramine

Review Video: Drug Suffixes
Visit mometrix.com/academy and enter code: 684170

Pharmacologic Interventions

Hormones Secreted by the Posterior Pituitary Gland

The **posterior pituitary gland** is responsible for the secretion of the hormones vasopressin/ADH and oxytocin. These hormones are synthesized in the hypothalamus, stored in the posterior pituitary, and secreted into the blood:

- Vasopressin/ADH
  - Works in the kidneys to retain more water in the blood; decreases urination and increases blood pressure.
  - Synthetic drugs: vasopressin, desmopressin, and lypressin (intranasal).
  - Uses: diabetes insipidus, hypotension, chronic ADH deficiency.
- Oxytocin:
  - Stimulates contractions of the uterus to initiate and sustain labor; also causes "let-down" reflex, releasing milk in response to infant's sucking on breast.
  - Synthetic: oxytocic drugs such as oxytocin.
  - Uses: induce labor, treat atonic uterus/postpartum hemorrhage, stimulate lactation.

Anticholinergics

Indication: Bradycardia, pre-op to reduce GI/respiratory secretions, COPD treatment, as anti-spasmodics, Parkinson disease, motion sickness, pesticide poisoning.

Mechanism of action: Interrupt parasympathetic nerve impulses in the central and autonomic nervous systems; block acetylcholine.

- Medications: belladonna alkaloids, atropine, scopolamine, trimethobenzamide, cyclizine, dimenhydrinate, meclizine, etc.

Side Effects: drowsiness, dry mouth, urinary retention, constipation, blurred vision, decreased sweating.

Teaching:

- Can chew sugarless gum/suck on ice or sugar-free candy to help alleviate dry mouth.
- Avoid overheating: saunas, yard work in hot weather, etc; decreased sweating increases risk of heat-related illness.
- Do not drive or perform other potentially dangerous tasks until you know how this drug will affect your vision.
- OD symptoms: hallucinations, seizures, rapid heart rate, coma.

A way to remember the effects of anticholinergics:

- Can't spit: dry mouth
- Can't pee: urinary retention
- Can't poop: constipation
- Can't see: blurred vision

Review Video: Cholinergic and Anticholinergic Drugs
Visit mometrix.com/academy and enter code: 770491

ANTIEPILEPTIC DRUGS/MOOD STABILIZERS

Indication: seizures, neuropathies, headaches, bipolar disorder, muscle tremors.

Mechanism of action: Depresses nerve cell excitation in the brain by altering ion movements into nerve cells; increases seizure threshold.

- Medications: carbamazepine, valproic acid, gabapentin
- Neurontin: diabetic nerve pain

Side Effects: changes in behavior, hepatotoxicity and pancreatitis (valproic acid), bone marrow depression (carbamazepine).

Teaching:

- Do not take carbamazepine with grapefruit (increases serum levels) or give valproic acid with carbonated beverages.
- Can reduce the effects of oral anticoagulants and oral contraceptives.
- Monitor serum levels of drugs, as well as liver function (divalproex sodium); platelets and hemoglobin (carbamazepine).

PHENYTOIN (DILANTIN)

Indication: epilepsy/seizures

Mechanism of action: Classified as a hydantoin (prototype: fosphenytoin); increases seizure threshold/decreased nerve cell excitability.

- Also works as cardiac antiarrythmic

Side Effects: drowsiness, confusion, dizziness; long term – gingivial hyperplasia, acne, hirshutism, osteoporosis.

Teaching:

- IV: *rapid administration can cause sudden cardiac arrest;* Administer no faster than 50 mg/min and flush at same rate.
- Will cause overgrowth of gums: use soft-bristled toothbrush and brush/floss often.
- Weakens bones over time; vitamin D supplement may be needed.
- Educate teenagers especially on importance of compliance; also counsel on body image, as this medication can cause alterations in self-esteem due to unpleasant cosmetic side effects.
- *Toxicity:* rapid eye movements (nystagmus), difficulty with speech, poor muscle coordination/tripping and falling, encephalopathy (neurological effects).

BARBITURATES

Indication: daytime sedation; insomnia; preop sedation and anesthesia; anxiety relief; anticonvulsant.

Mechanism of action: increase effect of GABA in CNS, reducing excitability and producing sedation.

- Medications: phenobarbital (prototype), secobarbital; *ends in -barbital*

Side Effects: respiratory depression, sedation, GI upset, hypersensitivity, angioedema, tolerance, psychological and physical dependence.

Teaching:

- Do not take with alcohol; do not drive or operate heavy machinery until you know how this drug will affect you.
- Decreases efficiency of oral contraceptives.
- Does not allow for REM sleep – this is the cycle of sleep where mental rejuvenation takes place; may result in increased agitation/decreased ability to deal with stress.
- Can cause paradoxical excitement in children and elderly.
- Phenytoin and valproic acid may increase toxic effects.

Cholinergics

Indications: treatment of myasthenia gravis, glaucoma (eye drops), post-op urinary retention and abdominal distention/atony.

Mechanism of action: Mimic acetylcholine and bind to muscarinic receptors; also, indirect-acting cholinergic drugs inhibit cholinesterase, which is the enzyme responsible for breaking down acetylcholine.

- Activates para-sympathetic nervous system: "rest and digest."
- Medications: edrophonium, prostigmine, pilocarpine, bethanechol, carbachol.

Side Effects: low heart rate, GI spasm, increased salivation and diaphoresis.

Teaching:

- Hold pressure on canthus for 60 seconds to prevent systemic absorption of cholinergic eye drops.
- Take 1 hr before or 2 hrs after meals (bethanechol).
- Antidote for cholinergic OD: atropine.
- Do not give to patients with asthma, urinary or bowel obstruction, or gastric ulcers.
- **Toxicity:** visual disturbance, bronchospasm, hypotension, cardiovascular collapse.

Atypical Antipsychotics

Indication: schizophrenia, bipolar

Mechanism of action: Block the dopamine and serotonin receptors; increase levels.

- Medications: clozapine, olanzapine, and risperidone, aripiprazole, lurasidone, quetiapine, and others.

Side Effects: weight gain, high cholesterol, dry mouth, blurred vision, drowsiness, tremors; persistent/painful erection (ziprasidone).

Teaching:

- Because of the decreased instance of extrapyramidal effects, atypical antipsychotics are becoming more widely prescribed.
- Suck on sugar-free candy/chew sugar-free gum for dry mouth.
- Need lab tests regularly to avoid blood issues/check cholesterol.

Typical Antipsychotics

Indication: schizophrenia, bipolar disorder, and other various psychoses.

Mechanism of action: Precise mechanism of action unknown; thought to work by affecting levels of dopamine and serotonin in the brain.

Medications: Haloperidol (oral or IM injection), fluphenazine, chlorpromazine, perphenazine, and others.

Side Effects: extrapyramidal symptoms, tardive dyskinesia (muscle twitching; strange, uncontrollable movements), serotonin syndrome (dangerously low levels of serotonin leading to coma and death).

Teaching:

- May take a few weeks to become effective; cannot stop taking suddenly.
- This classification is cheaper than atypical antipsychotics. While there is an increased risk of side effects, it may be more desired financially when long-term treatment is indicated.
- Report immediately: unusual muscle twitching, increased temperature or drooling, increased anxiety/agitation.

Review Video: Anti-Psychotic Drugs: Clozapine, Haloperidol, Etc.
Visit mometrix.com/academy and enter code: 240506

Lithium

Indication: mania (bipolar disorder), mood stabilizer; also used in headaches, depression, and neutropenia.

Mechanism of action: Unknown; acts in central nervous system as mood stabilizer.

Side Effects: drowsiness, dizziness, confusion, poor memory

Teaching:

- Serum lithium levels: 0.8-1.5 mEq/L; must check regularly.
- Critical to maintain an adequate level of sodium in diet: low-sodium diets lead to toxicity in these patients; also avoid overheating and excessive sweating to prevent sodium loss.
- Drink plenty of fluids to ensure adequate excretion.
- Do not take with haloperidol: encephalopathy could occur.
- *Toxicity (report immediately):* blurred vision, seizure, lack of appetite, N/V/D, ringing in ears, slurred speech, muscle weakness/decreased coordination, increased urination.

Benzodiazepines

Indication: agitation, anxiety, insomnia, seizures, alcohol withdrawal.

Mechanism of action: Decrease excitability in different areas of the brain, may interact with GABA receptors.

- Medications: temazepam, diazepam; *ends in -lam or -pam*

Side Effects: drowsiness, dizziness, headache, paradoxical excitement.

Teaching:

- Do not drive/operate heavy machinery or use alcohol while on this medication.
- Cannot use if pregnant or have narrow-angle glaucoma.
- Risk of addiction and abuse.
- **Overdose**: decreased level of consciousness, decreased reflexes, coma, respiratory arrest.
- Antidote: flumazenil.

Tetracyclic/Tricyclic Antidepressants

Indication: major depressive disorder; also used for migraine headaches, phobias, urinary incontinence, attention deficit disorder, ulcers, and diabetic neuropathy.

Mechanism of action: block reuptake of serotonin and norepinephrine.

- Medications: amitriptyline, amoxapine, imipramine, nortriptyline, etc.

Side Effects: dry mouth, constipation/urinary retention, sedation, orthostatic hypotension, diaphoresis, weight gain, serotonin syndrome.

Teaching:

- May take a few weeks to become effective
- *Increased suicide risk with initial treatment/change in dose*; monitor closely, especially with children and young adults (<25 y.)

Selective Serotonin Reuptake Inhibitors

Indication: depression, anxiety

Mechanism of action: Inhibits the reuptake of serotonin in the brain, resulting in increased levels of serotonin available for use.

- Medications: citalopram, escitalopram, fluexetine, paroxetine, sertaline.

Side Effects: N/V/D, dizziness, weight fluctuations, dry mouth, headache, agitation/nervousness, sexual dysfunction (decreased desire, erectile dysfuntion)

Teaching:

- Take with food/before bed to avoid stomach upset.
- Takes several weeks to become effective.
- Withdrawal symptoms if stop taking suddenly.
- Serotonin syndrome: report increase agitation, tremors, sweating, confusion, rapid heart rate immediately.
  - St. John's wort can cause serotonin syndrome if taken with an SSRI.
- SSS is a helpful mnemonic to remember the adverse effects of SSRIs: Stomach upset, Sexual dysfunction, Serotonin syndrome.

MAO Inhibitors

Indication: depression, anxiety, Parkinson disease

Mechanism of action: Inhibits monoamine oxidase, the enzyme that normally metabolizes norepinephrine and serotonin, making these neurotransmitters more available to the receptors.

- Medications: tranylcypromine sulfate, phenelzine sulfate, isocarboxazid, selegiline

Side Effects: dry mouth, headache, drowsiness, dizziness, N/V/D, constipation; weight gain, sexual dysfunction, paresthesia also possible.

Teaching:

- React with most medications: ask MD before starting any new medication or supplement.
- Interact with tyramine (amino acid in food), causing dangerously high blood pressure; must avoid all foods with this substance, including:
    - Aged cheeses
    - Fermented products (soy sauce, miso/tofu, sauerkraut, draft beer, wine)
    - Cured meats
- Serotonin syndrome: immediately report increased agitation, tremors, sweating, confusion, rapid heart rate.

Antiarrhythmics

Indication: Treatment of atrial and ventricular arrhythmias:

Mechanism of action: Divided into 5 classes (Vaughan Williams):

- *Class I:* Sodium Channel Blockers
    - **Ia**: quinidine, procainamide, disopyramide
    - **Ib**: lidocaine, phenytoin, mexiletine
    - **Ic**: flecainide, propafenone, moricizine
- *Class II:* beta-blockers (prototype: propranolol HCl)
- *Class III:* Potassium Channel Blockers (amiodarone, sotalol, dofetilide)
- *Class IV:* Calcium Channel Blockers (verapamil, diltiazem (Cardizem)
- *Class V:* Variable Mechanism – adenosine, digoxin, magnesium sulfate

Side Effects: varies by class; generally, risk of new or worsening arrhythmias, loss of appetite, diarrhea/constipation, change in taste, photosensitivity

Teaching:

- Monitor pulse while on these medications: report low heart rate or irregular rhythm to doctor.

Adenosine

Indication: acute treatment of paroxysmal supraventricular tachycardia; cardiac stress testing

Mechanism of action: temporarily decreases the conduction of impulses through the AV node; "resets" heart rhythm.

- Effective against reentry tachycardias (when an impulse depolarizes an area of heart muscle and returns and repolarizes it) that involve the AV node.

Side Effects: facial flushing, shortness of breath, dyspnea, chest discomfort.

Teaching:

- Patient MUST be hooked up to continuous heart monitor and the nurse should have the crash-cart nearby.
- IV Push: given quickly (1-3 seconds); nurse should expect a pause in heart rate—looks like a flat line on the machine, followed quickly by return to normal rhythm.
- If being used for scheduled stress test, the patient should not have any caffeine for the 12 hours before the test, including coffee, chocolate, tea, colas, or medications with caffeine.
- Not a long-term solution to arrhythmias.

Alpha-Adrenergic Blockers

Indication: hypertension, BPH (benign prostatic hypertrophy), heart failure, Reynaud phenomena, pheochromocytoma, skin conditions.

Mechanism of action: interrupts the actions of the catecholamines at the alpha receptors, resulting in relaxation of the smooth muscle in the blood vessels and increased dilation of blood vessels.

- Medications: doxazosin, prazosin, terazosin; *ends in -zosin*
- Tamsulosin: BPH

Side Effects: orthostatic hypotension, headache, dizziness, nasal congestion, decreased libido/impotence.

Teaching:

- "First-Dose Effect" – extreme drop in blood pressure with first dose; give at bedtime to avoid falls/injury.
- Men – educate about possible sexual side effects and treatment options.
- Do not stop taking abruptly – rebound hypertension could occur.

Beta-Adrenergic Blockers

Indication: heart attacks, angina, hypertension, hypertrophic cardiomyopathy, and supraventricular arrhythmias.

Mechanism of action: Prevent stimulation of the sympathetic nervous system by inhibiting the action of catecholamines at the beta-adrenergic receptors; cardioprotective.

- Propranolol, metoprolol tartrate - *ends in -olol*

Side Effects: bradycardia, respiratory depression, arrhythmia, bronchospasm, hypotension, fatigue.

Teaching:

- "Xanax for your heart": protects heart from harmful chemicals released after heart attack; crucial to keep taking.
- Check pulse – do not take if <60, call your doctor.
- Orthostatic hypotension: change position slowly to prevent dizziness and falls.
- Caution in diabetics: may block signs and symptoms of hypoglycemia.

Calcium Channel Blockers

Indication: hypertension, arrhythmias, Raynaud disease, migraines, angina pectoris.

Mechanism of action: affect the movement of calcium into the cells, relaxes blood vessels, reducing cardiac workload.

- Medications: amlodipine, nifedipine, verapamil, diltiazem, nicardipine

Ends in –dipine

Side Effects: hypotension, bradycardia, GI upset, edema, rash, flushing

Teaching:

- Monitor blood pressure and pulse; call doctor if unusually low.
- May be more powerful when taken with other blood pressure medications.
- Grapefruit juice may also potentiate effects.

Review Video: Calcium Channel Blockers
Visit mometrix.com/academy and enter code: 345329

Digitalis Glycosides

Indication: Heart failure, hypotension, supraventricular arrhythmias, paroxysmal atrial tachycardia.

Mechanism of action: Increases intracellular calcium at the cell membrane, thus increasing the force of the heart's contractions.

- "Positive inotrope, negative chronotrope"
- For arrhythmias, a loading dose is often given
- Medications: digoxin

Side Effects: bradycardia, headache, loss of appetite.

Teaching:

- Serum digoxin level: 0.5-2 ng/mL (very narrow therapeutic index).
- Check pulse before administration (Nursing: apical).
- Adequate potassium levels protect against toxicity. Ensure a diet that has a moderate amount of potassium, and do not take medications that would decrease levels (diuretics, steroids, theophylline, and amphotericin B) without potassium replacement.
- *Toxicity*: visual disturbances (green and yellow halos around lights/double vision), nausea/vomiting, diarrhea – report immediately.

Nitrates

Indication: Acute angina, myocardial infarction, hypertension

Mechanism of action: Dilates blood vesels, increasing blood flow to the heart and decreasing preload, afterload, and oxygen requirements of the heart.

- Medications: nitroglycerin, erythrityl dinitrate, isosorbide dinitrate, isosorbide mononitrate, pentaerythritol tetranitrate.

Side Effects: headache, hypotension, tachycardia

Teaching

- Nitroglycerin:
  - Lie down, and take 1 tablet under the tongue every 5 minutes until relief (max dose is 3 tablets in 15 min). If still no relief, call 9-1-1.
  - Store in dark container/protect from light; should feel a slight burning sensation under the tongue, means it is still working.
  - Can be given continuous IV infusion: monitor blood pressure closely, and titrate for pain relief/BP control.
- Headache is common, means medication is working; can take acetaminophen for relief.

NEVER take/give nitrates to patient with history of erectile dysfunction on medications such as sildenafil (PDE5 inhibitors); can cause severe, irretractable hypotension.

Cholesterol Medications

Statins

Statins (HMG-CoA reductase inhibitors) are cholesterol-lowering medications. Commonly used statins include lovastatin, pravastatin, simvastatin, atorvastatin, cerivastatin, fluvastatin, and rosuvastatin.

Mechanism of action: Statins reduce cholesterols levels by blocking the enzyme HMG-CoA reductase, which the liver requires to produce cholesterol.

Side effects: GI disturbance, rash, headaches, blurred vision, ophthalmoplegia, fatigues, insomnia, constipation, diarrhea, nausea, and myalgia/myopathy.

Patient teaching: Patients who experience myalgia/myopathy may progress to rhabdomyolysis, so they should be cautioned to immediately report any muscle pain. The medication should be used with caution with oral anticoagulants.

Fibric Acid Derivatives

Fibric acid derivatives (fibrates) are cholesterol-lowering drugs that primarily affect triglycerides but may also lower LDL and total cholesterol.

Mechanism of action: Fibrates activate lipoprotein lipase, an enzyme that breaks down cholesterol, cleaving triglycerides from LDL or VLDL and leaving just the lipoprotein behind.

Side effects: nausea, vomiting, diarrhea, gall stones, acute appendicitis, impotence, dysuria, hematuria, dizziness, rash, pruritus, alopecia, vertigo, headaches, and eczema. Increased risk of rhabdomyolysis if given with a statin.

Patient teaching: Fibrates may enhance the action of anticoagulants, increasing risk of bleeding. Patients should report adverse effects.

Antiplatelets

Indication: prevent arterial thromboembolism in patients at risk of MI, stroke, and arteriosclerosis, maintain patency of stents.

Mechanism of action: Inhibit platelet aggregation.

- Medications: aspirin, persantine, clopidogrel, ticlopidine, pentoxifylline, cilostazol.
- Pentoxifylline/Cilostazol: increases flexibility of RBCs, treats intermittent claudication with PAD.

Side Effects: bleeding, epigastric upset, dizziness, headache, neutropenia/agranulocytosis (ticlopidine).

Teaching:

- Along with lifestyle modification, will help prevent heart attack, stroke, stent occlusion.
- Report signs of bleeding immediately.
- Cannot be given to patients with hemorrhage, trauma, thrombocytopenia, or hemorrhagic stroke.

Aspirin

Indication: analgesic, anti-inflammatory (gout), antiplatelet - prevention of MI and stroke.

Mechanism of action: Salicylate: prevents platelets from sticking together and forming blood clots.

Side Effects: increased bleeding, bruising, stomach upset.

Teaching

- People at increased risks for bleeding should not use aspirin (e.g., hemophilia, severe liver disease, stomach ulcers).
- Aspirin should **NEVER** be given to children ≤15 years old, due to risk of Reye syndrome (potentially fatal liver disease in presence of viral infection, exclusively in this age group).
- **Toxicity:** dark, tarry stools (GI bleed); tinnitus (ringing in ears, metabolic acidosis).

Chemotherapy

Chemotherapy has been discussed as "bringing someone to the edge of death, to try and bring them back to life again." While this is a graphic description, it illustrates that fact that chemotherapy kills all types of cells in the body, normal and cancer cells alike. Normal cells typically recover when chemotherapy has stopped, so most side effects go away gradually after treatment stops, and the healthy cells can thrive normally. However, during chemotherapy, the patient should be prepared to experience any of the following side effects:

- Fatigue
- Nausea and vomiting
- Pain- drugs used for chemotherapy can cause some painful side effects
- Hair Loss or alopecia- is a common, but not guaranteed, chemotherapy side effect
- Anemia
- Increased infection risk
- Problems with Blood Clotting

- Sores in the Mouth and Throat
- Diarrhea or Constipation
- Infertility (potentially permanent)

The nurse should educate the patient on the importance of rest and adequate hydration during treatment, as well as on differing methods to help alleviate discomfort.

IMMUNOSUPPRESSANTS

Indication: organ transplant rejection prevention, autoimmune disorders, some cancer drugs.

Mechanism of action: exact mechanism of action unknown; may disrupt RNA synthesis, inhibit T cells.

- Medications: azathioprine, cyclosporine, lymphocyte immune globulin (ATG), muromonab-CD3, and tacrolimus. Cyclophosphamide; steroids are also considered immunosuppressants.

Side Effects: increased risk of infection, GI upset, increased blood pressure/cholesterol, insomnia, skin irritations, mood swings/insomnia.

Teaching:

- Avoid contact with sick individuals; wash hands frequently, avoid crowds.
- Report fever, foul-smelling urine, reddened wounds, nausea/vomiting, or any other signs of infection right away.

Review Video: Immunomodulators and Immunosuppressive Agents
Visit mometrix.com/academy and enter code: 411712

EPOETIN ALFA

Indication: normocytic anemia in ESRD, anemia in cancer patients and patients with HIV, and other anemias.

Mechanism of action: Stimulates RBC production in bone marrow.

- Trade names: Epogen, Procrit

Side Effects: hypertension, headache, GI upset, cough, fever, generalized pain, insomnia, irritation at injection site, weight loss, blood clots, allergic reaction.

Teaching:

- Subcutaneous Injection: store vials in refrigerator away from bright light; do not shake and do not reuse individual vials. Dispose of needles properly.
- May cause unsafe rise in hemoglobin or blood pressure; monitor both regularly.
- May need to take iron supplements/vitamins due to increased demand of body while making more RBCs.
- May notice increase in energy due to resolved anemia; however, still need to attend dialysis since actual issue is not resolved.
- Teach signs and symptoms of blood clots.

Folic Acid/Folate

Indication: folic acid deficiency in alcoholism, pregnancy, liver/kidney dysfunction, prevention of neonatal neural tube defects.

Mechanism of action: Supplement (vitamin B9); necessary for creation of blood in body.

- Medications: folic acid, vitamin B9, FA-8, folacin, folate

Side Effects: bitter taste, GI distress, headache, hypotension, skin issues (itching, rash, flushing, hypoglycemia, insomnia, decreased zinc levels).

Teaching:

- Large doses may counteract the effects of phenytoin, potentially leading to seizures.
- Found naturally in dark, leafy greens, fruits, organ meats, cereals, and tomato juice.
- Most effective in preventing neural tube defects in children if taken before pregnancy/during the first trimester. Woman seeking to become pregnant should begin taking a supplement with folic acid immediately.

Iron Supplements

Indication: iron deficiency anemia, low iron levels (pregnant women, toddlers, and teenage girls), hemorrhage, burns, hemodialysis.

Mechanism of action: mineral replacement; necessary component of blood (2/3 of iron in body).

- Medications: ferrous fumarate, ferrous gluconate, ferrous sulfate, iron sucrose, and iron dextran.

Side Effects: gastric irritation, dark stools; IV – allergic reaction, phlebitis, hypotension, orthostatic hypotension.

Teaching:

- Take with food to avoid gastric upset.
- Vitamin C increases iron absorption: take with orange or fruit juice.
    - Absorption is reduced by antacids, coffee, tea, dairy products, eggs, whole grains; avoid 1 h before/2 h after.
- Liquid: stains teeth; mix and drink through straw.
- Common cause of OD in chidren: keep away in locked cabinet.

Warfarin (Coumadin)

Indication: prevention of DVT/PE/stroke, atrial fibrillation, valve replacement.

Mechanism of action: inhibits clotting factors that rely on vitamin K (II, VII, IX, and X).

Side Effects: bleeding, increased bruising, GI effects (nausea, cramps).

Teaching:

- Monitor PT/INR: INR should be between 2-3 (a little higher for valve replacements).
- Avoid large doses of foods high in vitamin K (dark, leafy greens especially), as these inactivate warfarin's effects.

- Soft-bristled toothbrush, electric razor, avoid activities with high risk of injury; often taken in the evening before bed.
- May take a while to reach therapeutic levels, often "bridged" with heparin until INR is therapeutic.
- Antidote: vitamin K (phytonadione).

Review Video: Warfarin as an Anticoagulant
Visit mometrix.com/academy and enter code: 712643

Heparin

Indication: DVT prophylaxis, venous thromboemboli, atrial fibrillation, acute MI, used in lines and machines to prevent blood clotting (cardiopulmonary bypass, hemodialysis, etc.)

Mechanism of action: Inhibits conversion of prothrombin to thrombin, thus preventing clot formation (does not dissolve clots already present).

- Medications: heparin (IV or SQ), enoxaparin (SQ)
- SQ: abdomen @ 90-degree angle, do not aspirate or massage.

Side Effects: bruising, increased risk of bleeding, thrombocytopenia, rash, fever, heparin-induced thrombocytopenia (HIT); long-term use: hair loss and osteoporosis.

Teaching:

- Monitor aPTT; therapeutic when 1½ to 2½ times normal value.
- SQ injection: go over injection sites and proper needle disposal.
- IV heparin infusion: titrated to achieve goal pTT, must continuously monitor and adjust according to hospital policy.
- Do not take NSAIDs/aspirin: increased risk of bleeding.
- Use electric razor and soft-bristled toothbrush; avoid activities such as contact sports, ice skating, or anything that increases risk of falls or trauma.
- Antidote: protamine sulfate (works in 5 minutes).

Review Video: Heparin - An Injectable Anti-Coagulant
Visit mometrix.com/academy and enter code: 622056

Thrombolytic Drugs

Indications: embolism, acute MI, ischemic stroke, PE/DVT.

Mechanism of action: Intravenous medication that dissolves clots by activating conversion of plasminogen to plasmin, which breaks apart fibrin particles.

- Medications: alteplase (TPA), streptokinase, anistreplase

Side Effects: hemorrhage, allergic reaction, hematuria, hemoptysis, hematochezia, melena; hypotension, and dysrhythmias.

Teaching:

- These medications are generally given in emergency situations to dissolve clots and prevent further damage in MI and stroke; however, they must be given within 4-6 hours of onset of symptoms.
- Cannot give if patient has history of recent trauma, concussion/head bleed, surgery, post-partum, uncontrolled HTN, or abdominal bleed.
- Report immediately signs of bleeding such as bleeding from IV or old puncture wounds, coughing up blood, nose bleed, or blood in urine or stools
- Antidote: aminocaproic acid

Antihistamines

Indication: Acute allergic reactions, seasonal allergies, motion sickness, sleep aid

Mechanism of action: Histamine 1 (H1) receptor antagonists compete with histamine for binding to the H1 receptor sites throughout the body but cannot displace bound histamine.

- Medications: diphenhydramine, chlorpheniramine, prochlorperazine, loratadine, hydroxyzine hydrochloride, and hydroxyzine pamoate.

Side Effects: drowsiness, dizziness, dry mouth, nausea/vomiting, paradoxical excitement/agitation in children.

Teaching:

- Do not drive/operate machinery until you know how these medications will affect you.
- Since antihistamines cannot displace bound histamine, these medications are best when taken before symptoms appear/as soon as possible to prevent worsening.

Note: Loratadine may cause serious cardiac effects when taken with macrolide antibiotics (e.g., erythromycin), fluconazole, ketoconazole, itraconazole, miconazole, cimetidine, ciprofloxacin, and clarithromycin.

Antitussives

Indication: Used to treat a serious, *nonproductive* cough that interferes with a patient's ability to rest and perform ADLs; pneumonia, bronchitis, the common cold, and COPD; also, for diagnostic procedures.

MOA: Suppress or inhibit dry, nonproductive coughing.

- Medications: benzonatate, codeine, dextromethorphan hydrobromide, and hydrocodone bitartrate.
- Narcotic antitussives (codeine and hydrocodone) are used to treat the intractable cough associated with lung cancer.

Side Effects: nausea/vomiting, excitation, elevated temperature, increased blood pressure; narcotics may cause CNS depression.

Teaching:

- Do not take with productive cough; will prevent clearance of mucus from respiratory tract.
- Do not give to children younger than 6 years of age.
- These medications only provide symptom relief; do not "cure" anything. Drink plenty of fluids and get rest.

Decongestants

Indications: relieve the symptoms of swollen nasal membranes resulting from: hay fever, allergic rhinitis, vasomotor rhinitis, acute coryza, sinusitis, and the common cold.

Mechanism of action:

- Systemic: stimulate the sympathetic nervous system to reduce swelling of the respiratory tract's vascular network.
- Topical: same MOA, with quicker effects.
- Sudafed (pseudoephedrine), Sudafed PE (phenylephrine), Afrin (oxymetazoline).

Side Effects: anxiety/agitation, insomnia, increased blood pressure.

Teaching:

- Do not take nasal spray >3 days (rebound congestion).
- Increased CNS stimulation may occur when taken with other sympathomimetic drugs.
- Do not take with MOA inhibitors or alkalinizing drugs.

Expectorants

Indication: chest congestion, upper respiratory infection, bronchitis, influenza, sinusitis, bronchial asthma, emphysema, and other respiratory disorders.

Mechanism of action: Thin mucus so it is cleared more easily out of airways

- Medications: guaifenesin

Side Effects: Nausea/Vomiting

Teaching:

- Drink plenty of fluids; will thin mucus further and make it easier to cough up.
- Do not use for dry cough (ineffective); do not give to children younger than 6 years of age.

Methylxanthines

Indication: Used to treat breathing disorders, including asthma, chronic bronchitis, emphysema, and neonatal apnea.

Mechanism of action: Relax smooth muscle of bronchioles, resulting in dilation of airway.

- Medications: anhydrous theophylline, aminophylline, oxtriphylline, and theophylline sodium glycinate.

Side Effects: agitation, tachycardia, urinary frequency, gastrointestinal distress, seizures.

Teaching:

- Smoking increases elimination, decreasing serum concentrations and effectiveness.
- Avoid coffee, tea, chocolate, soda, and other foods or drinks containing caffeine, as these may result in additive adverse reactions.
- Theophylline: therapeutic serum level is 10-20 mcg/dL.

ANTACIDS

Indication: gastroesophageal reflux disease (GERD), heartburn, indigestion.

Mechanism of action: alkaline in nature, therefore is able to neutralize gastric pH.

- Medications: aluminum hydroxide, calcium carbonate, sodium bicarbonate (baking soda), magnesium hydroxide (Milk of Magnesia), etc.
- Aluminum hydroxide - reduces phosphorus (ESRD).
- Calcium carbonate: supplement to prevent osteoporosis.

Side Effects: rare; N/V/D; rebound increase in acid production.

Teaching:

- Do not cure issue, simply help manage symptoms.
- Talk to doctor before use if you have kidney disease, foul-smelling and painful diarrhea, or have heartburn that lasts longer than 2 weeks.
- Lifestyle modification: avoid spicy foods, stay upright for hour after meals, and avoid drinking large amounts of liquids with meals.

BILE ACID SEQUESTRANTS

Indication: high cholesterol; especially in cardiac and diabetic patients.

Mechanism of action: resins that trap bile acid in intestines and promote excretion through feces.

- Medications: cholestyramine (prototype), colestipol hydrochloride, colesevelam.

Side Effects: GI upset: constipation, nausea, heartburn, flatus, indigestion.

Teaching:

- Take other medications 1 h before/4 h after these drugs, as they can decrease absorption.
- Comes as a powder: can mix with water or other foods.
- Lifestyle modification: weight loss, low-fat diet, smoking cessation, and exercise are all effective ways to lower cholesterol.

SUCRALFATE

Indication: gastric, duodenal and oral ulcers, GI bleed, stress ulcer prevention.

Mechanism of action: forms a protective barrier on the GI mucosa, high affinity for areas of ulceration; local acid neutralization.

Side Effects: N/V/D, dry mouth, flatus, dizziness, rash.

Teaching:

- Must be given 1 h before/2 h after a meal.
- Do not give within 2 h of other medications; will decrease absorption.
- Decreased excretion in those with renal disease.
- Lifestyle Modification: avoid spicy, highly acid foods, as well as NSAIDs or other medications that could irritate the stomach lining.

Histamine (H2) Receptor Antagonists

Indication: duodenal ulcers, GERD, esophagitis.

Mechanism of action: blocks histamine's stimulation of gastric acid secretion.

- Medications: famotidine, cimetidine, ranitidine, and others.

Side Effects: headache most common, also diarrhea, dizziness, rashes.

Teaching:

- Take with a meal, often breakfast; can also take at bedtime.
- Wait at least 30 minutes between taking H2 blockers and an antacid.
- If required for more than 2 weeks, call doctor for further workup.
- Lifestyle Modification: avoid spicy, highly acid foods, carbonated beverages, citrus fruit, as well as NSAIDs or other medications that could irritate the stomach lining.

Proton Pump Inhibitors (PPIs)

Indication: heartburn, GERD, peptic ulcers.

Mechanism of action: Inhibits gastric acid production in the stomach.

- Medications: omeprazole, lansoprazole, esomeprazole, pantoprazole, and others.

Side Effects: nausea, headache, diarrhea, constipation, flatulence, osteoporosis, hypomagnesia.

Teaching:

- Take at least 1 hour before meals.
- Does not provide immediate relief of symptoms.
- May affect absorption of other drugs.
- Pantoprazole sodium IV: dilute and push slowly over 2-3 minutes.
- Lifestyle Modification: avoid spicy, highly acidic foods, as well as NSAIDs or other medications that could irritate the stomach lining.

Lactulose

Indication: hepatic encephalopathy (reduces blood ammonia levels), constipation.

Mechanism of action: synthetic sugar that binds to ammonia in the blood, pulling it into colon to be expelled.

- Names: Enulose, Generlac, Constulose, etc.

Side Effects: flatulence, bloating, diarrhea, hyperactive bowel sounds.

Teaching:

- Never hold dose due to diarrhea (means the drug is working).
- Monitor patient's mental status and level of consciousness, ammonia levels.
- May raise blood sugar in diabetics: monitor closely.
- Monitor patient for signs and symptoms of dehydration/fluid-electrolyte imbalance, especially elderly or pediatric patients.

Laxatives/Stool Softeners

Indication: constipation (treatment/prophylaxis), bowel surgery prep.

Mechanism of action:

- Osmotic: pulls in fluid; magnesium hydroxide (Milk of Magnesia).
- Bulk-Forming: swell in water to form gel that increases bulk and softens stool, increases peristalsis; Metamucil, Citrucel, MiraLAX.
- GoLYTELY: potent laxative used for bowel prep; patient drinks gallon over several hours, until stools are clear.
- Stool Softeners: reduce surface tension in the bowel increasing water absorption into stool; docusate (Colace.)

Side Effects: diarrhea, nausea, fullness/bloating; Milk of Magnesia - hypermagnesemia, renal dysfunction.

Teaching:

- Dependence can develop, especially in elderly patients. Do not take unless needed; educate that it is normal for bowels to slow with age.
- Lifestyle modification: increasing fluids, moderate exercise, eating high-fiber foods (prunes) are all ways to prevent constipation.
- Teaching - **Do not strain for stools:** can cause bradycardia and subsequent cardiac arrest secondary to vagal response.

Anti-Gout Drugs/Uricosurics

Indication: treatment of acute and chronic gout.

Mechanism of action: reduce the reabsorption of uric acid at the proximal tubules of the kidneys, increasing uric acid excretion in the urine.

- Medications: probenecid and sulfinpyrazone.
- Other gout medications:
  - Allopurinol and febuxostat: xanthine oxidase inhibitors block enzyme necessary for production of uric acid.
  - Colchicine: treats acute attacks; prevent worsening of symptoms during initial uricosuric/xanthine oxidase inhibitor treatment.

Side Effects: GI upset, rash (allopurinol), headache.

Teaching:

- Must take these medications regularly to prevent attack.
- Do NOT take these medications during a flare-up if you were not taking them before, as they could worsen symptoms initially.
- Lifestyle Management: stay hydrated and avoid alcohol to decrease risk of flare-ups.

Potassium-Sparing Diuretics

Indication: edema, diuretic-induced hypokalemia in patients with heart failure, cirrhosis, nephrotic syndrome, hypertension.

Mechanism of action: blocks aldosterone, which leads to an increased excretion of sodium and water; conserves potassium and hydrogen ions; may be used in conjunction with other diuretics.

- Medications: spironolactone (prototype), amiloride, and triamterene.
- Spironolactone is used to treat hyperaldosteronism and hirsutism.

Side Effects: frequent urination, stomach upset, rash, dizziness, headache, confusion, sexual dysfunction and gynecomastia (spironolactone), hyperkalemia.

Teaching:

- Frequent urination means drug is working, and should get better with time; take drug in morning to avoid nocturia.
- Lifestyle modification: avoid foods high in potassium (potatoes, orange juice, etc.) and limit sodium.
- Can cause hyperkalemia, especially when combined with ACE inhibitors.

Loop Diuretics

Indication: HTN, fluid overload in heart failure, liver/kidney disease.

Mechanism of action: blocks the resorption of sodium in kidneys, leading to increased excretion of sodium and water.

- Medications: furosemide (prototype), bumetanide, torsemide, ethacrynic acid.

Side Effects: hypokalemia, increased urination, dizziness, headache, N/V, diarrhea, hyperglycemia, blood issues, dehydration.

Teaching:

- Furosemide IV: push slowly (~20 mg/min) to avoid kidney damage and hearing loss.
- Eat foods high in potassium to counteract loss; MD may prescribe supplement.
- Increased risk of digoxin toxicity due to hypokalemia.
- Weigh daily, same time, naked, and before urination to determine effectiveness/spot early signs of heart failure.

Glucocorticoids

Indication: replacement therapy in patients with adrenocortical insufficiency, immunosuppression, anti-inflammatory.

Mechanism of action: Also known as "steroids"; inhibit immune response by:

- Decrease of leakage of plasma from the capillaries
- Suppression of the migration of polymorphonuclear leukocytes
- Inhibition of phagocytosis
- Decreased antibody formation in injured or infected tissues
- *Medications*: prednisone, cortisone, etc.; *ends in -sone*

Side Effects: weight gain, emotional liability, acne, "moon face," "buffalo hump," increase blood sugar and bruising, increased risk of infection; osteoporosis over time.

Teaching:

- Monitor blood sugar closely, especially diabetic patients.
- Increased risk of infection: wash hands frequently, avoid sick contacts, and stay hydrated.
- Must taper dose when therapy is completed – sudden cessation can cause adrenal crisis.

Insulins

Prior to 1921, insulin-dependent diabetes was a fatal disorder. However, with the discovery of insulin, diabetic patients can lead close to normal lives. Insulin works as a gateway protein to allow glucose to enter the cells of the body for fuel. There are several different types of insulin, each with unique properties. The nurse needs to be aware of these, especially the peak time of the insulin he/she is administering, as the risk of hypoglycemia is greatest during that time.

Type	Names	Onset	Peak	Duration
Rapid acting	Humalog/Lispro	5-15 min	1-2 hr	2-6 hr
Short Acting	Humulin/Novolin	30 min	1-4 hr	4-8 hr
Intermediate/Long Acting	NPH/Ultralente	1-3 hr	4-8 hr	8-24 hr
Long Acting	Lantus	1-2 hr	No peak	16-24 hr

Example: Samantha took her NPH insulin at 8:00 AM this morning. At what time should the nurse instruct her to be on the lookout for signs and symptoms of hypoglycemia?

Answer: Between noon and 4 PM.

Mixing Insulins

Sometimes patients/caregivers will be required to mix long-acting and short-acting insulin to acquire the desired blood sugar stabilization.

The process for mixing insulins is explained below:

1. Mix the insulin by gently rolling back and forth in the hands. Do not shake insulin or insulin products; air bubbles with alter dose.
2. Obtain syringe of appropriate size, draw up the same dose of air as insulin to be given.
3. Clean the tops of the insulin bottles with alcohol.
4. Inject the cloudy insulin with the air equal to the dose of insulin to be given.
5. Inject the clear insulin with air equal to the dose of insulin to be given.

6. Draw up the desired dose of clear insulin.
7. Insert the needle again into the cloudy insulin and draw the desired dose.

Remember:

- "Clear before cloudy" – prevents contamination.

Insulin is measured in units, and thus should ALWAYS be drawn up in insulin syringes; using any other type of syringe can lead to lethal medication errors.

- Insulin should be checked by two nurses prior to injection.

Oral Anti-Diabetics

Indication: Treatment of hyperglycemia in type II diabetic patients.

Mechanism of action:

- *Sulfonylureas:* stimulation of insulin production in pancreatic B cells; glipizide, glyburide, chlorpropamide, tolazamide, tolbutamide; name generally ends in -ase.
- *Biguanides:* decreases liver production of glucose, promotes weight loss in obese patients; metformin.
- *Thiazolidinediones*: facilitates glucose clearance; rosiglitazone.
- *Alpha-glucosidase inhibitors:* slows absorption of glucose in intestinal tract; acarbose.
- *Meglitinide*: increases insulin production; repaglinide.

Side Effects: hypoglycemia, renal impairment; individual side effects with each drug.

Contraindications: kidney dysfunction/recent IV contrast (metformin); must consult MD if drug is safe during pregnancy/breastfeeding.

Teaching:

- Patient should take regularly at same time every day.
- Patient should ask MD about taking if scheduled for imaging test.
- Weight loss, controlled diet, and regular exercise will help with blood glucose management.

Dermatology and Dermatological Pharmacology

The skin functions to protect, regulate temperature, and offer immune responses, biochemical synthesis, and sensory detection. When the skin has been altered, it loses one or all of these abilities. Therefore, skin integrity is a nursing priority. **Treatments for dermatological issues** vary widely, but may include:

- Oral steroids; often used in adjunct therapy for skin conditions.
- Ultraviolet radiation: psoriasis.
- Sunscreens: prophylactic.
- Vitamin D analogues, retinoids, and anthralin.
- Topical glucocorticoids: inflammatory conditions such as rash, pruritus, bullous disorders (e.g., herpes), collagen diseases such as systemic lupus erythematosus, and vasculitis.
- Antihistamines: rashes, allergic dermatitis.

SUCCINYLCHOLINE

Indications: Given as adjunct to anesthesia or for orthopedic manipulation to ensure relaxation of muscles and to facilitate intubation.

Mechanism of action: Prevents transmission of nerve impulses to certain muscles, resulting in muscle paralysis, by binding with cholinergic receptors at the motor endplates of nerves to produce depolarization and prevent repolarization. Skeletal muscle relaxant, depolarizing neuromuscular blocker, pregnancy risk category C.

Side Effects: arrhythmias, hyperkalemia, respiratory depression, anaphylaxis, malignant hyperthermia, rhabdomyolysis, rash, postoperative muscle pain and rigidity, and increased intraocular pressure.

Contraindications: angle-closure glaucoma, history (personal, family) of malignant hyperthermia, upper motor neuron injury, major burns, and penetrating eye injuries. Drugs should be used with caution in patients who are elderly or debilitated.

Teaching: If patient has prolonged muscle stiffness, talk to patient and reassure him/her that symptoms will subside.

ANTIBIOTICS

Indication: Treatment and prophylaxis of bacterial infections.

Types:

- *Penicillins*: end in –cillin.
- Cephalosporins: cef-/ceph-; cross-sensitivity with penicillins.
- *Tetracyclines*: ends in -cycline.
- *Aminoglycosides*: ends in -mycin.
- *Fluoroquinolones*: ends in -floxacin.
- *Sulfonamides*: begins with sulfa-/ends in –azole.

Side Effects: gastrointestinal distress, allergic reaction; some can cause nephro- and ototoxicity, photosensitivity.

Contraindications: Do not take with alcohol or with known allergy.

Teaching:

- Take all prescribed doses until complete to prevent bacterial resistance and recurrent infection.
- Take with food or milk to prevent stomach upset.
- If rash, swelling, or other signs of allergic reaction occur, stop taking and notify your doctor right away.
- Wear sunscreen when going outdoors (tetracycline and quinolones).

CARBAPENEMS

Indication: mixed aerobic and anaerobic infections, as therapy for serious nosocomial infections, or infections in immunocompromised hosts.

Mechanism of action: A class of beta-lactam; bind to cell wall interrupting growth.

- Medications: imipenem-cilastatin sodium and meropenem, ertapenem, doripenem.
- Broadest spectrum possible in an antibiotic; broader than any other antibacterial to date.

Side Effects: N/V/D; soreness/redness at injection site, headache, rash, fatigue, ringing in ears, paresthesias, secondary infections (candidiasis).

Teaching:

- Diarrhea is common, and could happen months after stopping medication; do not take anti-diarrheals without first consulting your doctor.
- Often given as an intramuscular injection.
- Report white coating over tongue, vaginal itching/discharge, and other signs of secondary infection.

Cephalosporins

Indication: Antibiotic used to fight infections, especially those in the respiratory and urinary tract, and skin and bone infections. Also used to prevent infections pre- and postoperatively.

Mechanism of action: Bacteriocidal: inhibits cell-wall synthesis; *begin in –cef/ceph.*

- First-generation: cefazolin, cephalexin; gram-positive organisms.
- Second-generation: cefoxitin, cefuroxime; gram-negative organisms.
- Third-generation: cefixime, ceftriaxone, cefotaxime; gram-negative and anaerobic organisms.
- Fourth-generation: cefepime; gram-positive and –negative organisms; widely effective.

Side Effects: gastrointestinal distress, nausea/vomiting, hypersensitivity (rash, itching, hives).

Teaching:

- Take all prescribed doses to prevent antibiotic resistance.
- Take with food or milk to prevent GI distress.
- Do not take with alcohol, as it can increase toxicity.
- Cross-sensitivity with penicillin; use caution in these patients.

Lincosamides

Indication: Bacterial infection; protozoal infections, toxoplasmosis, malaria, strep/staph, anaerobes, toxic shock syndrome (TSS).

Mechanism of action: Bacteriostatic; very powerful; inhibits bacterial protein synthesis by interfering with ribosomes.

- Medications: lincomycin, clindamycin, pirlimycin.

Side Effects: gastrointestinal upset, pseudomembranous colitis, bitter taste (IV), dizziness, headache, neutropenia/thrombocytopenia, allergic reaction.

Teaching:

- Because of the potential for serious toxicity and pseudomembranous colitis, use is limited to a few clinical situations in which safer alternative antibiotics are not available.
- Report diarrhea, bloody stools, abdominal cramps and fever immediately and do not take anti-diarrheals!
- May block neuromuscular transmission and may enhance the action of neuromuscular blockers.

MACROLIDES

Indication: bacterial infections, *H. pyloria* (stomach ulcers), respiratory infections, otitis media.

Mechanism of action: bacteriostatic; inhibit protein synthesis, stopping bacterial proliferation.

- Medications: azithromycin, clarithromycin, erythromycin.
- Erythromycin: Legionella pneumophila and Mycoplasma pneumoniae.

Side Effects: severe GI upset (cramping and pain), N/V/D.

Teaching:

- Take with food to decrease GI upset.
- Take all medication exactly as prescribed to prevent antibiotic resistance.
- Do not take with theophylline: increases levels, increasing toxicity risk.

SULFONAMIDES

Indication: bacterial infection, especially UTIs; also pneumonia in AIDS patients.

Mechanism of action: Bacteriostatic: stops manufacturing of folic acid by bacterial cells.

- Medications: sulfisoxazole, sulfamethoxazole and trimethoprim (SMX-TMP); *prefix sulf-*

Side Effects: urinary crystals, hypersensitivity, GI distress.

Teaching:

- Drink lots of water to help flush from kidneys and prevent stones (2,000-3,000 mL a day unless otherwise contraindicated).
- May increase the hypoglycemic effects of oral diabetic agents; be vigilant for Signs and symptoms of hypoglycemia.
- High incidence of allergy; alert MD right away if signs of reaction occur.

TETRACYCLINES

Indication: broad-spectrum antibiotic; gram-positive and -negative aerobic and anaerobic bacteria; spirochetes; mycoplasmas; rickettsiae; chlamydiae; and some protozoa.

Mechanism of action: Bacteriostatic – inhibits bacterial growth by inhibiting protein synthesis.

Side Effects: gastric distress, photosensitivity, GERD.

Teaching:

- Do not take with milk; aluminum, calcium, and magnesium antacids reduce absorption.
- Do not give at bedtime. When patients lie down it often causes gastric reflux.
- Can cause discoloration of the teeth of children, and fetuses when given to pregnant mothers.
- Wear sunscreen; more susceptible to sunburns
- *Toxic*: hearing loss, kidney dysfunction.

Fluoroquinolones

Indication: UTIs, upper respiratory infections, pneumonia, bone/joint/skin infections, gonorrhea, and others

Mechanism of action: Bacteriocidal; alter DNA

- Medications: ciprofloxacin, levofloxacin, trovafloxacin, ofloxacin

Ends in: -floxacin or -oxacin

Side Effects: GI upset, photosensitivity, headache, vertigo/seizures

Teaching:

- Take all medication exactly as prescribed.
- Wear sunscreen and sunglasses when outdoors.
- Take with food to minimize stomach upset; however, antacids decrease absorption, as well as zinc and iron.

Anti-Tubercular's

Indication: Treatment or prophylaxis if exposed to tuberculosis.

Mechanism of action: Alters DNA/RNA or lipid and nucleic acid synthesis; prevents growth of TB bacterium.

- Medications: isoniazid (INH; prototype), pyrazinamide (PZA), rifampin, rifapentine, rifabutin, streptomycin, ethambutol.

Side Effects: fever, liver dysfunction

- INH: hyperglycemia, rash, N/V, gynecomastia, peripheral neuritis
- Rifampin: orange-colored body fluids, inactivates oral contraceptives
- Ethambutol: retrobulbar neuritis, blindness

Teaching:

- Do not take alcohol with these drugs: severe liver damage.
- INH: take vitamin B6 to help with neuropathy, give before meals, and cannot take with phenytoin (toxicity).
- **Treatment can last >2 years**; must stress compliance to prevent multi-drug resistant strains.
- Teach signs and symptoms of liver dysfunction: unusual bleeding, jaundice, fever, N/V, loss of appetite, numbness/tingling in extremities.

Antiviral Drugs

Indication: Used to prevent or treat viral infections.

Mechanism of action:

- Work by disrupting viral replication.
- Acyclovir: herpes viruses and varicella-zoster virus.
- Foscarnet: cytomegalovirus (CMV) retinitis in AIDS patients.
- Amantadine/rimantadine: Parkinson disease.
- Ribavirin: nasal/oral: respiratory syncytial virus (RSV).
- Oseltamivir (Tamiflu): prophylaxis of influenza A or B, avian flu.
- Others: ganciclovir, famciclovir, nelfinavir, zidovudine, didanosine, and zalcitabine.

Side Effects: Vary widely; healthy cells often killed, so generalized malaise common

Teaching:

- Tamiflu – must be taken within 48 hours of onset of symptoms.
- No "cure" for viruses: simply control spread.
- Viruses use the body's own cells to replicate, so antivirals kill body cells; this means side effects are often worse with these drugs than with antibiotics.

Antifungals

Indication: systemic and local fungal infections, vaginal and oral candidiasis (thrush), ringworm.

Mechanism of action: binds to sterols in fungal cell membranes and alters the permeability of the membranes.

- Medications: amphotericin B, fluconazole, nystatin, itraconazole, griseofulvin; most end in -*azole.*
- Nystatin – "Swish and Swallow"; creams and mouthwash.
- Fluconazole – fewer side effects than amphotericin B.

Side Effects: Headache, N/V/D, abdominal pain, rash. Amphotericin: fever, hypotension, malaise, join and muscle pain. Griseofulvin: blood dyscrasias.

Treatment:

- Monitor for severe side effects/allergic reactions.
- Amphotericin B: pretreat with acetaminophen, antiemetic, and antihistamine for symptom management. Medication is light and time-sensitive: cover with foil and use within 24 hr.

Prevention: keep skin clean and dry; avoid excessive moisture and tight clothes: fungi thrive in moist, warm environments. Yeast infections can also be a side effect of antibiotic use.

Common Toxicity Reversal Agents and Important Therapeutic Drug Levels

Toxicity Reversal Agents

Acetaminophen	N-Acetylcysteine
Alcohol withdrawal	Librium
Ammonia	Lactulose
Warfarin	Vitamin K
Digoxin	Digibind
Heparin	Protamine Sulfate
Iron	Deferoxamine
Narcotics	Naloxone

Therapeutic Drug Levels

Digoxin	0.5-2 ng/mL
Lithium	0.8-1.5 mEq/L
Dilantin	10-20 mcg/dL
Theophylline	10-20 mcg/dL
Warfarin	INR levels of 2-3 (A-fib, MI, DVT, PE)
Warfarin	INR levels of 2.5-3.5 (for mechanical heart valves)

Blood Transfusions

Donor/Recipient Blood Compatibility and Transfusion Reaction Signs

RBC Compatibility

	Donor							
Recip.	AB+	AB-	B+	B-	A+	A-	O+	O-
AB +	YES	YES	YES	YES	YES	YES	YES	YES
AB-	NO	YES	NO	YES	NO	YES	NO	YES
B+	NO	NO	YES	YES	NO	NO	YES	YES
B-	NO	NO	NO	YES	NO	NO	NO	YES
A+	NO	NO	NO	NO	YES	YES	YES	YES
A-	NO	NO	NO	NO	NO	YES	NO	YES
O+	NO	NO	NO	NO	NO	NO	YES	YES
O-	NO	NO	NO	NO	NO	NO	NO	YES

Blood transfusion reaction: Remember AFH

- **A**llergic: facial flushing, hives, rash, anxiety, wheezing, decreased BP.
- **F**ebrile: high fever, headache, tachycardia, tachypnea, chills.
- **H**emolytic: decreased BP, flank pain, increased respirations, hemoglobinuria, chest pain, anxiety, fever, tachycardia, chills.

Review Video: Blood Transfusions
Visit mometrix.com/academy and enter code: 192415

CVADs

Central venous access devices (CVADs) are lines used for intravenous access that are long, thick, and end in the superior or inferior vena cava. CVADs include tunneled and non-tunneled catheters, peripherally inserted central catheters (PICCs) and ports. Tunneled catheters and ports are placed surgically, and used when IV access will be needed for an extended period of time. PICCs and non-tunneled catheters can often be placed at the bedside in emergency situations, and are used for therapy that is expected to last days to weeks instead of months.

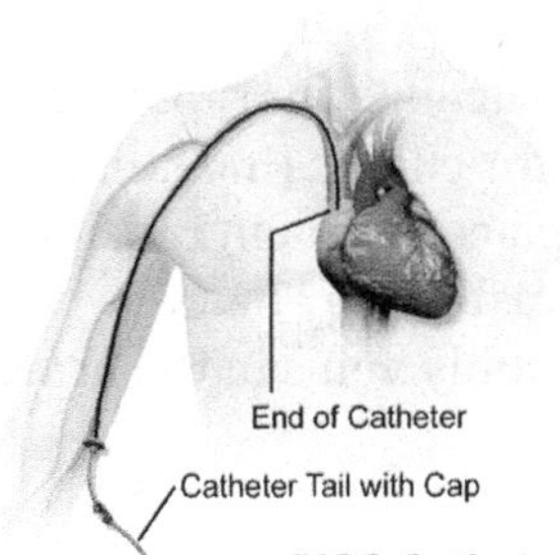

PICC Catheter

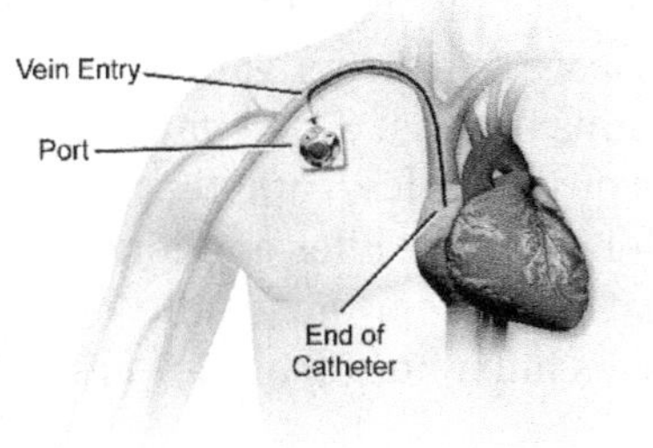

Venous Access Port

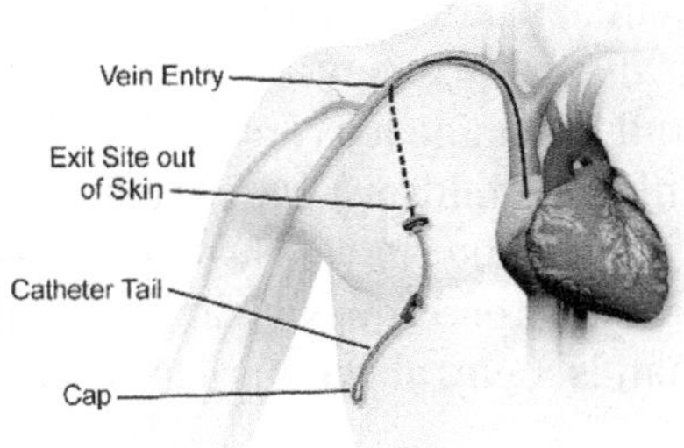

Tunneled Central Venous Access Device

Nursing Care Guidelines

There are a few guidelines a nurse should be aware of when dealing with **central venous access devices** (CVADs):

- **Central Line Associated Bloodstream Infections (CLABSI)**: CVADs greatly increase the risk of CLABSIs, which can be fatal. To prevent them, the nurse should maintain sterile technique when accessing the line. "Scrub the hub" for a minimum of 30 seconds before access and between uses. Change dressings weekly, or per hospital policy, using an occlusive chlorohexidine-impregnated dressing if available. Remove lines as soon as clinically possible, per MD order.
- **Medications**: Because CVADs are significantly longer than peripheral IVs, medications may take longer to reach the patient. *ALWAYS* flush the first 5ccs at the same rate as the medication, as this will prevent the patient from receiving medications too quickly. TPN, vasopressors, and other potentially irritating or harmful medications should be given exclusively through central lines to avoid extravasation and tissue necrosis.
- **Blood draws**: When drawing blood from a port, remember to flush and waste the first 10 mL, as this may contain medication or be diluted. Always flush after obtaining the sample with an additional 20 mL to avoid clotting off the catheter. If the catheter does become clotted, call the physician to obtain an order for a thrombolytic agent.

Considerations in the Administration of Blood Products

Administration of blood products is not within the scope of the practical nurse, though they can assist the registered nurse in monitoring the patient's response to this process, and therefore must be familiar with the process. Prior to **administration of blood**, the following must be verified/identified:

- Correct client, verified by at least two identifiers (wrist band, birthdate). The nurse should ask the client's name (if client alert and responsive), verify name by the wristband and room/bed assignment, and ask the birthdate.
- Correct prescription, checked against the blood bag to determine if names and ID numbers correspond.
- Correct type (including Rh status), verified by checking the cross-match report.
- Consent, signed with informed consent.

While protocols may vary, many require the use of large needles or catheters (18-20) for transfusions; however, studies indicate that larger gauges (14, 16, 18) are needed for rapid infusion and 20-gauge for routine transfusions but that 22-24 gauges can be used for clients (including infants/children) with small veins or if needles/catheters are already in place although the flow rate may be slower through smaller gauge needles and long PICCs. Transfusion may be administered through any vein that can accept the needle/catheter, commonly veins in the arms or hands. Central venous access devices must be at least 1.9 Fr.

Documentation of **administration of blood** must be completed by the registered nurse, and includes:

- **Before transfusion**: Medical record should include the reason for the transfusion and supporting laboratory findings, consent form, prescription that includes the component, dose or volume, the rate of administration as well as any special requirements. Ask client to urinate or empty urine drainage bag. Record any pre-transfusion medications and client education. Document insertion of catheter/needle or condition of IV site if already in place. Record baseline vital signs.
- **During and after transfusion**: Documentation must include time and date component received from the blood bank, verification of client ID and label match of client ID and blood label, time and date administration started and ended, donation number of the blood component and expiration date, method of administration, site and type of needle/catheter (including gauge), compatibility, volume of NS and blood component infused. Vital signs should be monitored at least at 5 minutes, 15 minutes, and 30 minutes for the first hour and then hourly or more often if indicated. Note any signs of reactions or negative response. Note changes with transfusions, such as stabilization of vital signs, improved color, changes in Hgb and Hct.

Intravenous Infusions

Calculation of Drip Rates of IV Medications

A nurse will use the type of tubing, total time of infusion, and total volume of infusion to determine drip rate. Drip rate is always rounded to the nearest whole number: The formula is:

$$\frac{\text{Total volume infused} \times \frac{\text{drops}}{\text{mL}}}{\text{Total time of infusion in minutes}} = \text{drops per minute}$$

Example: The order is for 1 liter (1000 cc) of normal saline (NS) to be administered over 8 hours, with the use of an administration set that will deliver ten (10) drops (gtt)/cc. What will the drip rate be for this fluid?

$$\frac{1000 \times 10}{8 \times 60} = \frac{10,000}{480} = 20.8 = 21\ \frac{gtt}{min}$$

Example: The order is for 2 liters (2000 cc) of 5% dextrose to be administered over 12 hours, with the use of an administration set that will deliver fifteen (15) drops (gtt)/cc. What will the drip rate for this be?

$$\frac{2000 \times 15}{12 \times 60} = \frac{30,000}{720} = 41.7 = 42\ \frac{gtt}{min}$$

Note: Micro drip tubing delivers 60 drops/mL.

Review Video: IV Drip Rates
Visit mometrix.com/academy and enter code: 278763

Intravenous Fluids

Intravenous fluids are classified according to whether the total osmolality is the same as blood (isotonic), less than blood (hypotonic), or greater than blood (hypertonic):

- **Isotonic fluids**: These fluids expand extracellular volume because they diffuse rapidly from the blood into the ECF, so 3 L is needed to replace 1 L of blood. Isotonic fluids include dextrose 5% in water, normal saline, and lactated Ringer's solution (which is NS with potassium and chloride added).
- **Hypotonic fluids**: These fluids are used to replace cellular fluids and treat hypernatremia and hyperosmolar conditions. Excessive hypotonic fluids may result in hypotension, edema, and intravascular fluid depletion. Hypotonic fluids include 0.45% NS and sterile water.
- **Hypertonic fluids**: These fluids are used to treat hypovolemia and hyponatremia but may result in intravascular fluid volume excess, so they must be monitored very carefully. Hypertonic fluids include dextrose 10% in water, 3% saline, and 5% dextrose in NS. Solutions with concentrations of greater than dextrose 10% must be administered per central catheter.

Possible Complications Involving an Intravenous Access Site

While intravenous (IV) access sites are a valuable asset to nursing, there are some common complications that occur with their use. The nurse should assess for these every shift. Complications include:

- **Infiltration**: Infiltration occurs when the IV slips out of the vein and into the surrounding tissue. Common symptoms of infiltration include swelling, tenderness at site, decreased or no infusion rate, blanching of the skin and surrounding tissue, and the site may be cool to touch. Certain medications are necrotic to the tissues, so if infiltration occurs, the physician should be notified immediately.
- **Phlebitis:** Phlebitis is inflammation of a vein, sometimes caused by irritating solutions or prolonged age of the IV. Common signs of phlebitis include a red line along the vein, erythema, heat, edema, and tenderness.
- **Accidental Removal:** This occurs when a patient (or practitioner) accidentally pulls the IV out of the skin.

Treatment includes:

- Infiltration/Phlebitis: discontinuation of the IV, and application of warm compresses.
- Infiltration of necrotizing substances: injection of antidote into tissue; cool compress.
- Accidental removal: apply pressure to stop the bleeding with a sterile gauze, and cover with a bandage.

IV Catheter Insertion

The procedure for IV catheter insertion is described below:

1. Identify appropriate vein, usually on dorsal surface of hand or arm (most distal site on nondominant side if possible), and apply tourniquet above site, palpate to locate insertion site.
2. Release tourniquet, apply gloves, prep site with antiseptic and let dry, and reapply tourniquet (4-6 inches above site).
3. Stretch skin and insert venous catheter with bevel up (10-30-degree angle), note flashback of blood.

4. Lower catheter until almost level with insertion site and advance catheter about 0.5, then loosen and remove stylet.
5. Continue to slowly advance the catheter only into the vein until the hub rests against the skin.
6. Release tourniquet with one hand while stabilizing the catheter with the other, then apply gentle pressure about 3 inches above insertion site and connect tubing or saline lock.
7. Flush catheter with NS or begin infusion.
8. Secure according to protocol with tape and/or catheter stabilization device and apply dressings, such as transparent or gauze.
9. Loop at secure extension tubing, label dressing according to protocol.
10. Safely dispose of sharps and supplies and remove gloves.
11. Educate client regarding safeguarding catheter and signs of adverse reactions (infiltration, infection) to report.

Review Video: Starting an IV
Visit mometrix.com/academy and enter code: 848550

PCA Pumps

Patient-controlled analgesia (PCA) allows the client to control administration of pain medication by pressing a button on an intravenous delivery system with a computerized pump. The device is filled with opioid (as prescribed) and must be programmed correctly and checked regularly to ensure that it is functioning properly and that controls are set. The most-commonly administered medications include morphine, meperidine, fentanyl, and sufentanil. Most devices can be set to deliver continuous infusion of opioid as well as patient-controlled bolus. Each element must be clarified by the physician's order and set by the registered nurse:

- **Bolus**: Determines the amount of medication received when the client delivers a dose.
- **Lockout interval**: Time required between administrations of boluses.
- **Continuous infusion**: Rate at which opioid is delivered per hour for continuous analgesia.
- **Limit (usually set at 4 hours)**: Total amount of opioid that can be delivered in the preset time limit.

Settings should be documented and checked at least every 2 hours. The practical nurse is responsible for monitoring PCA use and side effects. With Authorized Agent Controlled Analgesia (AACA), people who are trained and authorized (such as nurse, family member, and caregiver) may administer the medication as well as the client.

Pain Management

Pain Assessment

Assessment of pain is essential as part of overall evaluation and should be carefully documented, including the location, duration, and cause of the cause. Pain is categorized as:

- **Acute**: Usually associated with a specific injury or condition and lasting no more than 6 months. Acute pain usually responds to opioids, NSAIDs, or acetaminophen.
- **Chronic**: Constant or intermittent pain that lasts 6 months or longer. The cause of the pain may not be evident. Chronic pain is often very debilitating and is more difficult to control than acute pain because traditional pain medications are often ineffective. Patients may respond to complementary therapies (such as relaxation and acupuncture), local anesthetic agents, TCAs (such as amitriptyline), or anti-seizure medications (such as phenytoin).
- **Cancer-related**: May be acute or chronic and directly related to tumor growth or secondary to treatment. Pain control must be titrated to individual needs.

Assessment should include the characteristics of the pain, the intensity, the timing, the location, aggravating factors, alleviating factors, and the patient's response.

Pain Assessment/Pain Scales

The types of pain assessment/pain scales are as follows:

- Visual Analog Scale (VAS) (non-numeric): used to determine baseline pain.
- Numeric Pain Intensity (1 to 10 scale): for adolescents and adults to assess level of pain.
- Patient Comfort Assessment Guide: to assess pain status and pain relief, response to medications.
- Wong-Baker FACES: graphic depictions of pain through different facial expressions. Appropriate for children, non-English speakers, and some illiterate patients or patients with cognitive impairment. FACES has a pediatric version and an adult version.
- Brief Pain Inventory: assesses the effect pain has on activities.
- CRIES (crying, requires O_2, increased vital signs, expression, sleepiness): Assesses pain in neonates.
- FLACC (face, legs, activity, cry, consolability): appropriate for children to 3 years of age and older children with cognitive impairment.
- CPOT: Used in critical care settings (ventilated patients).
- Pain Assessment in Advanced Dementia Scale (PAINAD): appropriate for adults with cognitive impairment.

Controlled Pain Management Substances

Controlled substances (narcotics/opioids) must be stored in locked and secured carts, drawers, or cabinets (computerized preferred). Only those authorized to administer controlled substances may carry keys or have access to a computer code. Prior to administration, the nurse should verify that the count/volume is correct according to the inventory report, which should contain a record of all substances used or wasted and remaining. For each dose retrieved, the nurse should record the client's name, the date and time, the name of the medication and the dosage as well as the nurse's signature. If a partial dosage remains (such as a small volume in a vial), a second nurse must witness disposal (according to established facility protocol), and both nurses must sign the inventory record. The medication should be administered immediately and not stored for later use or administration delegated to another nurse. For administration, the date, time, medication, dosage, type of administration (SQ, IM, IV, PO) recorded, and site (for parenteral) must be recorded as well as response in 5 minutes, 15 minutes, 30 minutes, and 60 minutes.

Nonsteroidal Anti-Inflammatory Drugs (NSAIDs)

Indication: relief of acute/chronic pain, inflammation

Mechanism of action: prevent release of prostaglandins, inhibiting pain and inflammatory response.

- Medications: Ibuprofen (Motrin, Advil), Naproxen (Aleve), ketoprofen, indomethacin.

Side Effects: gastric upset, stomach ulcers, increased risk of bleeding, nephrotoxicity, hypersensitivity.

Teaching:

- Take with food or milk to decrease GI upset.
- Works well for muscle strain/spasms; works best if taken early to prevent pain.
- Overdose: renal failure. Do not take more than daily recommended amount/amount prescribed by MD.
- Report: dark, tarry stools, blood in vomit, gum bleeding, increased bruising, severe stomach pain, difficulty breathing, etc.
- May be given with misoprostol, which reduces gastric acid secretion, thus preventing NSAID-related ulcers; though this medication may increase menstrual bleeding *(contraindicated in pregnancy – causes miscarriage).*

Review Video: NSAID Effects
Visit mometrix.com/academy and enter code: 569064

Muscle Relaxants

Indication: acute injury, spasms caused by anxiety, inflammation, pain, trauma.

Mechanism of action: Central acting; work in central nervous system to potentiate effects of GABA (amino acid).

- Medications: baclofen, cyclobenzaprine.
- Dantrolene: acts directly on muscles to decrease excitability; spasticity, as well as malignant hyperthermia.

Side Effects: drowsiness, loss of coordination, dizziness/ lightheadedness, euphoria, constipation, hepatotoxicity (dantrolene).

Teaching:

- Do not take with alcohol, will potentiate CNS depression.
- Increased risk of injury: monitor ambulation, do not allow to operate heavy machinery while on this mediation.

Opioid Analgesics

Indication: Strong pain relief; adjunct treatment of MI (morphine)*

Mechanism of action: Naturally derived from the opium plant, opioids bind to opioid receptors - the specific proteins on cell surfaces in the spinal cord, brain, and gastrointestinal tract. In doing so, the drugs interfere and prevent the transmission of pain signals to the brain. Secondly, in the brain, they alter the pain sensation. Opioids do not eliminate the pain, but they do decrease and change the patient's perception of it.

Side Effects: euphoria, drowsiness, nausea/vomiting, constipation, dilated pupils and respiratory depression, CNS depression, emotional liability, risk of addiction.

Contraindications: respiratory depression, known allergy, suspected gallbladder disease (morphine).

Teaching:

- Teach not to drive or operate machinery while taking these drugs.
- Do not take with alcohol; take only as directed.
- Patient cannot sign consent while under influence of opiates.
- Educate on addiction, drug-sharing; other forms of pain relief.

*Morphine is often used in treating pain accompanying an MI. It decreases preload in the heart, relieving ischemia and allowing oxygen to perfuse the cells.

Intravenous Nutrition

TPN

Total parenteral nutrition (TPN) is a form of nutrition that is maintained exclusively by intravenous routes. The purpose of TPN is to bypass the gastrointestinal system while still providing adequate calories and nutrition to the body. TPN is also used to maintain a positive nitrogen balance for healing as well as to replace lost electrolytes, vitamins, and minerals to the body. The administration of TPN is generally via a peripherally inserted central catheter (termed a PICC line), or any other type of central line (chest port, intrajugular central, etc.); TPN should **never** be infused through a peripheral catheter, unless expressly ordered, and should be administered through a designated line or lumen that is solely for TPN. State laws vary regarding the LPN's ability to administer TPN, but LPN's are responsible for monitoring and caring for the patient receiving TPN.

Nursing considerations are as follows:

- These patients are at a considerably high risk of infection; TPN bag and tubing must be changed daily and any time a new bag is hung. Monitor patient for fever, chills, malaise, or other signs of infection.
- Hypoglycemia is another risk of TPN infusion: monitor blood glucose frequently. If TPN runs out before another bag can be obtained, run dextrose 10% in water until new bag is hung.
- **NEVER** run any other medications in the same line as TPN, and do not try to "catch up" infusion if delay occurs.

Reduction of Risk Potential

Abnormal Vital Signs

NORMAL VITAL SIGN RANGES

Age	Heart rate	Resp	BP (mm Hg)
Neonate (newborn)	100-220* (avg 140-160)	30-40**	Systolic 70-90
Toddler (12-36 mo.)	80-130	20-30	Systolic 70-100
Pre-school (3 to 5)	80-120	20-30	Systolic 80-110
School-age (6-12)	70-110	20-30	80-120/60-80
Adolescence (13-18)	55-100	12-20	110-131/64-84
Early adulthood (19-40)	60-100 (avg 80)	12-20	100-119/60-79 to 140/90 (high)
Mid. Adulthood (41-60)	60-100 (avg 80)	12-20	100-119/60-79 to 140/90 (high)
Late adulthood (61+)	60-100 (avg 70)	12-20	100-119/60-79 to 140/90 (high)

* HR begins to slow after ~3 months.

** RR is 40-60 for the first few minutes, before slowing to 30-40.

CAUSES OF ABNORMAL OXYGEN SATURATION AND RESPIRATORY RATE

Possible causes of **abnormal findings** include:

- **Oxygen saturation**: Levels should range from 95-99%. Levels may drop in the presence of hypoxia, and may also be less than normal as a result of lung disease (COPD, pneumonia, pulmonary edema, severe bronchitis, lung cancer, tuberculosis, and emphysema). Additionally, oxygen saturation levels may drop if there is inadequate hemoglobin to carry oxygen, such as may occur with anemia. When evaluating oxygen saturation and an unexpected drop, the first action should be to reposition the pulse oximeter and assess function.
- **Respiratory rate**: A decrease in respiratory rate may result from sedation (such as from narcotics, illegal drugs, anesthesia, overdose, or alcohol), central sleep apnea, liver failure/cirrhosis (because of increase blood ammonia), or damage to the brain stem (such as from a tumor). An increase in respiratory rate may result from exercise and anxiety as well as many health conditions (especially those affecting the heart or lungs), including diabetic ketoacidosis, pneumonia, pleural effusion, heart failure, COPD, laryngospasm, asthma, allergic response, foreign body aspiration, and pulmonary embolism.

Invasive Monitoring

Pulmonary Artery Pressure

Pulmonary artery pressure (PAP) is measured by a catheter usually fed through the right ventricle to the main pulmonary artery, measuring systolic, diastolic, and mean pressures, with the client in supine position ≤45° elevation:

- **Normal values:** PA systolic 20-30 mm Hg, diastolic 6-15 mm Hg. Postoperative rates should be <25 mm Hg. PAP is usually about 25-34% the systemic blood pressure rate. Oxygen saturation is usually about 80%.
- **Increased** pressure may indicate pulmonary obstruction or embolus, left to right shunt, left ventricular failure, pulmonary hypertension, or mitral stenosis, pneumothorax, lung/alveolar hypoplasia, hyperviscosity of blood, or increased left atrial pressure.
- **Decreased** pressure may indicate a decrease in intravascular volume or cardiac output, or obstruction of pulmonary blood flow. On the diagram, **A** represents systole; **B**, diastole; **C**, peak systole; and **D** (dicrotic notch), closure of pulmonic valve. The pulmonary artery catheter may have a balloon that can be inflated in the pulmonary artery to provide a measurement of pulmonary artery/capillary wedge pressure (PAWP/PCWP) to evaluate pulmonary hypertension, left ventricular failure, and mitral stenosis: Normal values 4-12 mm Hg. Increased pressure may indicate left ventricular failure, mitral insufficiency, or mitral stenosis.

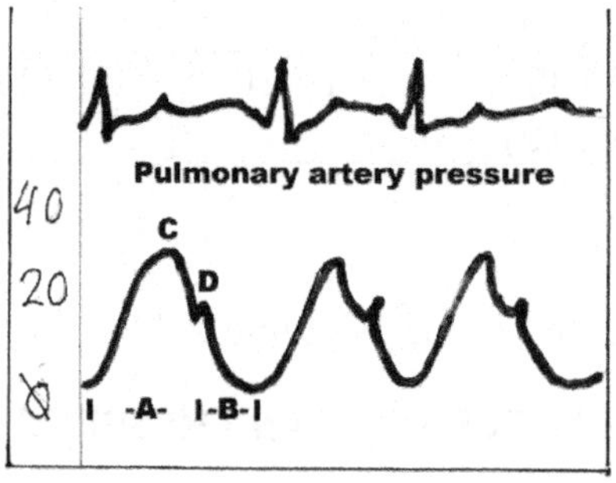

ICP

The **intracranial pressure (ICP) monitoring device** may be placed during surgery or a ventriculostomy performed in which a burr hole is drilled into the frontal area of the scalp and an intraventricular catheter threaded into the lateral ventricle. The intraventricular catheter may be used to monitor ICP and to drain excess CSF. Less accurate devices include the intracranial pressure monitor (subarachnoid) bolt, epidural monitors and fiberoptic monitors. CSF may be drained continuously or intermittently and must be monitored hourly for amount, color, and character. For ICP measurement, the client's head must be elevated to 30 to 45° and the transducer leveled to the outer canthus of the eye. Normal ICP is 0-15 mm Hg on transducer or 80-180 mm H_2O on manometer.

Diagnostic Procedures

CT Scan

The **computed tomography (CT)** scan offers imaging of sections of the body from various angles. CT assists in early diagnosis of disease and disease processes. The CT is approximately 100 times more sensitive than the normal x-ray. CT can be performed with or without contrast dye (media). Contrast offers enhanced views of the organs and structures being examined; an example is increased visibility of small tumors or abnormalities. The CT is used for viewing the brain, head, chest, abdomen, pelvis, spine, and bones of the body; it is used most often in determining coronary artery disease or lesions of the head, liver, and kidney. CT also assists in the diagnosis of tumors, edema, abscesses, infection, metastatic diseases, vascular disorders, stroke, and bone destruction and deformity. CT is also used to locate and identify foreign object within soft tissue.

Nursing Considerations: Use caution with contrast dye in patients with renal impairment. Ensure patient can lie still during test. Not an MRI – open machine. MD may order patient to be NPO before procedure.

Procedure: Patient will lie still on a table and move in and out of a hollow machine.

EEG

The **electroencephalography (EEG)** is a reading of the electropotentials within the brain. The electroencephalogram measures electrical impulses of brain cells, and is an assistive tool for diagnosing seizure disorders, neoplasm of the brain, cerebral vascular accident/strokes, trauma of the brain, and infectious processes of the brain and nervous system. Electroencephalogram is also used to determine brain death, and may also be useful in diagnosis of intracranial hemorrhage and intracranial abscess. The normal findings of an EEG are the same for the adult or child. Normal tracing and regular short waves are the expected findings of the EEG.

Nursing Considerations: Avoid sedatives, alcohol, and stimulants (caffeine) for 24-48 hours before the test; wash the hair with normal shampoo (do not condition); use of hairspray/products/oil in hair will alter test; *will not be painful*. Patient will simply rest quietly with electrodes placed on scalp. Can wash gel out of hair afterwards.

Procedure: Electrodes with gel will be placed on different areas of the scalp, and then patient will lie in quiet room for 1-3 hours; video may be taken during test.

Bladder Imaging Tests

The following are bladder imaging tests:

- **X-ray**: May show kidney stones, tumors, and size and shape of prostate.
- **Intravenous pyelogram (IVP)**: X-rays are taken after administration of IV contrast agent to show how the dye moves through the kidneys, ureter, and bladder. Can demonstrate problems resulting from urinary retention or reflux.
- **Cystoscopy**: Endoscopic examination of the bladder provides direct visualization of the urethra, bladder, and ureteral orifices.
- **Cystography**: Contrast dye is instilled into the bladder per catheter and then x-rays are taken to outline the bladder and show any perforations.
- **Voiding cystourethrography**: Contrast dye is instilled into the bladder and fluoroscopy utilized while the bladder is full and during urination. Frequently used to diagnose vesicoureteral reflux.
- **Ultrasound**: Shows the urinary tract and abnormalities as well as tumors and urinary retention.
- **CT**: Can show the presence of stones, cysts, injuries, and tumors, but not adequate for diagnosis of malignancy.
- **MRI**: Provides detailed images of the urinary organs and shows tumors or other abnormalities.

Gastrointestinal Series

A **gastrointestinal series** is an examination using x-ray. The gastrointestinal series uses fluoroscopy to visualize the esophagus, stomach, and small intestine. The patient will be asked to ingest oral contrast such as barium meal or meglumine diatrizoate. The contrast media is observed under fluoroscopy while it passes through the digestive tract. The gastrointestinal series is used to determine and diagnose inflammation, ulcerations, and tumors, and also to detect and diagnose hiatal hernias, pyloric stenosis, gastroenteritis, gastric polyps, foreign bodies, and malabsorption of the gastrointestinal system. Esophageal varices, obstructions, and strictures are also visible using a gastrointestinal series.

Laboratory Values and Samples

Obtaining Blood Samples

Options for **obtaining blood samples** include:

- **Venipuncture**: The vein of choice for both adults and children is generally the median cubital vein, which is large and well-anchored so it is less likely to roll. If not accessible, then the cephalic vein (thumb side) or basilic vein (5th-finger side) may be used. For neonates and children under 2 years, a dorsal vein on the hand may be used.
- **Central line**: (Note that protocols may vary slightly.) Infusions should be stopped for at least one-minute prior to obtaining a blood sample. The line must be flushed with approximately 10 mL of NS or heparin solution (according to protocol) and a sample of 5 mL blood obtained for discard before the actual laboratory sample is collected. The line should again be flushed with 10 mL NS or heparin solution to clear blood.
- **Venous access device**: Procedures are essentially the same as for central lines except that a needle must be attached to the syringes for implanted ports, and the ports should be used for obtaining a blood sample only if peripheral veins are not readily accessible because frequent use increases the risk of CLABSI.

Obtaining Stool Specimens

Stool specimens are obtained by placing a stool collection device in a toilet or in a bedpan. The specimen is then placed in a clean specimen container, or if for cultures, in a sterile container. Different types of containers may be used, with or without preservatives, depending on the type of tests being conducted. The sample is transferred using a tongue blade to the fill-line indicated on the container. If an additive is in the container, the sample should be shaken to mix contents. The container should be properly labeled and sealed in a biohazard bag for transport. For a stool culture, the specimen should be collected before the client begins antibiotics. The stool specimen is placed in a sterile container or a cotton-tipped swab is inserted into the rectum and rotated to obtain a fecal sample. Then the swab is inserted into a sterile tube. Stools specimens should be processed as soon as possible or stored at 4 °C if delay of more than two hours before processing. In the case of diarrhea and/or incontinence, stool may be collected via syringe and then distributed into the appropriate specimen cup. This is a common method when testing for bacterial infections such as *C.diff.*

Obtaining Wound and Nasopharyngeal Secretion Specimens

Wound specimens are generally obtained for culture and sensitivities when there are signs of infection in a wound or no progress in healing over a two-week period. The culture should be done with sterile technique prior to the administration of antibiotics, which may interfere with the results. A culture of the area may be done, taking the sample from clean tissue rather than exudate, which may give a false report, showing organisms in the area but not in the tissue itself. There are 3 methods of culturing:

- Swabbing the area is the most common method used but the sample is easily contaminated by surface flora.
- Needle aspiration of fluid adjacent to the wound may result in underestimation of organisms.
- Culturing by tissue biopsy is often most effective method, but not all labs can process these samples and the process disrupts the wound and increases pain.

Nasopharyngeal secretions are collected with swabs of the nasopharyngeal area. The client should be advised to open the mouth widely, and swabbing should avoid the back of the palate or the uvula to avoid the client's gagging. The swab is placed in a tube with transport medium.

Lab Levels Associated with Diabetes

There are two main labs that are used in diagnosis of diabetes: **HbA_{1c} and fasting blood glucose.** While other lab abnormalities are often seen, these two are considered diagnostic for the disease.

HbA_{1c} is the major determinant for glycosylated hemoglobin; it is used to determine blood sugar control over the last 90 days. This can be used to diagnose effectiveness of diabetic therapy or diagnose diabetes.

- **Normal HbA_{1c} is 2%-5%**; anything <7% considered controlled.
- Uncontrolled diabetes is >8%.

Fasting Blood Glucose (sugar): Glucose is formed from carbohydrates taken in with food and stored in the liver and skeletal muscles. Glucose levels are maintained by insulin production in the pancreas. Elevated glucose (hyperglycemia) indicates inadequate insulin production or utilization. Self-monitoring glucose is done with capillary blood or finger stick method.

- **Blood Glucose: 70-110 mg/dL**; panic level is <40 mg/dL or >400 mg/dL.

> **Review Video: Blood Glucose Pattern Management**
> Visit mometrix.com/academy and enter code: 626814

Thyroid Function Tests

Thyroid function tests are discussed below:

- **Thyroid-Stimulating Hormone (TSH)**: TSH is a hormone secreted by the pituitary gland that stimulates the production of T4 (thyroxine) from the thyroid gland. TSH is used in the diagnosis of thyroid and pituitary gland disorders.
    - TSH: 0.35-5.5 uIU/mL
- **Thyroxine (T4)**: T4 is the major hormone derived and secreted by the thyroid gland; used in the diagnosis of hypo- and hyperthyroidism.
    - T4: 4.5-11.5 ug/dL
- **Triiodothyronine (T3)**: T3 is a thyroid hormone that is always present in small amounts. Serum T3 is secreted in reaction to TSH; also used to diagnose altered thyroid function.
    - T3: 80-200 ng/dL

- **Calcitonin**: Calcitonin is secreted by the thyroid gland and aids in the maintenance of serum calcium and phosphorus levels. Calcitonin is elevated with thyroid cancer, and hyperplasia of the adenoma.
    - Calcitonin: Male: <40 ng/L; Female: <25 ng/L

BMP

A **basic metabolic panel (BMP)** includes 14 different lab tests that are used to assess the body's metabolism. The components of the BMP and general reference ranges are listed below. Note that normal values may fluctuate slightly in different facilities due to calibration of laboratory machines.

- Sodium (Na): 135-145 mEq/L
- Potassium (K): 3.5-5.3 mEq/L
- Calcium (Ca): 9-11 mg/dL (total), 4.5-5.6 mg/dL (ionized)
- Chloride (Cl): 95-105 mEq/L
- Albumin: 3.9-5.0 g/dL
- Alkaline phosphatase (ALP): 44-147 IU/L
- ALT: 8-37 IU/L
- AST: 10-34 IU/L
- BUN: 7-20 mg/dL
- CO_2: 20-29 mmol/L
- Creatinine: 0.8-1.4 mg/dL
- Glucose: 70-100 mg/dL
- Total bilirubin: 0.2-1.9 mg/dL
- Total protein: 6.3-7.9 g/dL

Review Video: Lab Values
Visit mometrix.com/academy and enter code: 887465

CBC

A **complete blood cell count (CBC)** is a combination of red blood cells, white blood cells, erythrocyte indices, hematocrit, differential white blood cell count, and may even include the platelet count. CBCs are used as diagnostic tests to assist in determination of anemia, blood loss, blood values, and hydration status.

- **RBC:** Male is 4.5-6.0 μL; Female is 4.0-5.0 μL

↓ RBC may indicate hemorrhage, anemia, or overhydration; ↑ RBC may indicate dehydration and polycythemia vera.

- **Hgb**: Male is 13.5-18.0 g/dL; Female is 12.0-16.0 g/dL

↑ Hgb levels may indicate hemoconcentration/dehydration, and polycythemia vera. ↓ Hgb may indicate anemia, acute blood loss, and hemodilution.

- **Hct**: Male is 40%-54%; Female is 36%-46%

↓ Hct indicates anemia and folic acid deficiency. ↑ Hct may indicate dehydration and polycythemia vera.

- White Blood Cells (WBCs): 3.5-10 x $10^3/mm^3$

↑ WBC indicate infection, inflammation, tissue damage, or leukemia; ↓ WBC indicates leukopenia (caused by cancer treatments or other immune deficiencies), cancer, severe infection, or liver/spleen disease.

Coagulation Studies

ApTT (Activated Partial Thromboplastin Time): ApTT will reveal clotting deficiencies, and is used to determine effectiveness of heparin management.

- pTT: 60-70 seconds.

PT (Prothrombin Time): Prothrombin time measures the clotting ability of factors I, II, V, VII, and X; used to monitor warfarin.

- PT: 10-13 seconds.

INR (International Normalized Ratio): INR is used to monitor clotting time in patients taking warfarin.

- INR: 2.0-3.0.

Platelet count: The platelet count is used to determine basic elements of the blood that promote coagulation (clotting). A decreased platelet count of <50% of the normal value will cause bleeding; this decreased platelet count places the patient at risk of hemorrhage.

- Platelets: 150,000-400,000 μL

Factor assay: Factor assays are ordered to detect deficiencies of blood coagulation components. There are 12 factor assays and they are equally important for blood clotting; these are generally interpreted by a hematologist.

Cardiac Labs

Cardiac labs are discussed below:

- **Troponin**: a form of globular protein found in cardiac and skeletal muscle. Troponin is released with injury or necrosis of the myocardium. There are 2 cycles of troponin release: 4-6 hours immediately post-cardiac injury, and may still rise 7 to 10 days following a cardiac injury.
    - Troponin: <0.012 mcg/L
- **CK-MB**: an enzyme found in heart muscle. Elevated levels indicate acute MI/heart attack, severe angina pectoris, cardiac surgical procedures, cardiac ischemia, myocarditis, and hypokalemia.
    - CK-MB: 0-6%
- **Brain natriuretic peptide (BNP)**: a peptide that is released into the bloodstream (circulation) of individuals with heart failure. Can be falsely elevated in severe kidney disease.
    - BNP: <100 pg/mL

CHOLESTEROL, HDL, LDL, AND SERUM TRIGLYCERIDE LEVELS

Cholesterol is a blood lipid synthesized by the liver and found in red blood cells, cell membranes, and muscles. Serum cholesterol is used as an indicator of atherosclerosis and coronary artery disease. HDL is considered the friendly cholesterol and consists of 50% protein and assists with decreasing plaque deposits in blood vessels; high levels are desirable. However, LDL and triglycerides are associated with atherosclerosis and increased risk of MI; therefore, low levels are desired.

The following are **special considerations**:

- Client NPO for the 12 hours prior to the test.
- Aspirin, cortisone, and alcohol (<24 h before test) can alter the cholesterol level, causing an increase or decrease. Ventilators, hypoxemia, and hemolysis of the specimen can cause false elevations.

Reference values are as follows:

- Total cholesterol: <200 mg/dL; moderate risk: 200-240 mg/dL; high risk: >240 mg/dL
- High-density lipoprotein (HDL): 29-77 mg/dL
- Low-density lipoprotein (LDL): 60-160 mg/dL
- Triglyceride level: 10-190 mg/dL

RHEUMATOID ARTHRITIS LABS

Labs associated with rheumatoid arthritis are described below:

- **ASO (antistreptolysin O)**: created in response to streptolysin, an agent secreted by beta-hemolytic group A *Streptococcus* that is capable of lysing red blood cells (RBCs). ASO levels that are elevated can indicate rheumatic fever, acute glomerulonephritis, and recent streptococcal infections.
  - ASO: <100 Todd units
- **ANA (antinuclear antibodies)**: The ANA is a diagnostic tool for screening systemic lupus erythematosus (SLE) and other collagen disorders such as rheumatoid arthritis, scleroderma, leukemia, and infectious mononucleosis.
  - ANA >1:20 (titer).
- **ESR (erythrocyte sedimentation rate)**: ESR is the rate in which red blood cells settle in unclotted blood in millimeters per hour. Elevated in the presence of inflammation in the body.
  - ESR: 0-20 mm/h
- **CRP (C-reactive protein)**: appears 10 hours after the onset of an inflammatory process in which tissue destruction is involved. CRP is used to monitor acute inflammatory phases of rheumatoid arthritis and rheumatic fever; infections - *will only elevate with bacterial infections.*
  - CRP: negative.

- **Rheumatoid factor (RF)**: Rheumatoid factor is a test utilized to measure antibodies IgM, IgG, and IgA found with rheumatoid arthritis.
  - RF: <40-60 u/mL/1:80 titer

Review Video: Systemic Lupus Erythematosus (SLE)
Visit mometrix.com/academy and enter code: 729095

ABGs

Arterial blood gases (ABGs) are performed for patients with suspected blood or metabolic malfunction, as well as to evaluate the effectiveness of ventilation. The basic components and expected normal values are:

- PO_2 75-100 mm Hg
- PCO_2 38-42 mm Hg
- Bicarbonate 23-26 mEq/L
- pH 7.38-7.44
- Oxygen saturation 95% or greater

The following are **nursing considerations:**

- An *Allen's test* should always be performed before performing an ABG to ensure that the hand has adequate perfusion; this is done by occluding both the radial and ulnar arteries, having the patient clench fist a few times, then releasing the ulnar (pinky side) artery only and observing for the return of color to the hand.
- Blood drawn should be bright red; dark blood may indicate venous blood.

Review Video: Acid-Base Balance & Blood Gas Interpretation
Visit mometrix.com/academy and enter code: 949839

Review Video: Newborn Cord Blood Gases
Visit mometrix.com/academy and enter code: 434576

Liver Function Tests (Liver Panel)

Liver function tests are discussed below:

- **Alkaline Phosphatase (ALP)**: Alkaline phosphatase is an enzyme produced mainly in the liver and bone.
  - ALP Normal: 42-136 units/L
  - Elevated in elderly patients; bone growth
- **Alanine aminotransferase (ALT)**: assists in the detection of liver disorders such as viral (acute) hepatitis, cancer, necrosis, alcohol abuse, and drug or chemical toxicity.
  - ALT Normal: 10-35 units/L
  - Elevated in males, infants, and elderly patients
- **Aspartate aminotransferase (AST)**: Elevated levels assist in the determination of heart and liver muscle damage. ALT is also used in conjunction with CK and LDH in diagnosing an acute MI.
  - AST Normal: 8-38 units/L
  - Infants and elderly increased; females decreased

- **Bilirubin**: Byproduct of RBC destruction; increased levels cause jaundice in the patient. Indicates liver dysfunction/RBC hemolysis.
  - Bilirubin Normal: 0.2-1.3 mg/dL

Pancreatic Function Tests

Pancreatic function tests are described below:

- **Amylase**: an enzyme that originates within the pancreas, salivary glands, and liver that functions to change starch into sugar.
  - Amylase: 60-160 U/dL (Somogyi).
  - Elderly levels are slightly higher than that of younger adults.
  - The nurse should be aware that glucose in an IV may cause a false-negative amylase.
- **Lipase**: an enzyme secreted by the pancreas and digests fat. Acute pancreatitis is the most common cause of an elevated lipase level. Decreased levels may indicate late cancer, or hepatitis.
  - Lipase: 20-180 U/L

Renal Function Tests

Renal function tests are discussed below:

- **BUN (blood urea nitrogen)**: BUN is utilized to detect disorders of the kidney such as dehydration, liver damage, overhydration, kidney function (renal insufficiency), and sepsis.
  - BUN: 5-25 mg/dL.
  - Slightly elevated in elderly patients.
- **Creatinine**: Creatinine is a byproduct of muscle catabolism; creatinine production is proportional to muscle mass. Creatinine is filtered by the glomeruli and is excreted in the urine. Creatinine is elevated with acute and chronic renal failure. Low magnesium and high creatinine signals renal failure.
  - Creatinine: 0.5-1.5 mg/dL.
  - Females are slightly lower related to lower muscle mass.
- **Albumin**: Albumin levels are used to determine the amount of albumin circulating in the blood or urine. Decreased levels are associated with liver disease, burns, inflammation, shock, malnutrition, and renal disorders.
  - Albumin: 3.5-5 g/dL.

Urinalysis and Culture and Sensitivity

Urinalysis may be performed to detect problems with renal function, disease processes, urinary tract infections, diabetes, prenatal examinations, and routine examinations. The nurse should remember that drugs and foods can alter the color of urine.

Normal results are as follows:

- *Color: Straw* (cloudiness may be due to phosphates and urates and is considered normal).
- Turbidity: Clear.
- *Specific Gravity: 1.001-1.02* (low: sickle cell, DM, diabetes insipidus).
- *Dipstick*: pH 4.5-7.5.
- *Protein: Negative* (positive: nephritic syndrome, renal tubular disease, pyelonephritis, and polycystic kidney disease).

- *Sugar: Negative* (positive: diabetes or other endocrine disease).
- *Acetone/ketones: Negative* (positive: non controlled diabetes, alcoholism, starvation).
- *Bile*: Negative.
- *Hemoglobin: Negative* (positive: bleeding, kidney/bladder irritation).
- *Nitrite: Negative* (positive: indicates bacteria).
- Leukocyte Esterase: Negative.
- Urobilinogen: Positive.

Labs and Diagnostics of HIV and AIDS

HIV is the retrovirus that causes AIDS. The diagnosis of AIDS is determined by the CD4+ T-cell count (per the CDC), with AIDS currently diagnosed with a CD4+ count of <200 cells/mm^3. HIV is transmitted in bodily fluids.

Signs and symptoms: The primary infection stage occurs between the times of initial infection to the development of HIV-specific antigens. Then, HIV/AIDS is staged depending on CD4+ count and conditions:

- *Category A:* (CD4+ count <500). Asymptomatic or lymphadenopathy.
- *Category B:* (CD4+ count 200 to 499). Conditions include candidiasis, PID, bacillary angiomatosis, fever, diarrhea, herpes zoster, ITP, and peripheral neuropathy.
- *Category C* (AIDS): (CD4+ count <200). Invasive diseases common. Conditions include cervical cancer, candidiasis, CMV, encephalopathy, TB, *P. jiroveci* pneumonia, Kaposi sarcoma, toxoplasmosis, wasting syndrome.

Diagnosis: HIV antibody tests (ELISA) and Western blot assay, viral load tests (reverse transcriptase PCR).

Treatment: Antiretroviral agents (NRTIs, NNRTIs, protease inhibitors, fusion inhibitors, integrase strand transfer inhibitors, and multiclass combination products).

Potential Risks and Complications

Risks for Aspiration

Risks for aspiration include:

- **Feeding tubes**: Aspiration pneumonia is a common complication, and, because of reduced cough reflex, there may be no obvious signs. Older age, cognitive impairment, poor oral hygiene, altered level of consciousness, neurological deficits, and history of GERD are all risk factors. Feedings should be given with client sitting up to at least 45 degrees if possible, and the client should remain sitting for at least an hour after feedings.
- **Sedation**: Sedation impairs the ability to swallow, increasing risk of aspiration. Risk is lower if the client has been NPO so that the stomach is empty but may still occur with gastric secretions. Oral fluids should be withheld until the client is fully alert.
- **Swallowing difficulties**: Clients with dysphagia, especially those with older age and/or stroke, Parkinson's disease, or muscular dystrophies, are at risk for aspiration. Additionally, clients with mouth sores, esophageal blockage (cancer, stenosis), or a history of radiotherapy or chemotherapy for cancers of the neck or throat are also at increased risk. Clients may need to be on a dysphagia diet, such as with soft foods and thickened liquids, and should eat with supervision while sitting upright.

Risks for Insufficient Vascular Perfusion

Risk for **insufficient vascular perfusion** include:

- **Immobilized limb**: Usually the result of trauma, which may involve the muscles, bones, ligaments, tendons, vasculature, and nerves—all of which may result in insufficient vascular perfusion—so the limb must be assessed frequently for delayed capillary filling, pallor, edema, and sensory changes. Muscle mass may decrease rapidly even with isometric exercises, and the movement needed to promote adequate venous return is missing. In the case of extended generalized immobility, the client should be put on DVT prophylactic precautions such as a subcutaneous blood thinner (Heparin) and sequential compression devices or compression stockings to prevent clotting and promote perfusion.
- **Post-operative status**: Many conditions associated with surgical repair may result in insufficient vascular perfusion—hypoventilation, hyper- or hypovolemia, mechanical obstruction of blood flow, hypoxemia, and decreased hemoglobin resulting from bleeding. Capillary refill may exceed 3 seconds, and the client may exhibit dysrhythmias, dyspnea, abnormal ABGs, behavior changes, altered mental status, cooling and pallor of skin, weak/absent pulses, cyanosis, and edema as well as oliguria/anuria.
- **Diabetes**: Often associated with atherosclerosis, neuropathy, and hypertension, and peripheral arterial disease, increasing risk of ulcers because of impaired perfusion.

Indications of Output Changes from Baseline

Indications of **output changes** from baseline include:

- **NG tube**: Drainage per the NG tube should be light yellow/green but volume may vary so it's necessary to monitor both volume and electrolytes to determine what is normal for the client. Reddish or coffee-ground drainage may indicate bleeding, which may increase volume.
- **Emesis**: Clients should not have emesis, so the volume of any emesis must be recorded and steps taken to determine cause and treat.
- **Stool**: Fecal output may range from 3-4 daily to one every 2-3 days, so the client's normal output should be assessed through history. If diarrhea occurs, then the frequency and volume must be noted as the client may develop dehydration. Constipation lasting longer than several days can be common post-operatively or with a patient on narcotic pain medication, and may require a stool softener. This client should also be monitored for the possibility of an ileus.
- **Urine**: Normal urinary output varies from 800 to 2000 mL per day (with intake of 2000 mL), depending on age, condition, and intake. Careful I & O should be done to establish an output that is normal for the client so that variations can be detected.

Post-Procedure Complications After Cardiac Catheterization

Post-procedure complications of cardiac catheterization include:

- **Catheterization**: Dysrhythmias (ventricular arrhythmias, atrial fibrillation, conduction abnormalities, and bradycardia) may develop during or after cardiac catheterization caused by irritation of cardiac tissue. Incidence may vary depending on where the tip of the catheter lies. Risks are highest for clients with a history of congenital heart disease and history of ECG abnormalities. In most cases, these abnormalities revert to normal sinus rhythm, but they may require immediate intervention. Some may experience an allergic response to contrast medium.

- **Surgical/Insertion site**: Bleeding may occur at insertion site (hematoma/retroperitoneal bleeding), arterial tearing (development of pseudoaneurysm), clot dislodgement (resulting in myocardial infarction or stroke), arterial occlusion (especially of radial artery), and infection (at insertion site, endocarditis). The surgical site should be assessed frequently (per facility protocol) for any signs of bleeding.

Stages of Blood Loss/Hypovolemia

Stage	Blood loss	Indications
1	15% 750 mL	Client may appear pale but vital signs, urinary output, and capillary refill may remain within normal limits.
2	15-30% 1500 mL	Pallor may increase with skin becoming cool and clammy. Diastolic blood pressure may increase and heart rate to >100 beats per minute. The client may appear anxious. Capillary refill is delayed but urinary output remains at 20 to 30 mL per hour.
3	30-40% 5000-2000 mL	Client becoming increasingly confused with altered mental status and diaphoresis. Systolic BP drops to below 100 and tachycardia increases to >120 beats per minute. Client is dyspneic with respirations >30 per minute. Capillary refill remains delayed but urinary output remains about 20 mL per hour.
4	>40% >2000 mL	Client increasingly lethargic and may become comatose, remains diaphoretic but skin mottling may be evident. Pulse is thready at >140 beats per minutes and systolic BP falls to below 70. Respirations are very shallow and rapid. Capillary refill is absent and urinary output is negligible or absent.

Procedures That Require Specific Positioning Post-Operatively

Procedures that require specific **post-operative positioning** to prevent complications include:

- **Angiography**: If an extremity is used, place restraint to keep the extremity straight for 6 to 8 hours.
- **Bronchoscopy**: Place in in semi-Fowler's position to prevent aspiration.
- **Myelogram**: With air contrast, place in Trendelenburg position; with oil contrast, place flat for 6 to 8 hours; with water-based contrast, place with head of bed elevated for 8 hours.
- **Liver biopsy**: Position on right side with pillow placed beneath the puncture site.
- Arteriovenous fistula formation: Elevate extremity.
- **Abdominal aneurysm**: Elevate head of bed to ≤45 degrees.
- **Ear irrigation**: Position client on affected side to promote drainage.
- **Lumbar puncture**: Keep flat for 4 to 12 hours.
- **Appendectomy**: Place in Fowler's position.
- **Cataract removal**: Place in semi-Fowler's or Fowler's position on back or opposite side of surgery.
- **Kidney transplant**: Place in Semi-Fowler's position on back or turned to opposite side of surgery.
- **Mitral valve replacement**: Place in semi-Fowler's position.
- **Thyroidectomy**: Place in high Fowler's or semi-Fowlers.
- **Tonsillectomy**: Prone or side-lying.

- **Amputation of leg (AK, BK)**: Elevate limb for 24 hours. Place in prone position at least two times daily.
- **Insertion nasogastric tube**: Keep head elevated to at least 30 degrees.

Insertion and Removal of NG/OG Tube

Procedure for **insertion and removal of nasogastric or orogastric** tube:

1. Gather PPE and equipment (stethoscope, lubricant, syringe, tape, suction if ordered, and pH strips) and carry out hand hygiene.
2. Assess nostrils for patency (if NG tube), abdomen for bowel sounds, and level of consciousness for ability to follow directions.
3. Position client at 45 to 90 degrees if possible.
4. Measure NG/OG tube from tip of nose to ear and from ear to xiphoid process and mark tube.
5. Apply clean non-sterile gloves. Flush tube with water or lubricate 3-4 inches with water-soluble lubricant. Curl tube in circles around fingers and then release to ensure proper curvature.
6. Ask client to drop chin down and breathe orally if NG tube. Insert NG tube (curved side down) into nostril and guide downward. Guide OG tube along back of tongue and downward with client breathing through nose. Twist tubes slightly if resistance encountered.
7. Ask client to sip water (if allowed) or dry swallow while tube is advanced nasally or to swallow only if using OG tube.
8. Secure with tape and aspirate contents for pH testing (should be <5).
9. Verify placement with x-ray. If properly placed, measure length of NG/OG tube from where it leaves the nostril/mouth to end.

To remove NG/OG, gather supplies, carry out hand hygiene, clear NG/OG tube by injecting 10-20 mL air, remove any tape and clips, ask client to take and hold a deep breath, and gently pull out in one steady motion.

Procedures for Insertion and Removal of Urinary Catheter

Procedure for **inserting and removing urinary catheter**:

1. Gather supplies (catheter insertion kit), perform hand hygiene, and place waterproof pad under client, ensure light source is adequate to view urinary meatus.
2. Place female on back with knees flexed and male in supine position.
3. Apply gloves and wash perineal area with soap and water, rinse, and dry.
4. Remove gloves and wash hands. Prepare drainage bag and tubing if indwelling catheter to be inserted.
5. Using aseptic technique, place catheter kit near client or between legs, open and apply sterile gloves from kit.
6. Apply drapes, cleanse urethral meatus with antiseptic from kit.
7. Insert catheter with drainage end attached to bag or in collection tray. For males, insert 7.5-10 cm and for females 5 to 7.5 cm or until urine flows freely.
8. Indwelling catheter, inflate balloon to required volume with sterile water.
9. Secure catheter and connect to tubing and drainage back if not already connected.

REMOVAL: Straight catheter—remove by pulling out slowly. To remove indwelling catheter, deflate the balloon using the appropriate port and gently pull the catheter out.

Procedures for Insertion and Removal of Fecal Management System

Fecal management devices are used for incontinent clients with loose or watery stools in order to prevent skin breakdown, discomfort, odor, and contamination of wounds, and to control the spread of organisms, such as *Clostridium difficile,* in bedridden or immobile clients. A number of different devices, such as the Flexi-Seal® FMS, are available and work similarly. A typical management system includes:

- Silicone catheter, silicone retention balloon at end of catheter, a 45-mL syringe, and charcoal filter collection bags.

The application of the fecal management system is relatively simple: The catheter is manually inserted into the rectum and balloon inflated with water or saline (using the 45 mL syringe) to hold it in place and to block fecal leakage. Some systems, such as Flexi-Seal® FMS, have a pop-up button to indicate when the balloon is adequately filled for the size of the rectum. The catheter contains an irrigation port so that irrigating fluid can be instilled if necessary. The charcoal filter collection bag is attached to the end of the silicone catheter to contain fecal material.

Maintaining Patency of Tubes

Procedures for **maintaining patency of tubes** include:

- **NG tube**: Flush with 30 to 50 mL of warm water or NS every 4 to 6 hours and before and after feeding or medications. Ensure tubing is not kinked if attached to drainage and check clamp. Gentle milking or massaging the tube may help to loosen any residue.
- **Chest tube**: Ensure that tubes are not kinked or dislodged and that clamp is open and fluid has not collected in dependent loops. Keep chest drainage unit below level of client's chest. Ensure water levels are correct. Aggressive milking/stripping can result in negative pressure and damage to tissue and should be avoided. If clots are evident, gently squeezing and releasing the tube hand by hand along the length may prevent occlusion.
- **Percutaneous endoscopic gastrostomy tube**: Care is similar to that for the NG tube with tube flushed before and after feedings, medications, and every 4 to 6 hours.

Thromboembolism

Thromboembolism includes both the formation of a thrombus (such as in the heart with A-fib and in the deep veins with immobilization) and embolism in which a clot breaks off and travels through the circulatory system. While thromboembolism may cause a heart attack or stroke, the most common presentation is a pulmonary embolism resulting from deep vein thrombosis.

Signs and symptoms: generally asymptomatic; pain at the thrombus site, which may be swollen and erythematous, typically in the lower extremity. When the patient develops pulmonary embolism, the usual presentation is acute onset of dyspnea. Some patients may have frothy sputum, cough, fever, and/or hemoptysis as well.

Diagnosis: Includes laboratory tests (CBC, troponins, D-dimer, ABGs, and BNP), ultrasound, spiral CT, pulmonary angiography, and ventilation/perfusion scanning.

Treatment: Includes anticoagulants, thrombolytic therapy, oxygen, and thrombectomy.

Prevention: smoking cessation, regular exercise, discontinuation of birth control pills, early ambulation after surgery, SCDs/compression hose, control of high blood pressure, treatment for peripheral arterial disease, and avoiding prolonged sitting.

Review Video: DVT - Prevention and Treatment
Visit mometrix.com/academy and enter code: 352193

Endocarditis

Endocarditis is inflammation of the endocardium and heart valves, caused by fungi, virus, or bacteria. Factors that may contribute to infectious endocarditis include history of valvular disease, surgical procedures, immunosuppressive drug therapy such as steroids, and heroin addiction. Infectious endocarditis also may be caused by extensive indwelling catheters (PICC/central lines), and prolonged IV antibiotics.

Signs and symptoms: weakness/fatigue, fever, heart murmur, dyspnea, night sweats, Janeway lesions (red spots on palms), Osler nodes (painful lesions), joint pain, splinter hemorrhages in fingernails.

Diagnosis: CBC, ESR, ECG, blood cultures, TEE, MRI, physical exam.

Treatment includes:

- IV antibiotics; plasmapheresis.
- Surgery may be indicated for valve replacement.
- Monitor the patient for jaundice, arrhythmias, CHF, glomerulonephritis, emboli.

Prevention: needle-exchange programs, *take antibiotics before dental procedures if high-risk (e.g., history of heart valve replacement.).*

Potential Sources of Infection for Transplant Patients

Infections pose a serious threat to **transplant patients**, especially during the first year. While opportunistic infections have decreased, nosocomial infections have increased, most related to bacterial infections. Transplant patients consistently show higher rates of infection than other patients. There are numerous potential sources:

- **Donor-infected organs** can transmit HBV, HBC, herpesvirus, HIV, and human T-cell leukemia virus type I. Additionally, donors who are immunocompromised prior to harvesting of the organs may have nosocomial bacterial or fungal infections that can be transmitted. Organs can also become infected during harvesting.
- **Health care workers** may transmit pathogens through droplets, airborne particles, or contact, frequently transmitting pathogens on their hands or clothing.
- **Blood and blood products** can transmit CMV, but transmission is rare. HCV transmission has been reduced to <1%.
- **Environmental reservoir sources** can include the water system, demolition activities, equipment, and surfaces. Some pathogens, such as MRSA and VRE, may be endemic to the hospital environment.

Common Viral Pathogens in Transplant Patients

Several **viral infections** are more likely to occur in transplant patients due to their immunocompromised state:

- **Cytomegalovirus (CMV)**: the most common pathogen related to transplant infections, affecting 40%-90% of recipients.
- **Herpes simplex virus**: reactivated/new - may disseminate to liver.
- **Human herpesvirus-6** – mostly reactivation, newer strain.
- **Varicella-zoster virus**: new – may disseminate to viscera.
- **Hepatitis B and C viruses**: causes liver failure; also affects kidney transplant patients.
- **BK virus (BKV)**: causes renal dysfunction; transmission unknown.
- **Adenoviruses (AdV)**: bone marrow transplant; can become systemic.

Prevention is as follows:

- **Serologic matching** can prevent primary transmission but the limited supply of organs may make this impractical.
- **Early diagnosis** with serum assay for targeted treatment.
- *Antiviral prophylaxis* in high-risk patients can be effective.
- **Immunization** has proven to be safe and highly effective, reducing the incidence of infection and the severity.
- **Immunoglobulin** is given to susceptible transplant patients exposed to certain viruses.
- Reduction in immunosuppressive medications if possible.
- **High-dose acyclovir** for some viruses may reduce severity of infection.
- Targeting patients at the highest risk of disease through surveillance and using proper transmission-based precautions are the most practical methods of infection control.

Common Bacterial Infections After Transplant Surgery

Staphylococcus aureus is the most common cause of bacterial infection in liver, heart, kidney, and pancreas transplant patients. Intravascular cannulas cause about 54% of MRSA infections, but nosocomial transmission occurs.

Vancomycin-resistant enterococci (VRE) causes 10%-15% of liver failures, according to recent studies. Nosocomial transmission occurs frequently, especially with prolonged hospitalization and ICU stay. VRE colonization puts patients at continued risk of infection and poses a reservoir for nosocomial infections.

Nocardia is found in the soil and decaying vegetation, and transmission is through inhalation. Lung, heart, and intestinal transplants have the highest rates of infection. Mortality rates are high for those who are infected. Risk factors include high-dose cortisone, high levels of immunosuppressants, and CMV infection within 6 months.

Infection control strategies include:

- *Handwashing* and basic clean technique are still the best methods of infection control in these patients.
- Environmental monitoring.
- Antibiotic prophylaxis is effective.

Electroconvulsive Therapy

Electroconvulsive therapy is administered in the morning with the client NPO to reduce the risk of vomiting and subsequent aspiration and with short-acting anesthesia and muscle relaxant intravenously. Electrode pads are placed on the side of the head and the shock, lasting 1-2 seconds, can be administered unilaterally or bilaterally, causing a brief seizure. After ECT, the client usually awakens within 5-10 minutes. A few hours of confusion are common, so the client must be carefully monitored and reoriented. Once completely awake, the client may dress, eat, and return home or to the hospital room. Immediately after treatment, side effects may include headaches, transient confusion, muscle soreness, nausea, and vomiting or jaw pain. ECT can also cause some memory loss, which may worsen over the course of treatment and may include retrograde amnesia, causing partial or complete memory loss of for events occurring days, weeks, months or occasionally years before the procedure. The client will need reassurance and support. The amnesia will usually resolve within a few months after treatment ends. ECT may cause tachycardia, hypertension, and in rare cases, death, so the client should be monitored carefully after treatment.

Aspergillus Fungal Infection After Transplant Surgery

Aspergillus infections primarily involve pneumonia and sinusitis, but 25%-35% disseminate systemically, and *Aspergillus* pneumonia infections have mortality rates up to 85%. *Aspergillus* is a serious fungal infection in immunocompromised transplant patients, especially lung transplant patients with 8% infection rates within 9 months of surgery. Liver transplant patients have infection rates of 1%-4% but disease occurs earlier, within 2-4 weeks. Heart transplant infection rates are 1%-6% with disease within 1-2 months. Aspergillus affects renal transplants the least with <1% infection rates. Prophylaxis with antifungals has not proven to be effective.

Infection control strategies include:

- *Monitoring environment and improving air filtration* with HEPA filtration or use of laminar air flow rooms for patients at high risk.
- *Construction precautions* to prevent dust and debris from circulating in patient care areas.

Standard precautions include high-resolution CT scans for early diagnosis rather than chest x-rays so treatment with voriconazole (drug of choice) can begin.

Infection Control Strategies for Spinal Cord Injuries

Infection control strategies for neurology/spinal cord injuries target the most common types of infection:

- **Urinary tract infection***:* Patients should be monitored for fever and/or changes in spasms or voiding habits that may indicate infection. When possible, intermittent catheterization (sterile rather than clean while in the hospital) should be used rather than continuous. Antibiotic prophylaxis has not proven to be effective but bacterial interference, colonizing of the urinary tract with nonpathogenic *E. coli* 83972, has shown promising results.
- **Decubital ulcers***:* Procedures for regular monitoring of skin condition, turning patients, and avoiding friction to prevent pressure from developing are critical. Both staff and patients must be educated about prevention, skin care, and cleanliness. Nutrition and hydration must be adequate to maintain integrity of the skin.
- **Respiratory infections**: Proper use of ventilation equipment must be monitored. Assisted coughing, such as through respiratory therapy and postural drainage, can reduce infections. Prophylactic antibiotics are not recommended, but patients should receive immunizations for pneumonia.

System-Specific Assessments

ASSESSMENT OF THE NEUROLOGICAL SYSTEM

Assessment of the neurological system should begin by evaluation of the patient's mental status and speaking ability to determine if the patient is oriented, as well as level of consciousness (alert, lethargic, obtunded, stuporous, or comatose). The physical examination should continue with examination of the cranial nerves (I–XII), which includes assessment of smell, visual abilities, facial movement, hearing, swallowing, voice, and speech. Then the motor system is assessed, including evaluation of position of the body, involuntary movements, muscle strength, muscle tone, flexion, extension, stability, and gait. Assessment of the sensory system includes evaluation of pain, temperature, position, vibration, light touch, position, and discrimination. The reflexes are assessed and graded on a scale of 0 (no response) to 2+ (normal) to 4+ (hyperactive). Reflexes include biceps reflex (evaluates C5 and C6), triceps reflex (C6 and C7), brachioradialis reflex (C5, C6), knee reflex (L2, L3, L4), ankle reflex (S1), and plantar response (L5, S1).

NEUROLOGICAL EXAM

The **neurological exam** helps determine the person's neurological health, and diagnose dementia/delirium/brain stem injury, and many other disorders. It includes:

- **Level of Consciousness (LOC)**: most important piece of the neurological exam, and often the only level of exam completed on a regular basis during nursing assessments.
  - *Arousal/Level of Alertness:* Assess as you walk into the room; may require noxious stimuli (sternal rub, nail-bed pressure).
    - Alert → Lethargic → Obtunded → Stuporous → Comatose
  - *Awareness*: Patient's orientation to person, place, and time.
- **Advanced Neuro Screening:** this is used for patients with known or suspected neurological deficit (e.g., stroke) who can respond to questions. May include NIH Stroke Scale in some facilities. Assessments may include:
  - *Orientation* to time, place, person, and purpose of visit.
  - *Following commands*/the use of language (fluency of spontaneous speech).
  - *Naming objects* such as a pen or watch; repetition of rhymes (e.g., "Mary had a little lamb"); checking for slurred speech and dysarthria.
  - *Short-term/long-term memory* (ask the patient to recall three items, such as, "rose, umbrella, truck," minutes after hearing the words).
  - Bilateral strength and coordination testing.

GLASGOW COMA SCALE AND GRADING OF DEEP TENDON REFLEXES

The **Glasgow Coma Scale (GCS)** is used to measure level of consciousness (LOC) and extent of brain injury. There are 3 components:

1. **Eye opening**: Spontaneous 4, To voice 3, To pain 2, None 1.
2. **Verbal response**: Oriented 5, Confused 4, wrong words 3, unintelligible 2, None 1.
3. **Motor response**: Obeys commands 6, Localizes pain 5, Withdraws from pain 4, Flexion (decorticate) 3, Extension (decerebrate) 2, None 1.

   Scoring guide (3-15): Mild, ≥13; Moderate, 9 to 12; Severe, ≤8.

Reflexes are graded 0 to 4, where 0 is absent, 1 is reduced, 2 is normal, 3 is increased, and 4 is clonus. Reflexes are tested over the biceps, triceps, brachioradialis, quadriceps, and Achilles tendons.

- *Reflexes graded 0 and 1* indicate lower motor neuron damage (ie, damage to anterior horn cell, anterior nerve root, peripheral nerve, or neuromuscular junction of muscle).
- *Reflexes graded 3 and 4* indicate an upper motor neuron damage (ie, in the cerebrum, brain stem or spinal cord).

Babinski Reflex

Babinski reflex occurs when the great toe flexes toward the top of the foot and the other toes fan out after the sole of the foot has been firmly stroked. This reflex is normal in infants, disappearing at the age of 2.

In people older than 2 years, the presence of a Babinski's reflex indicates damage to the brain/nervous system. The reflex can be temporary or permanent depending on the extent of the damage. Any condition in which there is suspected neurological insult warrants testing for a Babinski reflex; if found, further testing should be done immediately to determine the cause and extent of the damage.

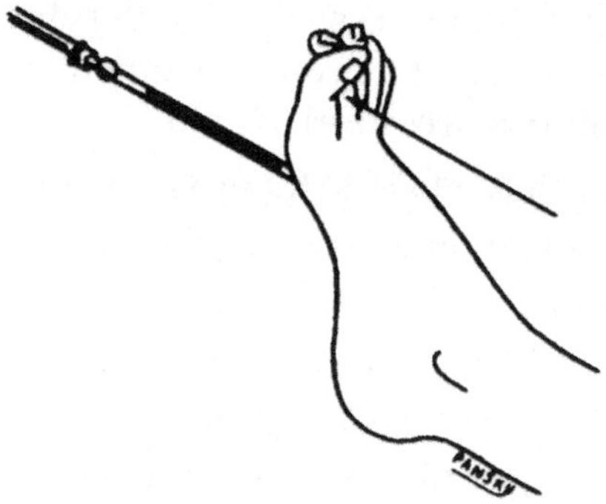

Positive (+) Babinski sign
(dorsiflexion of big toe)

Decorticate and Decerebrate Positioning

Decorticate and **decerebrate** posturing are caused by varying levels of damage to the brain/brain stem. If either of these postures is observed, it should be considered a medical emergency and reported immediately.

Decorticate (Flexion) Posturing

The patient will have the following: flexion of the head and trunk, adduction and internal rotation of the arms, pronation and flexion of the forearm, flexion of the wrists and fingers, flexion of the hips, knees, ankles, and toes, internal rotation of the legs, and inversion of the feet.

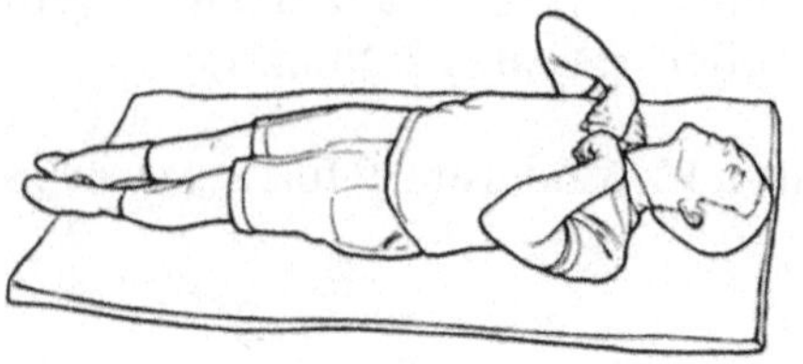

Decerebrate (Extension) Posturing

The patient will have the following: extension and internal rotation of all four extremities and may also show extension of the body and head (**opisthotonus**). Decerebrate posturing indicates a lesion of the midbrain or lower. It is also associated with a mortality rate of 70%.

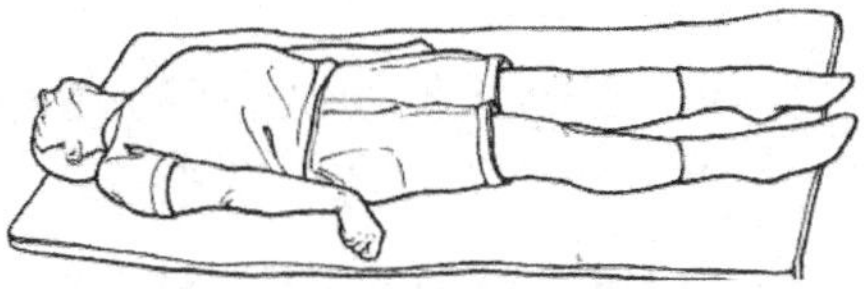

Assessment of the Cardiovascular System

Assessment of the cardiovascular system should begin with a health history and evaluation of any chest pain, including the location, duration, severity, and aggravating/alleviating factors. Topics to review include medications, nutrition, activities, exercise, emotional status, and sleep patterns. Physical assessment should include evaluation of the patient's general appearance and skin condition and color (noting any pallor, ecchymosis, or cyanosis). BP should be taken in supine and sitting position with 1-3 minutes between readings. Pulse rate should be evaluated both peripherally and per auscultation, noting the pulse quality on a scale of 0 (absent) to 4+ (bounding and strong), configuration, and rhythm. The heart sounds should be assessed for normal sounds (S1 and S2) and abnormal sounds (S3, S4, opening snaps, clicks, and murmurs). Jugular venous distention should be noted. The extremities should be examined with capillary refill time and any vascular changes noted, including weak or absent peripheral pulses. Edema should be evaluated by applying firm pressure for 5 seconds and then assessing on a 0 (absent) to 4+ (pitting >8 mm) scale.

Review Video: Cardiovascular Assessment
Visit mometrix.com/academy and enter code: 234630

Normal Blood Flow Through the Heart

Normal blood flow through the heart is described as follows:

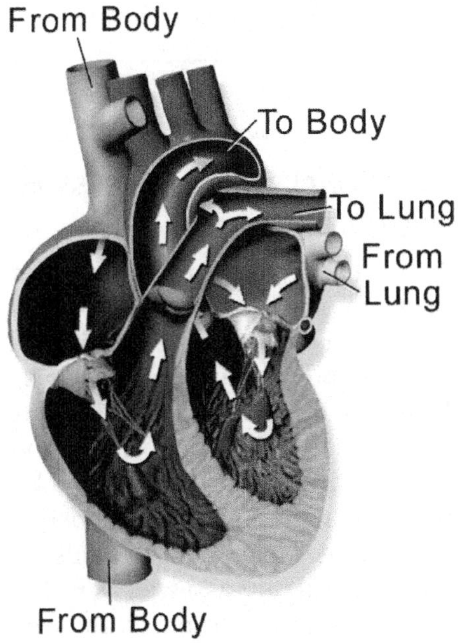

- Deoxygenated venous blood returns to the heart per the superior vena cava, inferior vena cava, and coronary sinus (bringing blood from the coronary arteries) into the right atrium.
- When the atrium is full, it contracts and the blood flows through the tricuspid valve into the right ventricle.
- When the right ventricle is full, it contracts and blood flows through the pulmonic valve into the pulmonary artery and to the lungs.
- The oxygenated blood then flows from the lungs through the pulmonary veins and into the left atrium. When the left atrium is full, it contracts and blood flows through the mitral valve into the left ventricle.
- Once full, the left ventricle contracts and the blood flows through the aortic valve and into the aorta and the coronary arteries and general circulation.

After blood flows through the valves, the valves close to prevent backflow. Both atria and both ventricles contract simultaneously.

Review Video: Heart Anatomy and Physiology
Visit mometrix.com/academy and enter code: 257818

Review Video: Heart Anatomy Mnemonics
Visit mometrix.com/academy and enter code: 258105

Review Video: Heart Blood Flow & Heart Anatomy Review
Visit mometrix.com/academy and enter code: 256281

Interventions for Circulatory Complications

Interventions for **circulatory complications** include:

- **Hemorrhage**: Identify and treat the cause. Apply pressure to site of external bleeding; administer blood, blood products, autotransfusion, colloids (such as plasma protein fraction), and/or crystalloids (such as normal saline); provide oxygen; utilize intubation and ventilation if necessary; monitor VS, hemoglobin and hematocrit; and administer medications, such as vasopressors (dopamine).
- **Embolus** (lung and brain are common sites): If lungs, position with head elevated, administer oxygen, monitor respiratory status and VS carefully, administer anticoagulants or thrombolytics (embolectomy may be indicated if client remains unstable), provide supportive care (such as compression stockings and moderate exercise) to prevent DVT. If brain, monitor VS and physical signs (paralysis, weakness), provide IV fluids, and administer thrombolytics.
- **Shock**: Identify and treat underlying cause, determine type of shock, monitor VS, provide rapid fluid administration (usually with 0.25-0.5L NS or isotonic crystalloid as needed to 2-3 L or blood products (if hemorrhaging), administer vasopressors (such as dopamine), provide oxygen through intubation and ventilation if necessary.

Review Video: Ventilators
Visit mometrix.com/academy and enter code: 322835

Additional System Assessments

Pulmonary System

Assessment of the pulmonary system should begin with a health history focusing on respiratory problems, such as dyspnea, cough, sputum production, chest pain, wheezing, hemoptysis, and lifestyle choices that are risk factors, such as smoking. The upper respiratory structures (nose, sinuses, mouth, pharynx, and trachea) should be examined and palpated. The patient's chest should be exposed and the patient in supine position for examination of the anterior thorax and in sitting position if possible, for examination of posterior thorax. Assessment includes observation of the rate, rhythm, depth, and effort of breathing and the patient's color. The fingers should be examined for clubbing and skin for cyanosis. Examination should include inspection, palpation, auscultation, and percussion of the lung fields. Normal breathing sounds (vesicular, bronchovesicular, bronchial, and tracheal) are assessed as well as abnormal sounds (fine or coarse crackles, wheezes, sibilant rhonchi, sonorous rhonchi, and friction rubs). Pulse oximetry is used to determine oxygen saturation.

Gastrointestinal System

Assessment of the gastrointestinal system should begin with a health history focused on GI problems, such as constipation, diarrhea, abdominal pain, nausea, flatus, and change in bowel habits. The mouth should be examined (removing dentures), including lips, gums, and tongue, using a tongue blade to depress the tongue so that the back of the mouth can be viewed. The abdomen should be examined with the patient in supine position with knees flexed. Auscultation is used to assess bowel sounds (*normal* are sounds every 5 to 20 seconds, *hypoactive* is less frequent, and *hyperactive* more frequent.). Percussion is used to assess internal organs and determine the presence of masses. Light palpation is utilized to determine areas of tenderness and deeper palpation to assess masses. The patient may be placed in knee-chest, left lateral, or standing with hips flexed positions for a rectal examination. A digital rectal exam should include asking the patient to bear down so that abnormalities, such as hemorrhoids, are easier to detect.

Review Video: GI Diagnostic Procedures
Visit mometrix.com/academy and enter code: 683920

Genitourinary System

Assessment of the genitourinary system should begin with a health history that includes sexually transmitted infections, urinary infections, incontinence, pain, dysuria, and sexual history including dysfunctions such as impotence and ejaculatory disorders. The external genitalis should be examined. The female reproductive system is usually assessed as distinct from the urinary system and requires a breast examination and pelvic examination. The genitourinary system includes the male genitals because of their proximity and dual function as part of the reproductive system and the urinary system. Physical assessment of the male should include a testicular and digital rectal examination. Assessment of the urinary system should begin with palpation of the bladder (which can usually only be felt if distended) and kidneys (although usually only part of the right kidney can be palpated in normal kidneys). Any tenderness in flank areas should be noted. If bladder percussion yields a dull sound following the patient's urination, this can indicate incomplete emptying of the bladder.

Integumentary System

Assessment of the integumentary system should begin with health history that includes history of any allergic skin disorders, skin conditions, and skin cancer and direct observation of the entire skin area, including inspection of the inside of the mouth, the scalp, and the nails. The nurse should wear gloves if any rash or lesions are present. Skin color should be assessed, noting erythema, jaundice, cyanosis, or other discolorations. If the patient has a rash or pruritus, the area involved should be carefully examined, noting any differences in skin texture or elevations (such as may occur with a rash). Skin lesions should be carefully documented, including size, shape, and appearance. Vascular changes, such as petechia, ecchymosis, and angiomas should be noted. Both fingernails and toenails should be examined for changes, including ridging or hypertrophy, and signs of paronychia noted. The angle between the nail and its base should be assessed (normal is 160 degrees). Hair should be examined (while wearing gloves) for color, texture, distribution, and loss.

Review Video: Integumentary System
Visit mometrix.com/academy and enter code: 655980

Peripheral Edema

Edema is usually checked by pressing the index finger into the tissue on top of each foot, behind the medial malleolus, and over the shin, starting distally and moving proximally to the highest level of edema, comparing both legs:

- **Edema** is rated on a 1-to-4-point scale:
  - 1+ slight pitting to about 2 mm (persists 10-15 seconds).
  - 2+ moderate pitting to about 4 mm (persists 10-15 seconds).
  - 3+ moderate-severe pitting to about 6 mm (persists >1 minute).
  - 4+ severe pitting to 8 mm or more (persists 2-5 minutes).
- **Venous edema**: edema from ankle to knee and may involve some limitation in ankle movement. Dependent pitting edema occurs, but may become non-pitting in chronic disease. Treatment includes diuretics, elevation, and compression stockings.
- **Lymphedema**: usually unilateral non-pitting hard edema from toes to groin or fingers to shoulder. In advanced disease, elephantiasis with huge enlargement of extremity may occur. Treatment includes massage, light exercise, compression garments, and pneumatic compression.

Delayed Wound Healing

Delayed wound healing occurs when a wound does not progress at a predictable rate through homeostasis, inflammation, proliferation, and remodeling. Wounds with healing by first intention (wound completely closed) should heal more rapidly than those left all or completely open. Indications of delayed wound healing include:

- **Scabs/Crusts**: May interfere with healing if forming over the wound. The wound should be kept moist with dressings that retain moisture to promote epithelialization.
- **Infection**: Slows the healing processes and may result in deterioration of wound. Wound must be observed carefully for signs of infection (erythema, edema, pain, purulent discharge) and appropriate wound care and/or antibiotic therapy initiated when needed to treat infection.
- **Necrotic tissue**: Slough and eschar must be removed for healing to take place adequately because they can cause the wound to breakdown further.
- **Pallor/Cyanosis**: Poor circulation to the area of the wound may result in poor healing because of inadequate blood supply and oxygenation.

Therapeutic Procedures

Alternate Wound-Closure Therapies

Described below are alternate wound-closure therapies:

- Whirlpool/Hydrotherapy
  - Vasodilation: blood flow brings oxygen, nutrients, white blood cells, and antibiotics to the tissues and removes metabolites.
  - Mechanical effects of whirlpool stimulate granulation tissue formation; also softens necrotic tissue/aids phagocytosis.
  - Sedation and analgesia are induced by the warm water.

- Used for: necrotic/wounds with heavy exudate or debris; tissue that can tolerate increased circulatory perfusion. **Contraindications:** edema, altered LOC, infection, fever, maceration, phlebitis, compromised cardiovascular/pulmonary function, renal failure, and incontinence.

- Vacuum-assisted closure/negative-pressure wound therapy
  - Special foam dressing with an attached evacuation tube is inserted into the wound and covered with an adhesive drape in order to create an airtight seal; removes excess fluid/reduces edema.
  - Increases vascularity/promotes formation of granulation tissue.
  - **Used for:** pressure ulcers/chronic wounds; surgical wounds/large and open wounds with excess exudate or drainage.
- Hyperbaric oxygen therapy
  - Systemic therapy where a patient enters a pressurized room or chamber to breathe 100% oxygen.
  - Increases the blood plasma levels of dissolved oxygen, which, in turn, delivers increases oxygen delivery to body tissues via perfusion.
  - **Used for**: dry/gas gangrene, skin grafts/flaps, crush injury, wounds not responding to more conservative treatment. Also used for decompression sickness, air or gas embolism, and carbon monoxide poisoning.

Caring for a Client Recovering from Anesthesia

Responsibilities when caring for a client **recovering from anesthesia** include:

- **Local**: Check for signs of swelling, hematoma. Check peripheral circulation if procedure in extremity. Note degree of numbness and level of pain. Provide pain medication if indicated when pain first begins rather than waiting for anesthesia to completely wear off.
- **Regional** (epidural, spinal, nerve block): Maintain client in flat position for spinal/epidural blocks for several hours (usually about 6) to prevent spinal headache from leakage of spinal fluid from the meninges. (An epidural blood patch may be applied to the epidural space if headaches persist.) Monitor vital signs. Note degree and extent of numbness and sensation. Evaluate lower extremities for circulation (color, capillary refill, edema, temperature, pulses). Position client carefully.
- **General**: Monitor vital signs, level of consciousness, and respiratory status. Monitor level of pain and administer analgesic as indicated. Position clients with nausea in side-lying position but maintain positioning required by the procedure (for example, keep the head elevated for those with brain surgery).

Care Measures for Musculoskeletal Conditions

Appropriate care measures for **musculoskeletal conditions** include:

- **Logrolling**: Requires two nurses positioned on the same side of the client. Place arm on side that the client is to turn above head or over chest. Place the other arm across the chest. Stand close to client. The nurse near the head reaches across client and grasps the shoulders and the mid-trunk while the second nurse grasps hips and legs. On count of three, they turn the client in one smooth move.
- **Abdominal pillow**: Used to provide support by holding against the abdomen when coughing and sneezing after abdominal surgery, such as C-section, cholecystectomy, gastric surgery, and hernia repair. May contain pockets for cold or hot packs to help to relieve discomfort.

- **Casted extremity**: Observe for signs of drainage penetrating cast, smell for unusual or foul odor, and feel for areas of cold or heat. Pain should be noted and area pinpointed. Examine fingers/toes for color, edema, and capillary refill as well as sensation of touch. Note peripheral pulses, including absence or presence and strength.

DIALYSIS

Dialysis is a process by which the blood is artificially filters to get rid of waste products. It is mainly used for patients with partial or total kidney failure, using one of two processes.

In the **hemodialysis process**, blood is taken from the patient via an access site, most often a fistula or graft in the arm. The blood runs through a machine called a dialyzer, which removes waste products then returns it to the patient through the same access site. Most patients that require hemodialysis go to a hospital or specialized hemodialysis center three days a week.

During **peritoneal dialysis**, a cleansing solution is placed into the abdominal cavity, where it is kept for some time to absorb waste. After a catheter is surgically installed in the abdominal wall, the patient can begin cycling cleansing solution in and out of the abdominal cavity, usually 3-5 times per day. When this process is done autonomously by the patient, it is known as continuous ambulatory peritoneal dialysis (CAPD). When done by a machine, it is known as continuous cyclic peritoneal dialysis (CCPD). Because there is a higher risk of infection involved with peritoneal dialysis, the patient should report bloody (if not menstruating) or cloudy dialysate, or symptoms of abdominal cramps, chills, or fever immediately.

LITHOTRIPSY

Lithotripsy is a procedure that utilizes extracorporeal shock waves to break up stones, usually kidney stones, although it may be utilized for gallstones as well. The procedure is usually carried out with some type of anesthesia (local, general, regional) and takes 45 to 60 minutes. The patient is positioned in a tub of water or more commonly on a special cushioned table through which the shock waves pass. This procedure is more effective for small stones than large. Patients often experience some discomfort and hematuria after the procedure as the fragments of fractured stones make their way through the urinary tract and are excreted in urine. In some cases, the procedure must be repeated. Lithotripsy is used less often now in favor of ureteroscopy, which directly removes the stones. However, there are more complications, such as bleeding or perforation, which may occur with ureteroscopy.

Physiological Adaptation

Alterations in Body Systems

Side Effects of Radiation Therapy

Delayed-onset side effects of radiotherapy depend on the type of radiation, dosage, and area of the body irradiated. Typical problems include:

- **Skin irritation**: Ranging from mild redness and itching to blistering, peeling, and severe burns and ulcerations. Onset is usually within 7-14 days of beginning radiotherapy. Management includes bathing with warm (not hot) water, patting dry, and avoiding applications of heat or cold to irradiated areas. Clients should wear loose clothing. Topical antibiotics may be needed for infection. Aloe gel, RadiaCare Gel®, topical steroids, and Aquaphor may help soothe skin between treatments.
- **Fatigue**: Onset is within a few weeks of beginning radiotherapy. Management include adequate rest periods and avoid over-exertion.
- **Head/neck issues**: Dry mouth may lead to dental problems. Dysphagia may result from fibrosis, edema, or narrowing of the throat. Management includes, mouth rinses for dry mouth, avoidance of whitening toothpastes, small soft meals for dysphagia, moisturizer, soft-bristled toothbrushes and avoidance of dental floss.
- **Chest issues**: Problems can include taste changes, pulmonary fibrosis, heart failure, anorexia, and radiation pneumonitis. Management includes: Sleeping with head of bed elevated to relieve dyspnea, fans to move air, oxygen for severe dyspnea.
- **Abdominal issues**: Problems can include nausea and vomiting, diarrhea, enteritis, indigestion, gas, gastric ulcers, and renal damage. Management includes dietary modification, antiemetics, and antidiarrheals.
- **Pelvic issues**: Problems can include rectal bleeding, incontinence (urine and stool), enteritis, painful urination and defecation, fertility problems, and sexual problems (including erectile dysfunction). Management includes monitoring urinary output, fertility preservation measures, absorbent pads and good skin care for incontinence.
- **Anemia**: May result from radiation to large body areas or pelvic, extremity, or chest bones, especially if chemotherapy is given concurrently. Management may include transfusions, nutritional supplementation.

Chronic and/or permanent side effects of radiation therapy vary according to radiation target and include:

- **Breast/chest**: Skin may darken and become dry and thin. Telangiectasias may be evident. Breast swelling or fibrosis may occur. If radiation is to the left chest, the cardiac muscle may be damaged. Radiation may result in damage to the lungs as well. Peripheral lymphedema may occur.
- **Head/Neck**: Hypothyroidism may occur because of damage to the thyroid gland. Some clients may experience long-term or permanent mental changes and emotional problems, especially with radiation to the brain. Xerostomia and increased risk of tooth decay may be a chronic problem. Peripheral neuropathy may occur. Thrombocytopenia may occur, especially if chemotherapy is given concurrently. Damage to the taste buds/salivary glands may affect the ability to taste.

- **Bones**: Osteoporosis may result in fractures.
- **Pelvis**: Infertility may be permanent. Early menopause may occur. Bladder irritation may result in urinary incontinence. Peripheral lymphedema may occur.

Central Line Placement

Central lines may be placed into the internal jugular vein (right preferred), subclavian vein, or femoral vein (usually avoided) and fed to the superior vena cava or right atrium to help determine hemodynamic therapy (central venous pressure, pulmonary artery pressure, pulmonary capillary wedge pressure). Indications include hypovolemic shock, post-operative monitoring, and confirmation of right-sided heart failure. CVP can be monitored manually with a manometer or electronically with a transducer that displays a continuous waveform on a monitor. Normal pressure ranges from 2-6 mm Hg but may be elevated after cardiac surgery to 6-8 mm Hg. Incorrect catheter placement or malfunctioning can affect readings. The central line may also be utilized for infusions and for drawing blood samples. The client must be carefully monitored for complications, such as pneumothorax, dyspnea, infection, and hematoma. Intake and output should be monitored carefully and vital signs routinely assessed. The catheter should be carefully examined at each shift to ensure all connections are secure and the catheter is intact.

Thoracentesis

A **thoracentesis** (aspiration of fluid or air from pleural space) is done to make a diagnosis, relieve pressure on the lung caused by pleural effusion, or instill medications. A chest x-ray is done prior to the procedure. A sedative may be given. The client is positioned sitting and leaning onto a padded bedside stand, straddling a chair with head supported on the back of the chair, or lying on the opposite side with the head of the bed elevated 30-45° to ensure that fluid remains at the base. The client should avoid coughing or moving during the procedure. The chest x-ray or ultrasound determines needle placement. After a local anesthetic is administered, a needle (with an attached 20-ml syringe and 3-way stopcock with tubing and a receptacle) is advanced intercostally into the pleural space. Fluid is drained, collected, examined, and measured. The needle is removed and a pressure dressing applied. A chest x-ray is done to ensure there is no pneumothorax. The client is monitored for cough, dyspnea, and hypoxemia.

Review Video: Thoracentesis Procedure
Visit mometrix.com/academy and enter code: 320503

Maintaining Optimal Temperature of Hypothermic Clients

Many clients with **hypothermia** (core body temperature <35° C.) are intoxicated with alcohol or drugs but some suffer from cold exposure. Symptoms of hypothermia include pallor, cold skin, drowsiness, alterations in mental status, confusion, severe shivering. Methods of maintaining **optimal temperature** may vary but may include:

- **Stage I** (mild) hypothermia (CBT 32-35° C): Support airway, breathing, and circulation as needed. Treat by ensuring clothes are dry and warm, and provision of passive external warming, such as warm drinks, warmed blankets, at warm baths at 40° C, and physical activity.

- **Stage II** (moderate) hypothermia (CBT 28-32° C.) **and stage III** (severe) hypothermia (24-28° C) with passive and active warming, such as warm intravenous fluids (at 38-42°C), warm humidified oxygen or air inhalation, warming with extracorporeal circuit, and internal (bladder, peritoneal pleural, GI) lavage, depending on condition. The client's cardiac status, vital signs, and oxygen saturation must be monitored continually. With severe hypothermia, active rewarming of the trunk should occur before the extremities to avoid afterdrop of CBT as cold blood from the extremities returns to central circulation, and the client should avoid physical activity.

Maintaining Optimal Temperature of Hyperthermic Clients

Hyperthermia occurs when heat accumulation in the body outpaces dissipation, resulting in increased temperature and dehydration, leading to thermoregulatory failure and multiple organ dysfunction syndromes. Most hyperthermia relates to environmental exposure but some may occur because of infection, drug intoxication, or poisoning. Classifications:

- **Heat stress**: Indications include dehydration, peripheral edema, itching, sunburn, heat syncope (pale moist skin, hypotension), heat cramps, and heat tetany (respiratory alkalosis). Remove from heat, cool, hydrate, and replace sodium.
- **Heat exhaustion**: Involves water or sodium depletion. Indications include flu-like aching, nausea and vomiting, headaches, dizziness, and hypotension with cold clammy skin and diaphoresis. Temperature may be normal or elevated but <41° C. Cool and replace sodium and fluids promptly. Monitor carefully as reactions may be delayed.
- **Heat stroke**: Involves failure of the thermoregulatory system with temperatures that may be >41° C and can result in seizures, neurological damage, multiple organ failures and death. Exertional heat stroke often occurs in young athletes who engage in strenuous activities in high heat. Young children and the elderly are susceptible to non-exertional heat stroke from exposure to high heat. Use evaporative cooling, rehydration, and supportive treatment according to organ involvement.

Caring for Ventilated Clients

Responsibilities for **ventilated clients**:

- **Oral care**: Provide mouth care at least every 8 hours with head elevated to 30 degrees. Suction excess secretions with flexible catheter with tonsil tip (usually every 2-4 hours). Brush teeth with soft toothbrush (or swab) for 3-4 minutes with antiseptic (such as chlorhexidine). Avoid the use of lemon-glycerine swabs or tongue scrapers. Use a water flosser or interdental stick for flossing if indicated. Rinse with sterile water (not tap) or mouth wash (alcohol free). Moisturize lips and mucous membranes with water-based moisturizer.
- **Suctioning (ET tube)**: Auscultate lungs and hyperoxygenate before suctioning. Perform tracheostomy care every 2 to 4 hours, Don PPE. Procedure:
    - Suction catheter should be 50% the size of the tracheostomy tube to allow ventilation during suctioning.
    - Vacuum pressure: 80-100 mm Hg.
    - Insert catheter ≤0.5 cm beyond tube to avoid damage to tissues or perforation.
    - Avoid irrigation as it may increase risk of aspiration.
    - Insert catheter without suction and used intermittent suction on withdrawal.

- **Respiratory assessment**: Auscultate lungs and ensure all lobes are ventilating. Notify the registered nurse or the physician of any abnormal sounds (wheezing, rales), and note synchrony with ventilation and any asynchrony, which may indicate insufficient sedation or improper setting.

WOUND ASSESSMENT

Wound margins and the tissue surrounding the wound should be carefully assessed and described with correct terminology:

- **Color** should be described using color descriptions and such terms as blanched, erythematous (red), or ecchymosed (purple, green, yellow).
- **Skin texture** may be normal, indurated (hardened), or edematous (swollen). Note if there is cellulitis or maceration evident.
- **Wound** edges may be diffuse (without clear margins), well defined, or rolled. A healing ridge may be evident if granulation has begun. Note if the wound is closed (as with a surgical incision) or open (as with dehiscence or ulcerations). Note if wound edges are attached or unattached (indicating undermining or tunneling).
- **Tunneling or undermining** should be assessed by probing the wound margins with a moist sterile cotton applicator, using clock face locators (toward the head is 12 o'clock, for example). Tunneling may be described as extending from 3 o'clock to 4 o'clock. A large area is usually described as undermining. The size should be measured or estimated as closely as possible.

BASIC REQUIREMENTS FOR DRESSINGS

The **basic requirements of dressings**, regardless of the type, are the following:

- Maintain a moist environment in order to promote healing.
- Absorb wound drainage and preventing leakage.
- Increase wound temperature to promote healing.
- Provide a protective barrier to prevent mechanical injury to the wound.
- Provide a protective barrier to prevent colonization and infection with microorganisms.
- Allow exchange of gases and fluids.
- Retain and absorb odor of wound or drainage.
- Remove easily without causing additional trauma to the wound or disrupting the healing process.
- Debride wound of dead tissue and exudate.
- Provide protection without toxicity or causing sensitivity reactions.
- Provide a sterile protective covering for the wound.

The dressing that directly covers the wound may be inadequate to absorb large amounts of drainage, so sometimes additional secondary dressings are needed.

DRESSING PRODUCTS

There are a wide variety of **dressing products**, and there is not one dressing that can suffice for all wounds. Dressings should be chosen according to the type of wound and the function of the dressing. A series of different types of dressings may be used during the healing process. There are

3 main types of dressings to consider when determining which will be the most effective for a particular type of wound:

- Traditional topical dressings that are used primarily to cover the wound, such as gauze and tulle.
- Interactive dressings, such as polymeric films, are generally transparent so that the wound can be observed and are permeable to water vapor and oxygen but provide an effective barrier for microorganisms, such as hyaluronic acid, hydrogels and foam dressings.
- Bioactive dressings provide substances that directly promote wound healing and may absorb drainage, such as hydrocolloids, alginates, collagens, and chitosan.

Stoma Assessment

Stoma assessment includes the following:

- Type of stoma may be fecal or urinary and constructed from small intestine, colon, bladder, or ureters. Diversion may be continent or incontinent.
- Characteristics of stoma include moist mucosa. Color depends on tissue used in construction. Stoma from intestines is red and beefy looking; from ureter or bladder, pale pink.
- Edema is usually present, so stoma should be measured routinely to determine changes.
- Shape and size may vary depending upon surgical technique and effects of peristalsis. Some are round; others, oval.
- Protrusion of stoma should be slightly above skin to provide for proper pouching, but stomas may retract below the skin or prolapse.
- Function depends upon type of ostomy and position. Urostomies produce urine immediately, but colostomies may not excrete stool for 4-5 days and ileostomies, 24-48 hours.
- Peristomal skin should be clear of irritation and intact with intact suture line.

Stoma Care for One- or Two-Piece Pouching Systems

Stoma care with one- or two-piece pouching systems is explained below:

1. Assemble supplies/equipment.
2. Empty pouch into toilet.
3. Gently remove pouch, working from the top down, using one hand to pull the pouch away from the skin and the other to push down on skin. Save clamp and place used pouch in a plastic bag.
4. Cleanse skin with water and examine for irritation or lesions. Dry. Shave if necessary, with electric shaver.
5. Examine stoma and measure if necessary.
6. Cut appliance to fit if necessary or use precut appliance if stoma is round. Remove paper backing from appliance. Apply starting from the bottom, fitting under the stoma first and then smoothing upward so the warmth of the hands helps the appliance to adhere. If two-piece appliance, apply pouch to skin barrier.
7. Apply tape at corners of pouch if necessary.
8. Place ostomy deodorant in fecal pouch if desired and then apply clamp/close spout.

Bronchoscopy

A **bronchoscopy** is an inspection of the interior of the tracheobronchial tree for either diagnosis, biopsy, or foreign body removal. A bronchoscopy can be used to visualize the larynx, trachea, and bronchi. With utilization of a bronchoscopy, the patient may have examinations of tissue, secretion removal, or specimen collection done. Normal findings of a bronchoscopy include normal structure and normal lining of the larynx, trachea, and bronchi.

Nursing Considerations

Educate the patient on the procedure, including anesthetic and relaxation techniques. Ensure consent is witnessed and on the chart; remove dentures, glasses, jewelry, and contact lenses. Monitor breathing and lung sounds post-procedure; keep NPO until they regain gag reflex/pass swallow screen. May give lozenges for sore throat after able to swallow; scant amount of blood after biopsy is normal.

Procedure

The nurse will obtain vital signs prior to the examination/procedure. Patient will be anesthetized, and a scope placed down trachea, and a small biopsy will be taken/ foreign object removed. Patient will not be unconscious during procedure.

Fluid and Electrolyte Imbalances

Magnesium Imbalances

Magnesium is a crucial extracellular ion that is vital to muscle and bone health. When imbalance occurs, it is crucial to identify and correct it quickly to prevent adverse effects.

Normal Range: 1.5-2 mEq/L.

Hypomagnesia:

- Causes:
    - Prolonged suction, vomiting, diarrhea, malnutrition
    - Diuretic therapy, diabetic acidosis, alcoholism,
    - High serum levels of calcium, aldosterone, ADH, T4/TSH
- Symptoms:
    - N/V, irritability, muscle cramps, hallucinations, seizures

Hypermagnesemia:

- Causes:
    - Magnesium overdose, renal failure, overdose of certain magnesium-containing medications (antacids, laxatives, etc.)
- Symptoms:
    - Diarrhea, lethargy, diminished reflexes, muscle atony, bradycardia, hypotension, coma.

Treatment for magnesium imbalance:

- Correct imbalance: magnesium replacement OR furosemide, IV calcium gluconate, or dialysis.
- Treat underlying cause (vomiting, alcoholism, etc.)

Potassium Imbalances

Potassium is a critical intracellular ion important for muscle function, cellular health, and especially cardiac conduction.

Normal Range: 3.5-5 mmol/L.

Hypokalemia:

- Causes:
  - Excessive diarrhea, malnutrition, diuretic use.
  - Alcoholism, hyperaldosteronism.
- **Symptoms**: weakness, CNS depression, disorientation, muscle weakness, cardiac arrhythmias.

Hyperkalemia:

- Causes:
  - Traumatic injury, burns, acidosis, renal failure.
  - Addison's disease, ESRD; potassium-sparing diuretics, excessive intake of salt-substitutes or foods high in potassium.
- **Symptoms**: muscle cramps, arrhythmias, neuropathies, respiratory distress.

Treatment of potassium imbalances:

- Correct imbalance: potassium PO/IV OR sodium polystyrene, IV insulin with dextrose, dialysis.
- Correct underlying cause: kidney failure, medications, etc.

Sodium Imbalances

Sodium (Na) is a critical extracellular ion important for nerve and brain function, as well as the regulation of the fluid balance in the body.

Normal Range: 135-145 mmol/L

Hyponatremia:

- Causes:
  - Diarrhea, excessive water intake/infusion of hypotonic fluids, burn patients (eschar, hydrotherapy, silver nitrate).
  - SIADH, pneumonia, heart failure – edema/fluid overload.
- **Symptoms**: weakness, dizziness, confusion, headache, muscle cramps, tachycardia.

Hypernatremia:

- Causes:
  - Dehydration, excessive intake, diarrhea/vomiting, rigorous exercise or fever (profuse sweating).
  - Diabetes Insipidus, hypertonic infusions, diuretics - excessive fluid loss.
- **Symptoms**: ascites, edema, dry mouth, decreased urine output, irritability/confusion, hypertension, low-grade fever.

Treatment of Sodium Imbalances:

- Correct Imbalance: infusion of hypertonic/hypotonic solution, sodium supplements/diuretics, diet/lifestyle modification.
- Correct underlying cause

DEHYDRATION

Dehydration occurs when fluid intake is not adequate for fluid loss. Dehydration may occur as the result of polyuria, diarrhea, high fever, vomiting, heat exposure, and excessive exercise, especially if coupled with high heat. Symptoms vary according to the severity of the dehydration, and young children and older adults may not exhibit typical thirst, making dehydration more difficult to diagnose.

- **Signs and symptoms**: Mild/Moderate—dry mouth, thirst, decreased urination, headache, constipation, dizziness, and lethargy. Severe—severe thirst, dry mucous membranes, irritability, confusion, decreased or absent urination, concentrated urine, sunken fontanels (infants), tearless crying, fever, poor skin turgor, tachycardia, tachypnea.
- **Diagnosis**: CBC, electrolytes, urinalysis, urine osmolality.
- **Treatment**: Mild/Moderate—increased fluid intake, including oral rehydration solutions for children and water or other liquids for adults (although carbonated beverages should be avoided). Salt pills are not recommended as they may result in hypernatremia. Severe—may require electrolyte replacement and intravenous fluids.

Review Video: Fluid and Electrolytes
Visit mometrix.com/academy and enter code: 806168

Hemodynamics

DECREASED CARDIAC OUTPUT

Cardiac output (CO) is the amount of blood is pumped through the ventricles during a specified period. Normal cardiac output is about 5 liters per minutes at rest for an adult. Under exercise or stress, this volume may multiply 3 or 4 times with concomitant changes in the heart rate (HR) and stroke volume (SV). Decreased cardiac output results in an increase in systemic vascular resistance (SVR) to compensate and protect vital organs. This, in turn, results in an increase of afterload in the left ventricle with increased need for oxygen. As the cardiac output continues to decrease, tissue perfusion decreases, coronary artery perfusion decreases, fluid backs up, and the left ventricle fails to adequately pump the blood, resulting in pulmonary edema and right ventricular failure, signs of cardiogenic shock. Decreased cardiac output and cerebral deoxygenation may result in severe agitation with combative behavior. Client may exhibit dyspnea, decreased urinary output, hypotension, thready pulse, tachycardia or bradycardia, increase JVP, peripheral edema, and metabolic acidosis.

PACEMAKER COMPLICATIONS

Pacemakers, transvenous, temporary, and permanent, are invasive foreign bodies and as such can cause a number of different **complications**:

- Infection, bleeding, or hematoma may occur at the entry site of leads for temporary pacemakers or at the subcutaneous area of implantation for permanent generators.
- Puncture of the subclavian vein or internal mammary artery may cause a hemothorax.

- The endocardial electrode may irritate the ventricular wall, causing ectopic beats or tachycardia.
- Dislodgement of transvenous lead may lead to malfunction or perforation of the myocardium. This is one of the most common early complications.
- Dislocation of leads may result in phrenic nerve or muscle stimulation (which may be evidenced by hiccupping).
- Cardiac tamponade may result when epicardial wires of temporary pacing are removed.
- General malfunctioning of pacemaker may indicate dislodgement, dislocation, interference caused by electromagnetic fields, and the need for new batteries or generator.
- Pacemaker syndrome.

Pacemaker Syndrome

Pacemaker syndrome can occur with any type of pacemaker if there is inadequate synchronicity between the contractions of the atria and ventricles, resulting in a decrease in cardiac output, and inadequate atrial contribution to filling of ventricles. Total peripheral vascular resistance may increase to maintain blood pressure, but hypotension occurs if it decreases.

Mild	Pulsations evident in neck and abdomen. Cardiac palpitations. Headache and feeling of anxiety. General malaise and unexplained weakness. Pain or "fullness" in jaw, chest.
Moderate	Increasing dyspnea on exertion with accompanying orthopnea Dizziness, vertigo, increasing confusion. Feeling of choking.
Severe	Increasing pulmonary edema with dyspnea even at rest and crackling rales. Syncope. Heart failure.

Review Video: Pacemaker Care
Visit mometrix.com/academy and enter code: 727655

Monitoring Pacemaker Function for Undersensing

The sensitivity is too low to detect the client's own cardiac depolarizations and triggers unneeded firing, competing with client's native rhythm. This may be related to dislodging of lead, incorrect positioning of lead, or low-amplitude cardiac signal. Undersensing leads to overpacing, risking R on T phenomena in which the pacer fires on the client's native T-wave, leading to dangerous arrhythmias such as V-tach or V-fib.

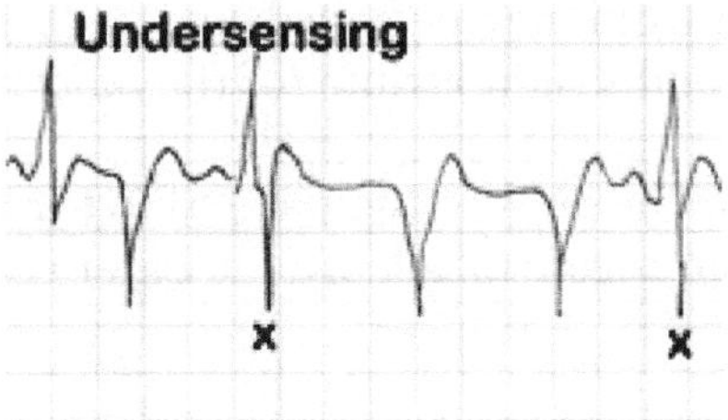

Monitoring Pacemaker Function for the Oversensing

The sensitivity is too high and misinterprets artifacts (such as muscle contractions) and non-depolarization events as contractions and fails to trigger, resulting in decreased cardiac output because of interruption in contractions. This may result from damage or disconnection of lead. Oversensing leads to underpacing.

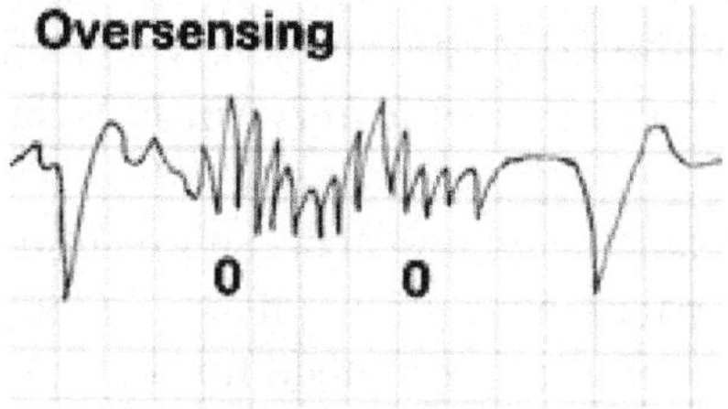

Monitoring Pacemaker Function for Non-Capture

The pacemaker fires, but does not trigger contractions. This may be related to settings, lead disconnection, low battery, or metabolic changes. Look for pacer spikes that are not followed by the appropriate P or QRS complex. In this case, the current (mA) must be increased.

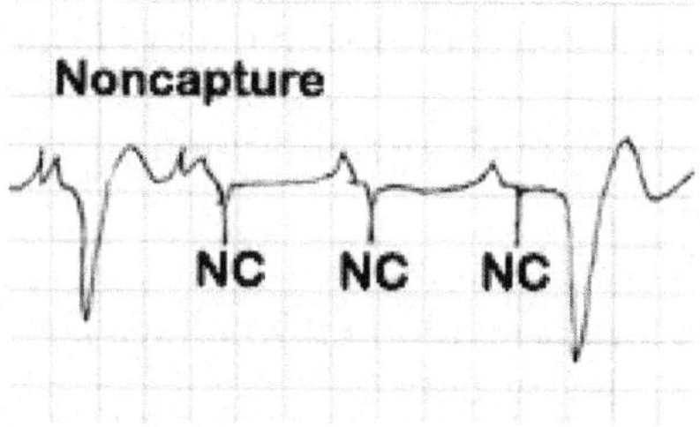

Arterial Line Maintenance and Interventions

Indications for an **arterial line** include hemodynamic instability, frequent ABG monitoring, placement of IABP, monitoring arterial pressure, and medication administration when venous access cannot be obtained. Sterile technique is utilized for arterial line insertion. Insertions sites include radial (most common), femoral (second choice), brachial, or dorsalis pedis arteries. The insertion site must be carefully monitored for signs of local infection (erythema, edema, pain, purulent discharge, heat), hemorrhage, and decreased/absent pulses distal to insertion site. Circulation in the limb must be continuously monitored (indicated by slow capillary refill) and catheter removed if circulation impaired. The client's temperature and vital signs must be monitored frequently for signs of bacteremia/sepsis. Continual infusion of NS (heparinized) is recommended over intermittent irrigation to maintain patency with infusion pump set higher than intra-arterial pressure. Indications of displacement include absence of normal arterial waveform, edema, bleeding, pallor, and pain of insertion area. If bleeding occurs because the catheter moves within the artery, a normal arterial waveform will be present and pressure applied may stop bleeding. Pressure readings and vital signs should be documented hourly. If the arterial line reading accuracy is in question, the line should be zeroed and re-read. The line should also be zeroed after patient movement or blood draws from the line have been made. Ensure that the transducer of the arterial line is lined up with the client's right atrium for the most accurate pressure reading.

Review Video: Nursing Care of Arterial Lines
Visit mometrix.com/academy and enter code: 259564

Illness Management

Shock

Shock is characterized by inadequate cellular metabolism due to poor tissue perfusion. There are four main types of shock:

- **Hypovolemic shock**: Decreased blood volume.
  - *Causes:* massive hemorrhage, dehydration.
- **Cardiogenic shock**: Heart cannot circulate blood adequately.
  - Causes: heart attack, heart failure, and arrhythmias.
- **Neurogenic shock**: Mass vasodilation, resulting in decreased venous return/cardiac output.
  - Causes include general anesthesia (deep sedation), injuries to the central nervous system, barbiturate intoxication, spinal anesthesia, and fainting.
- **Septic shock**: Toxic substances/infectious organisms cause inflammation and dilation blood vessels.
  - Causes of septic shock include gram-positive organisms such as pneumococci, staphylococci, and streptococci.

Signs and symptoms: First sign – tachycardia, hypotension, tachypnea, weak pulse, cool, clammy skin, altered LOC, decreased urine output.

Diagnosis: vital signs, clinical picture, blood work.

Treatment is as follows:

- Treat underlying cause; generally fluid resuscitation and vasopressors required.
- Can progress to uncompensated shock: fatal at this point.

Klinefelter Syndrome

Klinefelter syndrome is a genetic disorder of males in which the child is born with an extra X chromosome (usually 47XXY), and is a common cause of hypogonadism, androgen deficiency, and infertility.

Signs and symptoms: Boys often appear normal but begin to have problems in school because of delayed development of language and learning disabilities, such as auditory and verbal processing problems. Children often have normal intelligence but decreased ability to access information from memory. Onset of puberty is often delayed. Boys tend to be tall and thin with extra-long extremities and wide arm span. Testicular size is abnormally small and gynecomastia is common; adolescents develop less than normal facial and body hair. Some children may also have cardiac, respiratory, and dental abnormalities.

Diagnosis: Per chromosomal analysis.

Treatment: Testosterone replacement is started when the child is 11 to 12 years old with doses gradually increased to maintain adult levels of testosterone by age 15 to 17. This improves masculinization but does not alter infertility.

Phenylketonuria

Phenylketonuria (PKU) is an autosomal inherited recessive disorder related to the synthesis of phenylalanine, an essential amino acid required by the body. As byproducts of phenylalanine accumulate in the brain, the individual experiences developmental delays. The Guthrie test is done on all infants at birth to determine serum phenylalanine levels, as PKU was once a common yet preventable cause of intellectual disability.

Signs and symptoms: urine and sweat with a musty odor, eczema, fair skin and eyes, failure to thrive, emesis, microcephaly, hyperactivity, altered behavior patterns, convulsions, and developmental delay.

Diagnosis: blood work (Guthrie test, phenylalanine levels, etc.), genetic testing

Treatment includes the following:

- Diet low in phenylalanine/protein: Lofenalac formula is given to infants, avoid sugar-free products (aspartame), milk, cheese, beef, pork, chicken, fish and beans.
- Teaching: keep food diary/track protein intake, find support groups, take special formula for protein replacement, see doctor if pregnant—uncontrolled PKU during pregnancy will harm infant.

Wilson Disease

Wilson disease is an inherited autosomal recessive condition in which high levels of copper build up in various tissues throughout the body. The key organs affected are the eyes, brain, liver, and/or kidneys. It can be difficult to differentiate between Wilson disease and other liver diseases.

Signs and symptoms: gait disturbances, jaundice, tremors, abdominal pain/distention, dementia, speech problems, muscle weakness, splenomegaly, and confusion.

Diagnosis: bilirubin/PT/AST increased, albumin/uric acid production decreased, MRI, genetic testing, liver biopsy, Kayser-Fleischer rings in the eyes.

Treatment includes the following:

- Medications: penicillamine, trientine, zinc acetate.
- Lifestyle management: low-copper diet (avoid shellfish, nuts, chocolate, mushrooms, and liver).
- Monitor the patient for cirrhosis, muscle weakness, joint pain/stiffness, anemia, fever, hepatitis.

Legg-Calve-Perthes Disease

Legg-Calve-Perthes disease is a condition in which an anatomical anomaly results in poor blood supply to the superior aspect of the femur. It is most common in boys ages 4-10, with a 5 times higher incidence rate in boys than girls. The result of this condition is the femur ball flattens out and deteriorates, leading to impaired ambulation and pain. This condition is very similar to *slipped capital femoral epiphysis*, a common hip disorder in adolescents in which the ball of the femur separates from the femur along the epiphysis. Both are diagnosed and treated similarly.

Signs and symptoms: hip and knee pain, limited active and passive ROM, pain with ambulation, unequal leg length; may notice child wants to cross legs, keep affected limb across the body.

Diagnosis: x-ray, MRI, bone scan, test range-of-motion, clinical picture.

Treatment includes the following:

- Bracing/crutches/bed rest: keep weight off of affected hip.
- Physical therapy; strengthen affected ligaments and muscles.
- Casting: keeps legs apart, allow to heal for 4-6 weeks.
- Surgery: may need hip replacement/joint realignment if severe.

Cystic Fibrosis

Cystic fibrosis is an autosomal recessive disorder causing generalized malfunction of the exocrine glands, resulting in the excessive production of viscous mucus. It is caused by a genetic defect that affects sodium chloride movement in cells. People that have a family history of CF and are of Northern European descent are at an increased risk for CF. There is no cure for CF, but with early diagnosis and treatment, these patients often make it far into young adulthood.

Signs and symptoms: salty-taste to skin, recurrent respiratory infections, productive cough, steatorrhea (fatty, foul-smelling stool), constipation (newborn - intestinal blockage), poor weight gain; *Long-term* – pancreatitis, infertility, and diabetes.

Diagnosis: sweat test, physical exam, genetic testing.

Treatment includes the following:

- Medications: bronchodilators, mucolytics, possible prophylactic antibiotics to prevent URIs; pancreatic enzymes, vitamin supplements (A, D, E and K especially) for digestion.
- Diet: high calories/fat, increased amounts of sodium and fluids.
- Daily pulmonary hygiene.
- Teaching: encourage activities and support groups, good nutrition is vital, avoid sick people/wash hands, report infections immediately, take enzymes *before* every meal.

Wilms Tumor

Wilms tumor is traditionally a malignant tumor of the kidney characteristically diagnosed in childhood prior to the fifth year of life, and has traits of an inherited autosomal dominant disorder. Those with a family history of Wilms, of African-American descent, and born with other abnormalities such as hypospadias, aniridia, and undescended testicles have an increased risk of Wilms tumor. While it is rare, it often has a very good prognosis.

Signs and symptoms (often asymptomatic): palpable abdominal mass, fever, anemia, blood in urine, abdominal ascites, well-defined abdominal wall veins, and metastases to the gonadal area.

Diagnosis: blood work, CT/MRI, physical exam.

Treatment includes the following:

- Surgery to remove tumor and possibly kidney, followed by chemotherapy and radiation depending on staging of disease.
- Teaching: ensure family has adequate support, use language understandable to child and parents, frequent rest during chemo.

***NEVER** palpate the stomach of a child with diagnosed/suspected Wilms tumor—it could cause metastasis!*

Childhood Cancers

Childhood cancers usually originate in non-epithelial or embryonic cells, especially in preadolescent cancers. These cancers tend to be fast growing with the child rapidly deteriorating over a period of weeks or months. Childhood cancers may result from:

- **Congenital genetic abnormalities** (such as retinoblastoma and Wilms tumor).
- **Impaired immune system**, such as from AIDS or immunosuppression (increased risk of non-Hodgkin lymphoma, Hodgkin disease, leiomyosarcoma, Kaposi sarcoma).
- **Chromosomal abnormalities**, such as Down syndrome (trisomy 21) (markedly higher risk of leukemia).
- **External/Environmental carcinogens** resulting in genetic mutations (diethylstilbestrol, anabolic androgens, immunosuppressants, radiation exposure, and toxic chemicals) (may result in primary or secondary cancers).

While signs and symptoms vary according to the type of cancer, common findings include pain, palpable mass, cachexia, bruising, recurrent infections, anemia, and neurological impairment. Diagnostic tests include bone marrow biopsy, CBC, LP, and ANC, as well as CT, MRI, and ultrasound and surgical biopsy.

Infancy Through Adolescence

Incidence of **childhood cancers** varies according to the age of the child:

- **Infancy to younger than 5 years**: Acute leukemia is most common, followed by brain and CNS tumors, sympathetic nervous system tumors, and kidney tumors. Less common are soft tissue, eye, and other tumors, as well as lymphomas.
- **Ages 5 to 9 years**: Acute leukemia remains most common followed by brain and CNS tumors, lymphoma, and soft tissue cancers. Less common are bone, kidney, eye, and other tumors, as well as sympathetic nervous system tumors.
- **Ages 10 to 14 years**: Incidence of acute leukemia, lymphoma, and brain and nervous system tumors are relatively equal followed by bone cancer, carcinoma, soft tissue cancer, germ cell cancer, and others.
- **Ages 15 to 19 years**: Incidence shifts with lymphoma as the most common cancer, followed by carcinoma, germ cell cancer, and then acute leukemia. Less common cancers include sarcoma, bone cancer, and other.

Cerebral Palsy

Cerebral palsy (CP) is a non-progressive disorder of the nervous system in which the individual is unable to control voluntary muscles, present at birth or noted early in childhood (diagnosed within the first 3 years of life). CP can be acquired due to fetal injury or inherited, with males typically affected more often than females. There are 4 types of CP:

- Spastic cerebral palsy is characterized by increased muscle tone.
- Dyskinetic cerebral palsy is characterized by involuntary athetoid (constant slow) movements.
- Ataxic cerebral palsy is characterized by poor posture and decreased muscle control and coordination.
- Mixed: combination of any of the other three.

Signs and symptoms: poor respiration status, intellectual disability, spasticity speech and language deficits, delayed motor and sensory development, seizures, joint contractures.

Diagnosis: sensory/motor testing, spasticity, CT scan/MRI, EEG

Treatment includes the following:

- Medications: muscle relaxers (baclofen, diazepam), anticonvulsants.
- PT/OT/ST for functional deficits.
- Surgery: release contractures; if severe, can cut nerves to relieve symptoms (rhizotomy).

Scoliosis

Scoliosis is an abnormal curvature of the spine to one side, defined as a deviation of greater than 10 degrees. The curvature varies from slight to severe. The spine can bend either way at any point along the spine. The chest area (thoracic scoliosis) and the lower part of the back (lumbar scoliosis) are the most common regions. Scoliosis can develop at any time during childhood and adolescence. It is more common in girls than boys, most commonly occurring at the start of adolescence, though it can occur at any time during childhood.

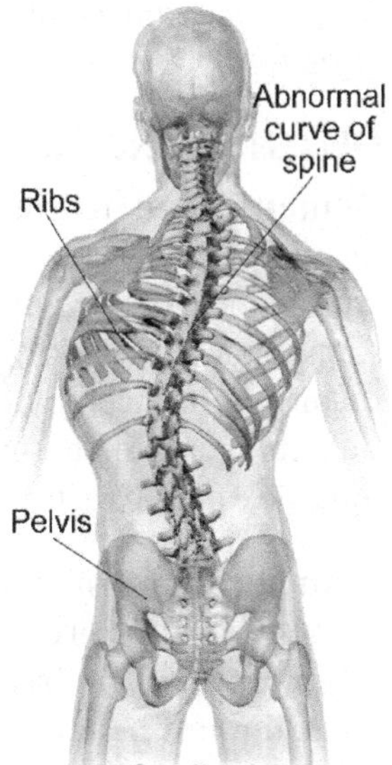

Scoliosis

Signs and symptoms: spinal curvature, sideways body posture, one shoulder raised higher than the other, clothes not hanging properly, local muscular aches and ligament pain.

Diagnosis: Physical exam (child stand in underwear facing away from examiner), x-ray.

Treatment includes the following:

- Bracing of the spine.
- Surgery (if severe); if mild, may just continue to watch for further development.
- Lifestyle Modification: educate family, encourage activity for strengthening, chiropractic/physical therapy may help.

Spina Bifida

Spina bifida includes any congenital defect involving insufficient closure of the spine. *Spina bifida occulta* occurs when the bones of the spine do not close, but skin usually covers the defect. **Myelomeningocele** is the most severe form of spina bifida. In this condition, the spinal cord and meninges (the membranes covering the spinal cord) protrude out of the child's back.

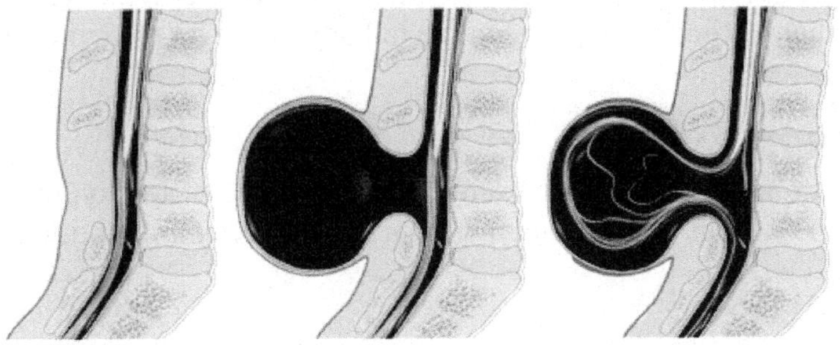

Signs and symptoms: Mild forms asymptomatic; may have hairy patch or birth mark over lower part of spine. Severe: neurogenic bowel/bladder, paralysis, sepsis, scoliosis, hydrocephalus.

Diagnosis: x-ray, CT scan, physical exam; can be detected in utero with ultrasound, blood tests, and amniocentesis.

Treatment includes the following: **(Myelomeningocele)**

- Cover with sterile, moist dressing to prevent infection; do not elevate to prevent increased pressure; requires surgery to fix (can be done in utero).
- May require placement of shunt to prevent/treat hydrocephalus.
- Physical and occupational therapy as child grows; be alert for learning difficulties.

Be aware; many children with spina bifida have latex allergy (avoid balloons, bananas, latex catheters).

Dementia and Delirium

Dementia and delirium are both alterations in mentation that result from some sort of physiological origin. Dementia is a chronic syndrome encompassing any disorder that is characterized by cognitive deficits that must include memory impairment. Examples include Alzheimer's, vascular, general medical conditions like HIV, Parkinson's disease; head trauma, or disorders induced by substance abuse or unknown origins. A key symptom of dementia is cognitive deficits including memory impairment plus at least one of the following issues: aphasia, agnosia, apraxia, or an executive functioning disturbing.

Delirium is a short-term consciousness alteration that cannot be explained otherwise by a dementia that is pre-existing or evolving. It usually fluctuates over the course of the day and affects attention span. Delirium is frequently accompanied by sleep-wake cycle disturbances and psychomotor behavior. It is important to note that the latter may be either increased or decreased. While a quietly delirious older person may be overlooked, delirium must be considered a RED FLAG, as it can signal many underlying pathological processes, including an MI, pneumonia, or UTI. It can also be superimposed on existing dementia; therefore, any sudden cognition changes in an individual with dementia should be evaluated for a potential underlying physiological cause.

Coma, Persistent Vegetative State, and Brain Death

Coma

A state of unconsciousness in which both wakefulness and awareness are absent. The patient cannot be aroused and does not display any purposeful reactions to noxious stimuli. The coma state is a continuum from light to deep and patients can fall anywhere on the continuum regarding their level of reactions.

Persistent Vegetative State

Wakefulness is present but awareness is absent. Sleep wake cycles and hypothalamic and brain stem functions are present but they are not aware of self or environment due to lack of cerebral function.

Brain Death

Complete, irreversible cessation of function of the entire brain and brain stem. Spinal reflexes may or may not be present. When brain death occurs, the patient is considered dead regardless of the presence of a heartbeat, or mechanical ventilator-assisted respirations.

Generalized Seizures

Generalized seizures are neurologic events of unknown origin that cause loss of musculoskeletal control and cognitive awareness in an individual. Seizures can be caused by numerous conditions; patients with repeated seizures of unknown origin are diagnosed with *epilepsy.*

- *Absence seizures* (petit mal) have abrupt onset characterized by episodes of staring, cessation of activities lasting approximately 30 seconds.
- *Myoclonic seizures* have a brief shock-like contraction of muscles. This may be limited to a certain limb or area or include the entire body.
- *Tonic-clonic* (grand mal) seizures involve loss of consciousness and sustained muscle contraction of entire body, with occasional jerking; may last 1-2 minutes.

Diagnosis: exam, EEG, PET scan, blood work, lumbar puncture

Treatment includes the following:

- Medications: lorazepam IV for emergency; long-term therapy:
    - Absence: valproate, and ethosuximide.
    - Myoclonic seizures: valproate.
    - Tonic-clonic seizures: carbamazepine, phenobarbital, phenytoin, primidone, and/or valproate.
- Instruct patients to NEVER stop taking medications.
- Avoid known "triggers": get rest, avoid flashing lights, etc.

Educate on first aid: lower to floor, never restrict/ put anything in mouth, place on side with pillow under head.

Meningitis

Epidemic meningitis, seen most frequently in college dormitories and military barracks, is an inflammation of the meninges of the brain and spinal cord. *Neisseria* and *Streptococcus* bacterium are often the cause, transmitted by airborne droplets. However, there are also viral and fungal forms of meningitis.

Signs and symptoms: headache, photosensitivity, nausea/vomiting, nuchal rigidity, fever, lethargy.

- *Brudzinski sign*: When the neck is flexed, flexion of the knees also occurs. Flexion of the neck is passive.
- *Kernig sign*: Flexion of the knee with the lower extremity in a "raised position" that causes pain.

Diagnosis: blood culture, x-ray/CT scan, lumbar puncture

Treatment includes the following:

- Medications: antibiotics (bacterial meningitis), steroids for brain swelling, pain medication.
- Supportive care: bed rest, fluids, seizure precautions.

Prevention: stay on schedule with vaccines, wash hands/practice good hygiene; if pregnant, avoid unpasteurized products such as raw cheeses, diary, etc. Cook deli meat and hot dogs thoroughly.

Multiple Sclerosis

Multiple sclerosis (MS) can range from relatively benign to devastating, as communication between the brain and other parts of the body is disrupted. In the case of MS, it is the nerve-insulating myelin that comes under assault. Such assaults may be linked to an unknown environmental trigger, perhaps a virus. Most people experience their first symptoms of MS between the ages of 20 and 40; often symptoms come and go in a relapsing/remitting pattern.

Signs and symptoms: vision abnormalities, paresthesia, generalized pain, difficulty with speech, tremors, dizziness, cognitive impairments, depression.

Diagnosis: blood levels, MRI, lumbar puncture

Treatment includes the following:

- No cure; symptom management.
- Medications, including corticosteroids for acute attacks, and beta-interferons and immunosuppressant drugs to prevent relapse.
- Lifestyle modification: avoid extreme heat (may precipitate relapse), take frequent rest periods, join support groups to prevent feelings of depression/isolation.

Myasthenia Gravis

Myasthenia gravis is an autoimmune disorder that results in sporadic, progressive weakness of striated (skeletal) muscles because of impaired transmission of nerve impulses. Myasthenia gravis usually affects muscles controlled by the cranial nerves, although any muscle group may be affected. Many patients also have thymomas.

Signs and symptoms: increasing weakness and fatigue that worsens throughout the day. Patients often exhibit ptosis and diplopia. They may have trouble chewing and swallowing and often appear to have masklike facies. If respiratory muscles are involved, patients may exhibit signs of respiratory failure. Myasthenic crisis occurs when patients can no longer breathe independently.

Diagnosis: Tests include electromyography and the Tensilon test (IV injection of edrophonium or neostigmine, which improves function if patient has myasthenia gravis). CT or MRI to diagnose thymoma.

Treatment: Anticholinesterase drugs (neostigmine, pyridostigmine) relieve some muscle weakness but lose effectiveness as the disease progresses. Corticosteroids may be used. Thymectomy is performed if thymoma present. Tracheotomy and mechanical ventilation may be needed for myasthenic crisis. Instruct patients to take medications at the same time every day, first thing in the morning.

Review Video: Myasthenia Gravis
Visit mometrix.com/academy and enter code: 715123

Bell's Palsy

Bell's palsy occurs when nerve impulses of the seventh cranial nerve (facial) are blocked because of an inflammatory reaction of the nerve, usually at the internal auditory meatus. Onset is rapid, but symptoms usually subside within 2 months, although the condition may recur on the same or opposite side. The causes may include infection, tumor, trauma, or hemorrhage, but the cause is often not clear.

Signs and symptoms: Sudden onset of unilateral facial weakness with mouth drooping, distorted taste perception, difficulty chewing and swallowing, facial pain, and incomplete eye closure on affected side.

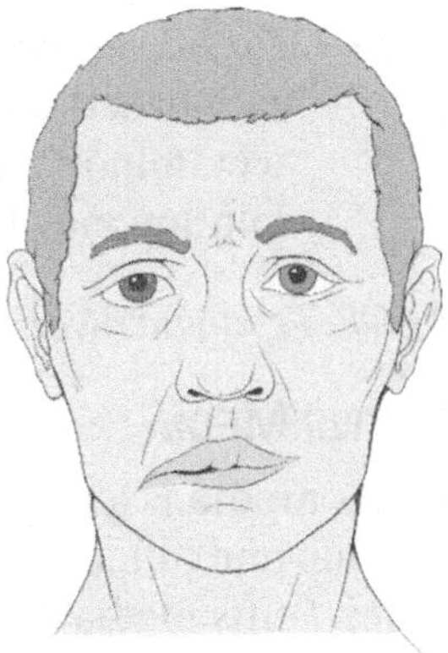

Diagnosis: Per assessment of signs and symptoms. Electromyography may help to confirm diagnosis and determine likely recovery time.

Treatment: Prednisone is usually administered to relieve inflammation for 2 weeks. Moist heat to affected area may relieve discomfort, and electrotherapy and massage may help to maintain muscle tone. The patient may need to wear an eye patch to protect the eye, especially if outside. Patients may need a modified soft diet, avoiding hot foods because of lack of sensation.

PARKINSON'S DISEASE

Parkinson's disease is a neurological disorder characterized by a lack of dopamine (a neurotransmitter) in the brain. The deficiency of dopamine may occur related to degeneration, vascular disorders, or inflammatory changes. It most often occurs in men older than 60, but rarely occurs in younger people as well.

Signs and symptoms: Rhythmic muscle tremors ("cogwheeling"), rigidity with movement, shuffling gait in which the trunk, legs, knees, and hips are flexed, but remain stiff, festination-quickened gait, droopy posture, tremors of the hands ("pill rolling"), mask-like facial expression, weight loss, difficulty with enunciation, small hand-writing (micrographia).

Diagnosis: Physical exam, neurological exam – no specific tests.

Treatment includes the following:

- Medications: levodopa/carbidopa, antidepressants.
- PT/OT/ST for functional deficits.
- Teaching: small frequent meals, increased amounts of liquid in the diet and increased fiber in the diet, ensure family has adequate support system.

TONSILLITIS

Tonsillitis is infection of the palatine tonsils, masses of soft tissue on each side of the throat. Tonsillitis may be a viral or bacterial. Strep throat, caused by *Streptococcus pyogenes*, may result in rheumatic fever if untreated.

Signs and symptoms: Severe sore throat with red swollen tonsils, sometimes with purulent drainage, rhinitis, difficulty swallowing, fever, headache, nausea, earache (from referred pain), and rash.

Diagnosis: per clinical examination and culture and sensitivities (if bacterial infection suspected).

Treatment includes the following:

- Viral tonsillitis usually clears within a few days without treatment.
- Bacterial tonsillitis, especially strep throat, may require antibiotic therapy.
- Other treatments are supportive and include gargling with salt water and NSAIDs and/or acetaminophen for fever and discomfort.

- *Tonsillectomy* may be indicated for repeated tonsillitis or enlarged tonsils that interfere with breathing or sleeping. Postoperatively, the patient should be given cool liquids, acetaminophen, and an ice pack to relieve swelling and pain. An oral viscous lidocaine solution may be used to relieve pain as well.

NOTE: Frequent swallowing is warning sign of hemorrhage!

Otitis Media

Otitis media is a common bacterial infection of the inner (middle) ear or tympanum causing fluid buildup and inflammation, often occurring in young children related to their short, wide eustachian tubes. Otitis media is often associated or accompanied by upper respiratory infections. Children in day care, bottle-fed babies, and those exposed to second-hand smoke are at an increased risk.

Signs and symptoms: ear pain, tugging/pulling at ears and irritability in infants, fever, altered or decreased hearing, vertigo, and/or loss of balance.

Diagnosis: physical exam (pneumatic otoscope), hearing exam, tympanometry.

Treatment includes the following:

- Medications: Tylenol for pain, antibiotics if bacterial or systemic symptoms, often "wait and see" approach taken first.
- May place tubes in ears if recurrent: tubes drain fluid, preventing ear infections; fall out on their own in ~6 months.

Prevention: wash hands/avoid respiratory infections, breastfeed/feed child in upright position, avoid second-hand smoke, vaccinate appropriately.

Review Video: Otitis Media
Visit mometrix.com/academy and enter code: 297773

Conjunctivitis

Conjunctivitis (also known as "pink eye") is the inflammation of the conjunctiva caused by viruses or bacteria. If it is viral, it is highly contagious. Conjunctivitis can also be caused by chemicals or allergic reactions. Recurring conjunctivitis can indicate a larger underlying disease process.

Signs and symptoms: inflamed, pink-colored eyes, purulent discharge from eyes, crusts, itching/burning eyes, blurred vision.

Diagnosis: physical exam, clinical picture.

Treatment includes the following:

- Antibiotic eye drops: place drops into eye without touching lashes, do not share bottle to avoid spread, do not use same wash cloth/eye drops between infected/non-infected eyes.
- Symptom management; warm cloths to the eye are helpful, as well as OTC "artificial tears" for irritation/burning, throw away contact lenses/eye makeup used during infection, wear glasses.

Prevention: wash hands frequently, do not share eye makeup/contact lenses, avoid touching eyes.

Glaucoma

Glaucoma is a condition in which the pressure inside of the eye is increased due to poor drainage of aqueous humor inside the eye, leading to damage to the optic nerve. The exact cause is often unknown, but a family history of glaucoma, diabetes, impaired vision, and increased age are all recognized risk factors.

Signs and symptoms: often asymptomatic; loss of peripheral vision, halos around lights, eye pain, headaches, hazy-looking eyes (infants).

Diagnosis: complete eye exam, including tonometry and vision test.

Treatment includes the following:

- Eye drops: Ensure pressure is held on the inner canthus of the eye for a minimum of 30 seconds to prevent systemic effects.
  - Prostaglandins: latanoprost (common)
  - Beta-blocker: timolol
  - Carbonic anhydrase inhibitors: end in -amide; also given as oral medications: acetazolamide
  - Adrenergic: brimonidine
  - Miotics: pilocarpine and carbachol
- Surgery: increases drainage out of the eye.
- Teach: Vision loss is irreversible, but early intervention and treatment can prevent further loss of vision.

Review Video: Glaucoma vs. Cataracts
Visit mometrix.com/academy and enter code: 937483

Cleft Lip and Palate

Cleft lip and/or **Cleft palate** are facial malformations that occur during embryonic development in which the soft palate of the mouth does not close completely, leaving a gap. These two conditions may appear separately or together. While the cause is unknown, it is possible that heredity, maternal medications, and viruses during the first trimester may play a role in the development of cleft lip/palate.

Signs and symptoms: obvious physical deformity of mouth/lips, difficulty feeding, ear infections/hearing loss, speech difficulty.

Diagnosis: prenatal ultrasound, physical exam.

Treatment includes the following:

- Surgery: close lip/tubes in ears by 12 months, palate by 18 months; may protect suture with Logan bow, use Z-plasty to minimize scar retraction.
- Feeding: generally, cannot breastfeed; must use special bottle that does not require high amounts of suction. Post-op: cannot put any objects in mouth; will be fed by syringe, no pacifier, wear arm restraints to prevent bringing objects to mouth

Hypertension

Hypertension is a condition in which the blood pressure of the body is elevated, generally about 120/80 mm Hg. It can be transient, such as in disease states, or prolonged. Prolonged hypertension is a leading cause of heart attack and stroke, and is associated with stenosis, peripheral vascular disease, and increased vascular resistance.

Blood Pressure (BP) = cardiac output (CO) x systemic vascular resistance (SVR)

Signs and symptoms: Often known as the "silent killer," patients with HTN are generally asymptomatic. However, with severe hypertension (SBP >170), the patient may experience a headache at the base of the skull, flushing, and blurred vision, sensation of pounding in head, neck, or chest.

Diagnosis: physical exam, blood pressure monitoring

Treatment includes the following:

- Medications: antihypertensives, diuretics such as hydrochlorothiazide.
- Lifestyle modification: low-sodium diet, regular low-impact exercise, stress management, and weight loss are all known to lower blood pressure.

Valvular Diseases

Common **valvular diseases** include:

1. **Mitral Stenosis**: A thickening and contracture of the mitral valve cusps of the heart. This thickening and constriction causes narrowing of the mitral valve and produces a resistance to diastolic filling of the left ventricle. The most common cause of mitral stenosis is rheumatic fever.
2. **Mitral Insufficiency**: An incompetent deformity of the mitral valve. Also termed valvular regurgitation and is characterized by valves that do not close completely, resulting in retrograde blood flow back up into the atrium from the ventricles.
3. **Aortic Valve Stenosis**: A narrowing of the opening between the left ventricle and the aorta. It is the most commonly caused by a genetic disorder, rheumatic fever, or atherosclerosis.
4. **Aortic Insufficiency**: Characterized by deformed flaps of the heart valves that prevent proper closure. Without proper closure, the blood flows back from the aorta into the left ventricle.
5. **Tricuspid Stenosis**: A restriction of the tricuspid valve.
6. **Tricuspid Insufficiency**: A regurgitation of the blood from the right ventricle to the right atrium that occurs during ventricular systole.

Heart Failure

Heart failure is a condition in which the heart becomes unable to adequately pump blood throughout the body. It encompasses ventricular dysfunction, ischemic cardiomyopathies, and systolic and diastolic dysfunction. Heart failure generally starts as left-sided, and proceeds to the right side as the condition worsens. There is no known cure for chronic heart failure, so treatments focus on symptom management and palliative care.

Signs and symptoms:

- *Right-sided*: generalized edema, jugular vein distention, and hepatomegaly.
- *Left-sided*: dyspnea on exertion, cough with blood-tinged or frothy sputum, orthopnea (difficulty breathing while laying down).

Diagnosis: Blood work (BNAP >100), echocardiogram, ECG.

Treatment includes the following:

- Furosemide/bumetanide: Loop diuretics to decrease fluid overload; thiazide diuretics may also be used.
- Blood pressure management: often use ACE inhibitor—relaxes blood vessels, decreasing workload of the heart; ends in "-pril."
- May also include beta-blockers, and digoxin for increased cardiac strength.
- Lifestyle modification: low-sodium and fluid-restricted diet, low level exercise, may require oxygen during end stages, weigh self-daily, same time, report >1-2 lb in a day/>3-5 in a week.

Review Video: Antihypertensives: ACE Inhibitors & ARBs
Visit mometrix.com/academy and enter code: 664767

ATRIAL ARRHYTHMIAS

Atrial arrhythmias include the following:

- **Atrial tachycardia**: AT is a supraventricular (arising above the ventricles) tachycardia with an atrial rate ranging from 150 to 250 bpm. AT may be transient and is sometimes associated with excess caffeine use, marijuana use, electrolyte imbalance, or physical or emotional stress. AT may also occur with cardiac disorders, such as MI or cardiomyopathy.

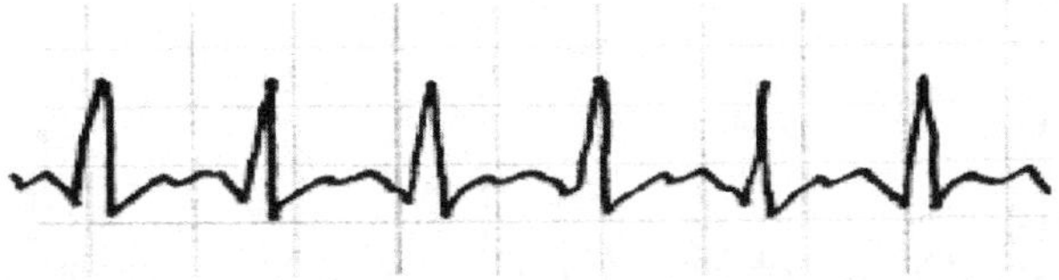

- **Atrial fibrillation**: results from chaotic electrical stimulation of the atria, resulting in an unpredictable irregular rhythm. The atrial rate may exceed 300 bpm but the AV node blocks some impulses so the ventricular rate is usually between 100 and 150 bpm.

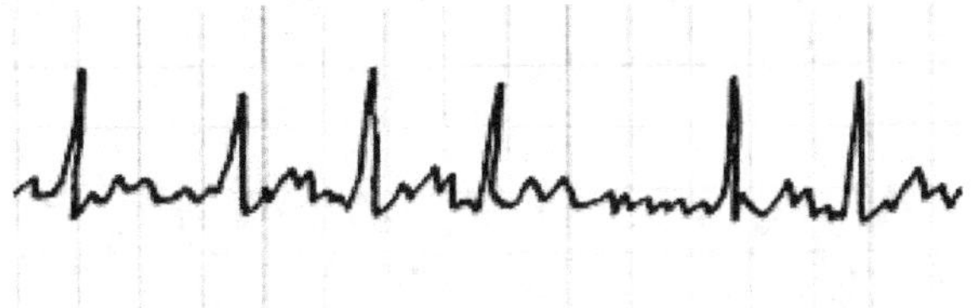

- **Atrial flutter**: AF is a supraventricular tachycardia with an atrial rate of about 300 bpm in a rapid but regular rhythm with a ventricular rate that is commonly 60 to 100 but may be 125 to 150. A common finding is a 2:1 conduction rate, which is an atrial rate of 300 bpm with a ventricular rate of 150 bpm.

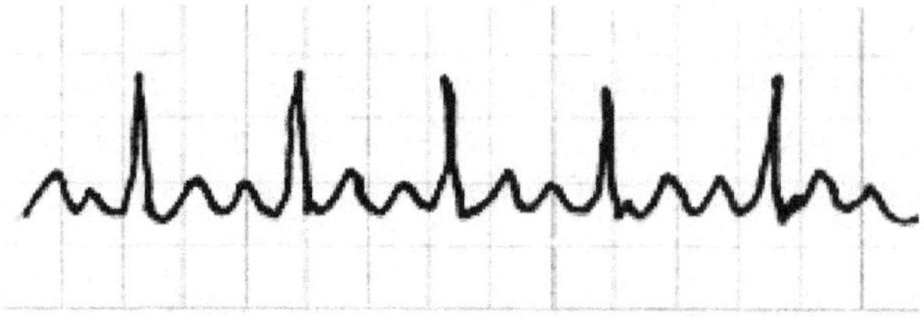

Review Video: EKG Interpretation: Atrial Fibrillation & Atrial Flutter
Visit mometrix.com/academy and enter code: 686212

Ventricular Arrhythmias

Ventricular arrhythmias originate from the ventricles, often detected by the lack of a discernible P wave. Three main types of ventricle arrhythmias include:

- **Premature Ventricular Contraction (PVC)** - A wide and bizarre, premature QRS complex, followed by compensatory pause.

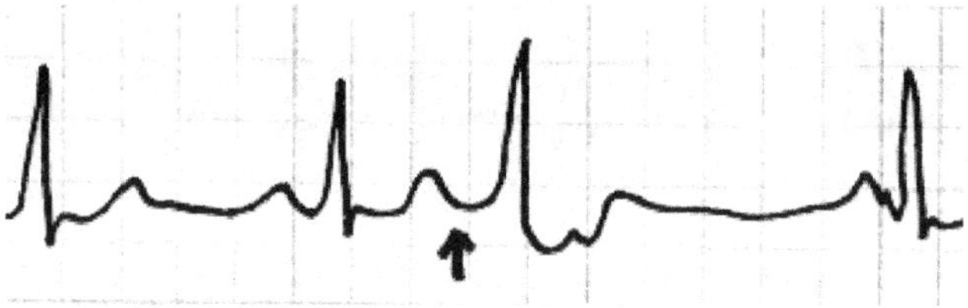

- **Ventricular Tachycardia** - Presence of 3 or more PVCs, rate of 150-200 bpm, possible abrupt onset. Possibly due to an ischemic ventricle or electrolyte imbalance.

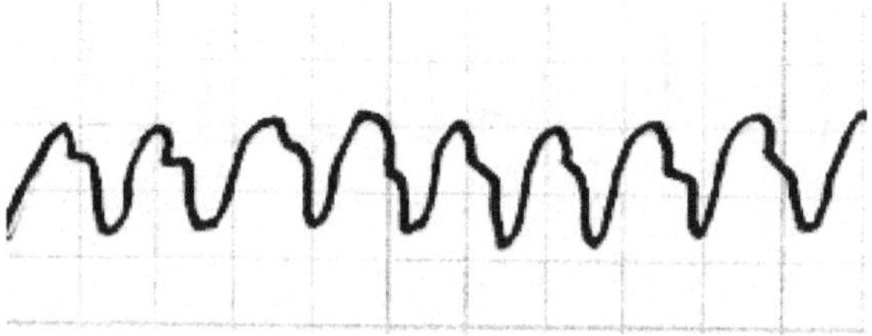

- **Ventricular Fibrillation** - Completely abnormal ventricular rhythm with no discernible QRS complex; ventricles are literally quivering. Requires emergency intervention.

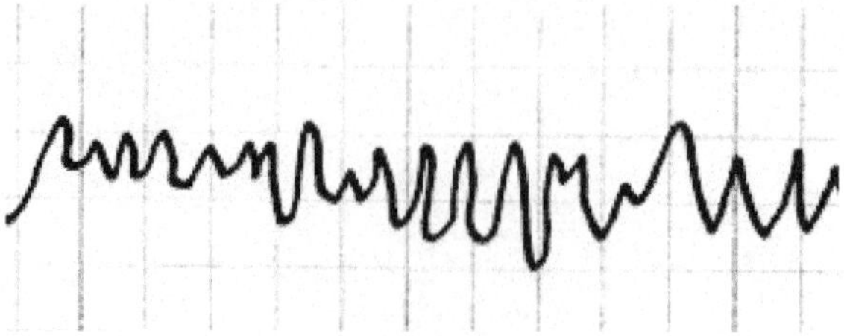

Diagnosis: ECG, physical exam, blood work (BMP).

Treatment includes the following:

- CHECK FOR PULSE; if no pulse, activate code and begin CPR.
- PVCs: occasional PVCs are common, especially with caffeine or stress. However, check electrolytes if frequent (>6/minute), as this increases risk of V-tach/V-fib.
- V-Tach: Use **LAMB** to remember treatment:
  - **L**idocaine
  - **A**miodarone
  - **M**agnesium/Mexiletine
  - **B**eta-Blocker

Review Video: EKG Ventricular Arrhythmias
Visit mometrix.com/academy and enter code: 677734

AV Block

The following are different types of AV block:

- **Atrioventricular (AV) block, first degree**: Conduction of impulses from the atria to the ventricles is delayed with block usually at AV node or bundle of His. Atrial and ventricular rhythms are regular.

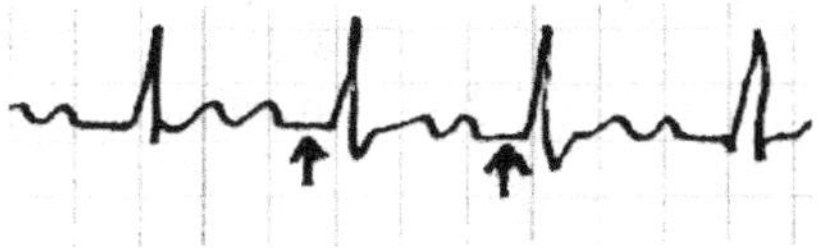

- **AV block, second degree, type I (Mobitz I)**: Some impulses are conducted and some are blocked, with each successive impulse from SA node delayed longer than previous until an impulse fails to be conducted, after which the pattern repeats. This block is usually secondary to drug effects or conditions (such as CAD or MI) and is usually transient.

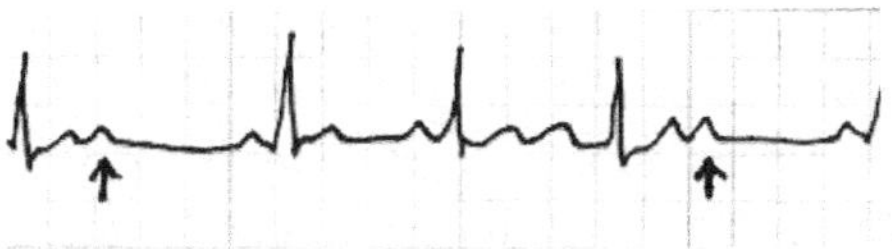

- **AV block second degree, type II (Mobitz II)**: Impulses from the SA node sometimes fail to conduct to the ventricles. Blocks, which may be consecutive, are below the AV node at the bundle of His or bundle branches.

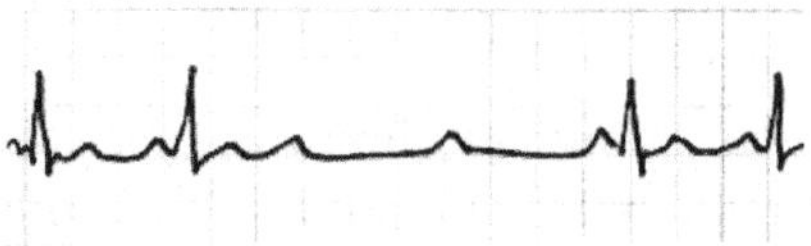

- **AV block, third degree**: This life-threatening complete heart block allows no impulses to reach the ventricle with block at the level of the AV node, the bundle of His, or the bundle branches.

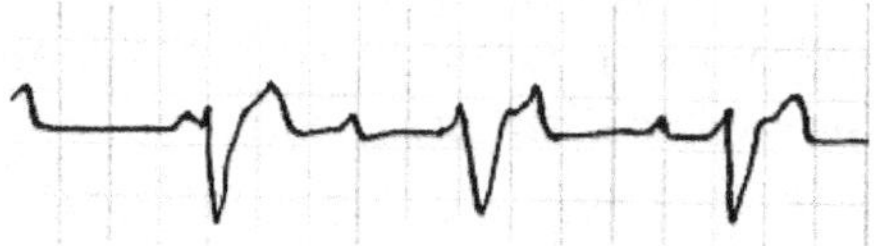

Review Video: AV Heart Blocks
Visit mometrix.com/academy and enter code: 636235

Acute Coronary Syndromes

Acute coronary syndrome (ACS) is a condition in which there is a sudden decrease of blood flow/oxygen supply to the cardiac tissue. The most common forms of ACS are *unstable angina* and *myocardial infarction*. Acute coronary syndromes develop when atherosclerotic plaque buildup lines the walls of the vessels, causing occlusion of the vessel. ACS can also be caused by an embolus or arterial vasospasm. Unstable angina that occurs as a result of occlusion is reversible ischemia. Irreversible ischemia causes myocardial infarction and muscle death and damage.

Signs and symptoms: chest pain/pressure, may radiate to left arm, jaw and shoulder; nausea/vomiting, diaphoresis, SOB/dyspnea on exertion.

Diagnosis: EKG, blood work (troponin and CK-MB), physical exam.

Treatment includes the following:

- Medications: nitroglycerin (angina), morphine for pain and decreases cardiac workload, aspirin, may use thrombolytic such as TPA if clot is suspected and cath lab not readily available.
- Place on oxygen, and bedrest.
- Cardiac Catheterization - to open vessels/ablate clot; may require open heart surgery (CABG) if disease is severe.
- Teaching: Angina – Causes (4 E's): **E**xertion, **E**ating, **E**motional Distress, **E**xtreme Temperature; weight management, low-cholesterol/low-sodium diet, monitor for signs and symptoms of heart failure/cardiogenic show.
- **MONA** for chest pain**: M**orphine**, O**xygen**, N**itroglycerin**, A**spirin**.**

**See Coronary Artery Disease teaching card for more information.*

Kawasaki Disease

Kawasaki disease is a short-lived childhood autoimmune disease of unknown origin that attacks the heart, blood vessels, and lymph nodes, causing widespread inflammation and damage. Generally, the child will make a full recovery with no long-term effects. However, these patients should be monitored for coronary aneurysm and heart attack/stroke during the acute phase of the disease, and should also have follow-up appointments to ensure there is no coronary damage.

Signs and symptoms: fever lasting longer than 5 days, joint pain, swollen lymph nodes, peripheral edema, rashes, papillae (small bumps) on the tongue, chapped and peeling red lips, hands and feet.

Diagnosis: primarily based on signs and symptoms; may also do blood work and echocardiogram.

Treatment includes the following:

- Immune globulin (human) infusion: prevents long-term complications.
- High-dose aspirin: decreases inflammation, pain, and fever.
- Education: early diagnosis and treatment is vital!

Cardiac Tamponade

Cardiac tamponade occurs when fluid, usually blood, accumulates in the pericardial sac. If the fluid accumulates rapidly, the walls of the pericardial sac do not have time to stretch to accommodate the fluid, so the patient may quickly develop pulseless electrical activity (PEA) with fluid accumulation of 50 to 250 mL. If fluid accumulates slowly, such as with pericardial effusions associated with cancer, patients may tolerate up to 2L of fluid before symptoms become acute. Cardiac tamponade compresses the heart and limits the venous return to the heart and blood flow into the ventricles, thereby reducing cardiac output.

Signs and symptoms: Beck's triad of symptoms typical to acute cardiac tamponade include decreased arterial blood pressure, increased jugular venous distention, and muffled heart sounds.

Diagnosis is per symptoms, ECG, chest x-ray, and/or echocardiography **Treatment** is pericardiocentesis to relieve pressure. In some cases, a drain may be placed in the pericardial sac or a window cut to allow drainage into the pleural cavity if there is a large effusion.

Thromboangiitis Obliterans

Thromboangiitis obliterans (Buerger disease) is an inflammatory process of the arteries and veins. Thromboangiitis obliterans occurs most often in young and middle-aged men, especially those who smoke. Thromboangiitis obliterans is characterized by occlusions of the extremities (both upper and lower) that are caused by inflammation and thrombus formations that occlude the vessels.

Signs and symptoms: ulcerations of the extremities, coolness and pallor in the hands and feet, increased sensitivity to cold, paresthesia, intermittent claudication in legs, cyanotic hands and feet.

Diagnosis: blood work, Allen test, angiogram, clinical picture.

Treatment includes the following:

- Smoking cessation is cornerstone of treatment to halt progress of disease; medications to dilate vessels; compression stockings.
- Monitor patient for infection and gangrene.
- **Note:** Do not confuse with *Raynaud disease*, a condition that most commonly occurs in young/middle-aged woman, caused by arterial vasospasm of hands and feet; similar symptoms, and often related to psychological illness.

Cancer

Cancers (neoplasms) are the uncontrolled or uncontrollable proliferations of abnormal cells. Cancer cells typically are immature, abnormal, and encapsulated, allowing for easy metastasis and invasion of surrounding cells. Causative factors associated with cancers include viruses, chronic irritation of skin or other tissues (e.g., sunburns), chemical exposure, high-fat /low-fiber diets, and/or genetics.

Signs and symptoms: CAUTION UP is a helpful mnemonic to assist you to remember the early warning signs of cancer.

- **C**hange in bowel or bladder
- **A** lesion that does not heal
- **U**nusual bleeding or discharge
- **T**hickening or lump in breast or elsewhere
- **I**ndigestion or difficulty swallowing
- **O**bvious changes in wart or mole
- **N**agging cough or persistent hoarseness
- **U**nexplained weight loss
- **P**ernicious anemia

Diagnosis: blood work, CT, MRI, PET scan, biopsy

Treatment includes the following:

- Chemotherapy; systemic agents that destroy cancer in the body.
- Radiation: using radioactive particles to destroy cancer; local.

Prognosis depends on cancer type and progression at diagnosis.

Review Video: Cancer Classifications & Metastasis
Visit mometrix.com/academy and enter code: 661160

Classifications of Neoplasms

Classifications of **neoplasms** include:

1. **Carcinoma**: Originates from the epithelial tissue of the skin, lung, gastrointestinal tract, breast and uterine lining. Carcinomas traditionally begin to spread via the lymph system, followed by the bloodstream. The two major types of carcinoma are the glandular (adenocarcinoma) and squamous cell carcinoma. *Squamous cell carcinoma is the most frequently diagnosed type of cancer.*
2. **Sarcoma**: A neoplasm of the connective tissue. Sarcomas have an increased risk of malignancy, and originate from an excessive proliferation of mesodermal cells. Sarcomas are common in bone and muscle, and are generally characterized by large masses that may or may not metastasize to other areas of the body.
3. **Lymphoma**: Neoplasms of the lymph or reticuloendothelial tissue. Lymphomas are typically solid tumors that traditionally appear in the lymph nodes, spleen, or any other organ tissue. Hodgkin disease is an example of lymphoma. Lymphomas are categorized according to cell involvement (B or T cells).
4. **Leukemia**: Both acute and chronic and encompasses the blood-producing organs. Leukemia is a progressive proliferation of abnormal leukocytes. Categorized by cell type and duration from initial onset to time of demise.

Review Video: Leukemia
Visit mometrix.com/academy and enter code: 940024

Lymphomas

Lymphomas are cancers of the lymphocyte cells that make up the immune system. Lymphoma is further classified as *Hodgkin* or *non-Hodgkin* lymphoma:

- Hodgkin lymphoma:
  - Identified by the presence of Reed-Sternberg cells.
  - More prevalent in 15-19 years of age; also in men >50.
  - May be sub-staged as "A" or "B," indicating presence of symptoms.
- Non-Hodgkin lymphomas (NHL):
  - More prevalent in children <14 years.
  - Approximately 60% of pediatric lymphomas are NHL.

Signs and symptoms: Stage A - asymptomatic. Stage B - persistent fever, night sweats, unexplained weight loss; enlarged, firm, nontender lymph nodes; itching, difficulty breathing, malaise.

Diagnosis: Blood tests, bone marrow biopsy, PET scan, chest x-ray

Review Video: Lymphoma
Visit mometrix.com/academy and enter code: 513277

Therapeutic management is as follows:

- Radiation/ Chemotherapy (alone or with radiation)
- Prognosis depends on severity/progression of the disease

Iron Deficiency Anemia

Iron deficiency anemia is a lack of circulating hemoglobin resulting from a lack of iron in the blood. There are several causes for this disease:

- *Inadequate supply*: rapid growth (prematurity, adolescence, pregnancy), poor eating habits.
- *Impaired absorption*: malabsorption disorders.
- *Blood loss*: hemorrhage, parasitic infections.
- *Hemodilution of pregnancy*: increased blood volume results in a relative deficiency of circulating hemoglobin and other components of the blood.

Signs and symptoms: pallor, poor physical/cognitive development (infants), infections, edema, irritability, tachycardia, fatigue, glossitis, spoon-shaped fingernails (termed *koilonychia*), PICA (eating non-food substances, such as ice chips or soap).

Diagnosis: complete blood cell count with differential; fecal occult blood.

Treatment includes the following:

- Increase dietary iron: dark, leafy vegetables, red meat, do not use cow milk for infants ≤1 year of age.
- Iron supplementation:
  - Oral - can cause darkening of stools and stomach irritation. Take with a meal.
  - IV – Do not give with other medications. Watch for extravasation, which will cause irritation of tissues.
- Blood Transfusion (severe cases)

Review Video: Pernicious Anemia
Visit mometrix.com/academy and enter code: 924752

APLASTIC ANEMIA

Aplastic anemia is characterized by a decreased production of red blood cells within the bone marrow, causing a decreased volume of circulating erythrocytes, leukocytes, or platelets in the blood. Causes of aplastic anemia include, but are not limited to, exposure to drugs and/or chemicals, anti-tumor agents, 6-mercaptopurine, antimicrobials, heavy metals, radiation, and pregnancy (rare).

Signs and symptoms: dyspnea, ecchymoses, petechiae, fatigue, fever, hemorrhage, menorrhagia, occult blood, epistaxis, pallor, palpitations, weakness, retinal hemorrhage, weight loss.

Diagnosis: blood work (CBC), bone marrow biopsy, physical exam.

Treatment includes the following:

- Blood transfusion, stem cells.
- Medications: immunosuppressants, bone marrow stimulants (epoetin alfa, sargramostim, filgrastim), antibiotics for infection.
- Lifestyle modification: wash hands frequently/avoid sick people, rest frequently, avoid contact sports/other things that increase risk of injury and subsequent bleeding.

HEMOPHILIA

Hemophilia is an inherited x-linked chromosomal disorder that results in impaired clotting of the blood. Because it is x-linked, hemophilia most often occurs in males, and is inherited from their mothers.

Types:

- *Hemophilia A*: "Classic hemophilia," deficiency of factor VII.
- *Hemophilia B*: "Christmas disease," deficiency of factor IX.
- *Hemophilia C*: mild form, occurs equally in males and females.

Signs and symptoms: mild to severe bleeding from minor wounds, joint pain, bruising, nosebleeds.

Diagnosis: Blood work (pTT/INR/blood clotting factors), physical exam.

Treatment includes the following:

- Medications: desmopressin, antifibrinolytics, replacement of missing factor, blood transfusions; cannot take NSAIDs or blood thinners.
- PT/OT for joint damage from bleeding; may require surgery if joint bleeding severe.
- Teaching: treat wounds immediately, report excessive bleeding, exercise regularly to strengthen muscles/must avoid contact sports; practice good oral hygiene to prevent gum bleeds, wear medical alert bracelet/educate caregivers.

SICKLE CELL ANEMIA

Sickle cell anemia is an autosomal recessive disorder that occurs primarily in African Americans. Patients have **sickle cell crises**, during which there is partial or complete replacement of normal Hgb with abnormal hemoglobin S (Hgb S). This results in elongated, "sickle"-shaped red blood cells that are rigid and obstruct capillary blood flow. These microscopic clots cause damage to organs of the body, especially the spleen. Patients are at increased risk of heart attack and stroke due to clots. Precipitating factors for a crisis are most commonly anything that causes hypoxia in the tissues, including trauma, infection, fever, physical and emotional stress, dehydration, increased altitude (even poorly pressurized airplanes), hypoventilation, and hypothermia.

Signs and symptoms: extreme pain, especially in joints/chest, shortness of breath; long-term effects include infections, delayed growth, swollen hands/feet.

Diagnosis: blood smear, sickle turbidity test, serum electrophoresis, newborn screening.

Treatment includes the following:

**Treat underlying cause of crisis!*

- Medications: antibiotics, analgesics* (will require high amounts due to tolerance.)
- Oxygen, IV fluids, moist heat for discomfort, possible routine blood transfusions.
- Surgery: splenectomy if recurrent splenic sequestration.
- Bed rest to maximize energy and improve oxygenation.
- Teach: stay hydrated, get adequate nutrition, and report signs and symptoms of infection immediately.

**Sickle cell pain is considered real pain on NCLEX, priority to treat.*

Review Video: Sickle Cell Disease
Visit mometrix.com/academy and enter code: 603869

Thalassemia

Thalassemia is an autosomal inherited recessive trait characterized by the abnormal formation and decreased life span of red blood cells that occurs primarily in the Asian, Middle Eastern, and Mediterranean populations. The decreased lifespan of RBCs leads to increased serum iron/increased bilirubin. There are two types of thalassemia, alpha and beta.

Signs and symptoms: pallor, jaundice, bronzed/freckled appearance, anorexia, hepatomegaly, splenomegaly, fatigue, decreased appetite and poor diet, altered growth patterns/delayed sexual maturation, dyspnea, gallstones (cholelithiasis), and pathologic (unexplained) fractures. Thalassemia may cause mongoloid faces in older children.

Diagnosis: blood work (CBC, BMP), family history, clinical picture.

Treatment includes the following:

- Blood transfusions: desired hemoglobin will be 9.3 g/dL at minimum.
- Folate may be given and iron chelation therapy (a mechanism of treatment to remove specific particles from the blood) may be utilized.
- Daily penicillin may be used as a prophylactic mechanism.
- The nurse should counsel the patient to avoid strenuous exercise, and also to avoid iron rich foods.

Note: Cooley anemia is beta-thalassemia major.

HUS and TTP

Hemolytic uremic syndrome (HUS) and **thrombotic thrombocytopenic purpura (TTP)** are characterized by microangiopathic hemolytic anemia (platelet-rich clots forming in capillaries and arterioles) and thrombocytopenia. The hemolytic anemia occurs when red blood cells pass through areas with thrombi and become fragmented by the turbulence. There are, however, some differences:

HUS	TTP
Affects primarily children younger than 5 or older adults Commonly results in renal impairment Cause is usually severe diarrhea from Shiga-toxin producing *E. coli* Signs and symptoms: Fever, dehydration, abdominal tenderness, acute renal failure, neurological impairment. Diagnosis: CBC, coagulation tests, stool cultures, kidney function tests. Treatment is supportive care and dialysis. Plasma exchange has not been as effective with HUS. Eculizumab for treatment of atypical HUS. Blood/platelet transfusions may be indicated.	Primarily affects adults Commonly results in neurological impairment Cause is genetic, autoimmune, or drug-induced Signs and symptoms: altered mental status, fatigue, petechiae, fever, and hemoglobinuria. Diagnosis: CBC, coagulation tests, assessment of von Willebrand factor–cleaving protease (ADAMTS13) activity Treatment is total plasma exchange with FFP. Platelet transfusions are usually avoided. Corticosteroids may also be administered. Refractory cases may respond to vincristine.

DIC

Disseminated intravascular coagulation (DIC) is a life-threatening coagulopathy that occurs secondary to other disorders that accelerate clotting, resulting in occlusions of small blood vessels and depletion of clotting factors and platelets with activation of fibrinolysis. This, in turn, results in hemorrhage. Clotting may impair functioning of the kidneys and other organs. Triggering factors may include various infections, obstetric complications, malignancies, tissue necrosis, heatstroke, toxins, fat embolism, blood transfusion reactions, cardiac arrest, and cardiopulmonary bypass.

Signs and symptoms: Abnormal bleeding of all types (GI, petechiae, oozing around IVs or from surgical incisions), cyanosis (especially of the extremities), impairment of renal function, nausea, vomiting, severe pain (back, abdomen, muscles), shock, and multiple organ failures.

Diagnosis: DIC panel with prolonged prothrombin and partial prothrombin times, increased D-dimer, thrombocytopenia (below 100,000/mcL), fragmented RBCs, and decreased fibrinogen and clotting factors.

Treatment: Identifying and treating underlying cause, anticoagulants, cryoprecipitate (to increase fibrinogen), coagulation inhibitors, and replacement blood products, such as FFP and platelets.

Rheumatoid Arthritis

Rheumatoid arthritis (RA) is a chronic autoimmune disease characterized by cartilage damage that results in inflammation, cartilage and bone deformities, and decreased mobility. Phagocytes (neutrophils and macrophages) form enzymes that cause inflammation and degrade synovial tissue and articular cartilage. This inflammatory process can result in hemorrhage, coagulation, and fibrin deposits within the synovial fluid.

Signs and symptoms: fever, fatigue, joint pain and swelling, decreased ROM, hand/feet deformities, numbness, skin color changes.

Diagnosis: rheumatoid factor tests, C-reactive protein, ESR, synovial fluid exam, x-rays of involved joints.

Treatment includes the following:

- Symptom management; no cure.
- Medications: corticosteroids, anti-malarial drugs, COX-2 inhibitors, NSAIDs.
- Physical therapy, moist heat, splinting for symptom relief.

SLE

Systemic lupus erythematosus (SLE) is an autoimmune disorder that causes widespread inflammation in the joints, skin, and various organ systems. Exacerbations and remissions are part of the disease process of SLE. Possible contributing factors include immunology, environmental factors, hormone abnormalities, and genetics. It is 9 times more common in females.

Signs and symptoms: "butterfly" rash - a red or pink rash spread across the nose and cheeks, weight loss, fever, hair loss, abdominal pain, mouth sores, fatigue, seizures, arthritis, nausea, joint pain, psychosis.

Diagnosis: CBC, chest x-ray, ANA test, Coombs' test, urine analysis, test for various antibodies.

Treatment includes the following:

- Medications: NSAIDs, cytotoxic drugs, hydroxychloroquine.
- Monitor the patient for seizures, anemia, myocarditis, infection, renal failure.
- Teaching: avoid sunlight, wear sunscreen and a hat while outside, contact health care provider if ill or suspect infection; conserve energy, and avoid stress as much as possible.

Respiratory Terminology

1. **Tympanic percussion:** Lung is hyper expanded with air as in asthma, emphysema, chronic bronchitis, and cystic fibrosis.
2. **Dull percussion:** Lung filled with fluid, pus (pleural effusion.)
3. **Decreased breath sounds:** Over obstructed areas (cancer), or decreased lung tissues (emphysema), atelectasis.
4. **Crackles:** Sounds like small, cracking/popping noises – indicates fluid in lungs, like that found in fluid overload or pneumonia.
5. **Rhonchi**: Rough, "course" lung sounds – indicates congestion.
6. **Wheezes:** High, musical sounds resulting when bronchi are narrowed (asthma, chronic bronchitis, cystic fibrosis, localized tumor.)

Review Video: Lung Sounds
Visit mometrix.com/academy and enter code: 447681

Alterations in Respirations

Alterations in respirations are described below:

- **Tachypnea**: respiratory rate >20 breaths per minute.
- **Hypopnea**: respiratory rate <12 breaths per minute.

- **Dyspnea**: shortness of breath, often accompanied by anxiety, gasping, and sitting upright.
- **Ataxic respirations**: completely irregular pattern of respirations with increasing periods of apnea, often associated with brain damage (stroke, TBI) and poor outcome.
- **Cheyne-Stokes**: The patient breathes shallowly at first and then progressively deeper and finally progressively more shallowly until breathing stops for periods of apnea that vary from 30 seconds to 2 minutes before the cycle repeats, associated with dying patients.
- **Biot's breathing**: pattern includes periods of regular but rapid respirations followed by periods of apnea, associated with damage to the medulla in the brain from stroke or tentorial herniation. May also be associated with long-term opioid use.
- **Kussmaul's respirations**: pattern of hyperventilation with the patient increasingly gasping for air, associated with metabolic acidosis/diabetic ketoacidosis.
- **Apneustic respirations**: Prolonged inspiration followed by markedly prolonged expiration, which may be apneic. Associated with damage to respiratory center of the brain.

Pulmonary Hypertension

Pulmonary hypertension (PH) is a condition in which the pulmonary arteries that carry blood from the right atrium to the lungs become constricted so that the pressure inside rises, causing the right atrium to apply increasing pressure in order to facilitate blood flow. This causes the right atrium to expand and weaken to the point it is unable to adequately pump blood to the lungs. PH may be primary or secondary (causes include sarcoidosis, metastases, vascular obstruction, COPD, and scleroderma). Primary hypertension is most common in females (20-40 years) and is usually fatal within 3-4 years.

Signs and symptoms: increasing dyspnea, weakness, syncope, and right heart failure (peripheral edema, jugular venous distention, hepatomegaly, and ascites.)

Diagnosis: ABGs, ECG, cardiac catheterization, pulmonary angiography, echocardiogram, 6-minute walk test, V/Q scan, and pulmonary function tests.

Treatment: includes diuretics (furosemide), anticoagulants (warfarin), inotropic agents (digoxin), oxygen therapy, monitoring of blood gases, daily weight, intake and output, bosentan (blocks endothelin, which constricts arteries), epoprostenol or treprostinil sodium (dilates pulmonary arteries), and sildenafil (relaxes smooth muscles). Definitive treatment is lung or heart/lung transplantation.

Pleural Effusion

Pleural effusion is the accumulation of fluid in the pleural space, usually secondary to other disease processes, such as heart failure, TB, neoplasms, nephrotic syndrome, and viral respiratory infections. The fluid may be serous, bloody, or purulent (empyema), and transudative or exudative.

Signs and symptoms: Depends on underlying condition but includes dyspnea, from mild to severe. Tracheal deviation away from affected side may be evident. **Diagnosis**: includes chest x-ray, lateral decubitus x-ray, CT, thoracentesis, and pleural biopsy.

Treatment: includes treating underlying cause, thoracentesis to remove fluid, insertion of chest tube, pleurodesis, pleurectomy or pleuroperitoneal shunt (primarily with malignancy).

Empyema

Empyema is a pleural effusion in which the collection of pleural fluid is thick and purulent, usually as a result of bacterial pneumonia or penetrating chest trauma. Empyema may also occur as a complication of thoracentesis or thoracic surgery.

Signs and symptoms: acute illness with fever, chills, pain, cough, and dyspnea.

Diagnosis: chest CT and thoracentesis with culture and sensitivity.

Treatment: antibiotics and drainage of pleural space per needle aspiration, tube thoracostomy, or open chest drainage with thoracotomy.

PNEUMONIA

Pneumonia is an infection caused by fluid in the lungs. There are several types of pneumonia, including viral pneumonia, "walking pneumonia," *Legionella* pneumonia, CMV pneumonia (AIDS), aspiration pneumonia, and atypical pneumonia. Pneumonia is a leading cause of death in hospitals, and requires rigorous attention to prevent and treat to avoid complications. Regardless of the cause, pneumonias are all treated similarly.

Signs and symptoms: fever, headache, difficulty breathing, feeling short of breath, cough, inspiratory chest pain.

Diagnosis: chest x-ray, CT scan, pulmonary perfusion scan, CBC, sputum culture, auscultation of crackles.

Treatment includes the following:

- Antibiotics if caused by a bacterial infection.
- Respiratory treatments to open airways.
- Steroids: decrease swelling in lungs.
- IV fluids; thin secretions to cough up, rehydrate.
- Supplemental oxygen and pain medication for discomfort.

Prevention: pneumococcal vaccine for high-risk individuals/those older than 65, incentive spirometry/teaching hospitalized patients to cough/deep breathe, early ambulation.

ARDS

Acute respiratory distress syndrome (ARDS) is inflammation of the lungs. In ARDS, the pulmonary neutrophils gather in excessive amounts at the site of inflammation, along with fibrin and platelets. Injury to capillaries from inflammation leads to edema. The fluid contains plasma proteins that can inactivate the surfactant of the alveoli, causing alveolar collapse. Fibrin clotting then causes obstructed airspaces. The result is decreased respiratory compliance, decreased function, decreased residual volumes, and dead airspace. The end result for the patient is ventilation perfusion mismatching, intrapulmonary shunting, and hypoxemia, and subsequent death. ARDS can be caused by trauma, chemical inhalation, pneumonia, or septic shock.

Signs and symptoms: respiratory distress, hypoxemia, cyanosis, hypotension, tachycardia progressing to bradycardia.

Diagnosis: arterial blood gases, chest x-ray, CBC, blood cultures, physical exam.

Treatment includes the following:

- Mechanical ventilation/intubation with high tidal volumes and PEEP.
- Treat the underlying condition; IV antibiotics, etc.
- Monitor the patient for pulmonary fibrosis, MODS, ventilator-associated pneumonia, and acidosis.

Asthma

Asthma is a chronic obstructive pulmonary disease of the airways that causes them to tighten. During acute attacks, the air supply to the lungs may be shut off completely. *Status Asthmaticus* is when the respiratory distress continues despite vigorous therapeutic measures.

Signs and symptoms: chest tightness, shortness of breath, wheezing, cough, wheezing followed by sudden silence (ominous sign.)

Diagnosis: physical exam, pulmonary function tests (PFTs)

Treatment includes the following:

- Emergency Medications: epinephrine IV (status asthmaticus) albuterol, ipratropium, oral/IV steroids.
- Long-term medications: corticosteroids, sympathomimetics (e.g., terbutaline), bronchodilators (e.g., salmeterol), theophylline (monitor serum levels), leukotriene modifiers (e.g., montelukast).
- Chest physiotherapy (CPT).
- Hyposensitization - allergy shots.
- Avoid exacerbation/allergens.
- Monitor function with peak flow meter.
- Regular exercise to promote pulmonary health.

Review Video: Asthma and Allergens
Visit mometrix.com/academy and enter code: 799141

COPD

Chronic obstructive pulmonary disease (COPD) is an umbrella term for diseases of the bronchi that cause irreversible narrowing of the airways, and forced expiration is decreased. COPD includes chronic bronchitis and emphysema most often, but also includes asthma, cystic fibrosis, and bronchiectasis.

- Chronic bronchitis: productive cough for at least 3 months over the span of 2 years; copious sputum production and cough, morning headache; "blue blowers" – cannot get enough oxygen in.
- Emphysema: overfilling/dilation of alveolar sacs, leading to decreased expiratory effort; minimal cough, wheezing and decreased lung sounds; "pink-puffers" – retain CO_2.

Signs and symptoms: difficulty breathing, dyspnea on exertion, wheezing/tight lung sounds, increased posterior-anterior chest diameter ("barrel chest"), weight loss.

Diagnosis: ABGs, pulmonary function tests (PFTs), clinical picture.

Treatment includes the following:

- Supplemental O_2; however, do not give more than 2-3 liters, as these patients have hypoxic drive to breath.
- Nutrition: hypermetabolic state (increased work of breathing) requires increased calories; however, may limit carbohydrates to limit hypercarbia.

- Teaching: frequent rest/ energy conservation, and pursed lip breathing to increase alveolar resistance, smoking cessation, and avoidance of respiratory irritants (aerosols, allergens, etc.).

**See COPD teaching card for more information*

Epiglottitis

Epiglottitis is an infection of the epiglottis (the flap of tissue that closes off the larynx during swallowing) and the area around the voice box (larynx) caused by *Haemophilus influenzae* type B (HIB). HIB is an aggressive bacterium that used to be responsible for many serious infections in children younger than 5. However, since vaccinations are routinely given, epiglottitis is much more rare, sometimes caused by burns in the throat, trauma, or other organisms.

Signs and symptoms: drooling/difficulty swallowing, sore throat, difficulty breathing, stridor (noisy breathing, "crowing" sound when inhaling), hoarseness, chills, shaking, fever, cyanosis.

Diagnosis: x-ray of throat/chest ("thumb" sign), blood/throat cultures, physical exam.

Treatment includes the following:

- Fluids, antibiotics, steroids for swelling
- Surgery: possible tracheotomy if severe respiratory distress
- Teaching – vaccinate children according to schedule, teach signs and symptoms of respiratory distress; wash hands frequently, do not share food/personal objects

NEVER stick anything into the mouth of a child who has suspected epiglottitis, or try to start IV/do anything distressing; could cause acute throat closure. Must ensure patent airway first.

GERD

Gastroesophageal reflux disease (GERD) is esophagitis caused by reflux of stomach acid back up into the esophagus. There is an increased risk of GERD with decreased sphincter tone with smoking, alcohol, and fatty meals. Reflux is also worsened with obesity, pregnancy, impaired gastric emptying, prone positioning, and peristaltic dysfunction.

Signs and symptoms: heartburn after meals, morning cough or hoarseness (irritation of larynx) less common. Often asymptomatic.

Diagnosis: Physical exam/clinical picture, EGD, pH monitoring.

Treatment includes the following:

- Medication: PPIs (esomeprazole, etc.)/H2 blockers (cimetidine, etc.), antacids (TUMS, etc.)
- Lifestyle modification: decrease irritating foods in diet (coffee, alcohol, carbonated beverages, fatty foods, citrus, tomatoes/tomato products, chocolate, etc.); stay upright an hour after meals, and raise head of bed when sleeping.
- Teach risk of prolonged exposure (especially nocturnal): mucosal damage, including ulceration, erosion, and Barrett esophagus (intestinal metaplasia; higher risk of cancer of esophagus) - may require surgery.

Review Video: What Is GERD
Visit mometrix.com/academy and enter code: 806648

Peptic Ulcer Disease

Peptic ulcer disease (PUD) refers to gastric or duodenal ulcers (erosions of mucosa), which may be associated with NSAID use, aspirin use, *Helicobacter pylori* infection, or chronic alcohol use. Peptic ulcers may be acute or chronic. Gastric ulcers tend to be superficial and associated with normal to decreased gastric secretions while duodenal ulcers are more likely to be penetrating and associated with increased gastric secretions. Both types may result in perforation, hemorrhage, or obstruction.

Signs and symptoms: Gastric ulcers—pain or burning in high epigastrium 1 to 2 hours after meals; Duodenal ulcers—pain, cramping, burning in mid-epigastrium, upper abdomen, and back; 2-4 hours after meals as well as between meals and middle of the night.

Diagnosis: Endoscopy and laboratory tests, including CBC and stools for blood. Barium studies if patient is unable to tolerate endoscopy. *H. pylori* test.

Treatment: Antibiotics if positive for *H. pylori*, H2-receptor blockers, cytoprotective drugs, and antacids. Some patients may benefit from TCAs to reduce stress.

Review Video: Peptic Ulcers and GERD
Visit mometrix.com/academy and enter code: 775788

Dumping Syndrome

Dumping syndrome is a rapid cycle of gastric emptying. When large volumes of food are placed into the small intestine too quickly, fluid is pulled from within the cells to accommodate digestion and hypovolemia occurs, causing the symptoms associated with dumping syndrome. Dumping syndrome is generally the result of gastric surgery, such as gastric bypass or surgery to remove stomach cancer.

Signs and symptoms (take place 30-60 minutes after a meal): flushing, diaphoresis, weakness, dizziness, nausea, abdominal cramping, diarrhea, and potential vasomotor failure (tachycardia, orthostatic or positional hypotension.)

Diagnosis: clinical symptoms, gastric emptying test, serum glucose.

Treatment includes the following:

- Avoid carbohydrates and simple sugars; eat high-fiber foods and protein.
- Do not drink water with meals; eat multiple small meals throughout the day.
- Lie down after eating to ease dizziness and slow gastric emptying.

Gastroparesis

Gastroparesis is a condition in which the muscles that cause peristalsis slow down or stop working all together, resulting in delayed gastric emptying and abdominal discomfort. Patients who have been diagnosed with diabetes have an increased risk of gastroparesis related to diabetic neuropathy of the vagal nerve that innervates the stomach area. Other high-risk patients include those with nervous system diseases, recent surgery, hypothyroidism, and certain cancer and other medications.

Signs and symptoms: bloating, feelings of fullness and/or nausea, vomiting, gastric pain, and heartburn.

Diagnosis: Esophagogastroduodenoscopy (EGD)/upper GI exam/barium swallow, gastric-emptying exam, breath test.

Treatment includes the following:

- Medications: metoclopramide for motility, ondansetron/ antiemetics for nausea/vomiting.
- Surgery: place feeding tube/gastric vent; generally temporary.
- Lifestyle modification: low carbohydrate diet, small, frequent meals are helpful; some patients find that low-fat/fiber, soft or liquid diets assist with food toleration, low-level exercise after eating.

IBS

Inflammatory bowel disease (IBS) is a chronic disorder of the large or small intestine with an unknown cause. *Chronic ulcerative colitis (CUC)* and *Crohn's disease* are designated as inflammatory bowel diseases. Crohn's disease occurs most often between 15 and 35 years, and CUC most often between the ages of 15 and 30 years or between 50 and 70 years. Patients will often experience remissions/exacerbations.

Signs and symptoms: constipation/diarrhea, weight loss, abdominal pain, fever, joint pain, GI bleeding, fistula formations, fat-malabsorption, enlarged colon (megacolon), and obstruction of the bowel.

- *Ulcerative colitis*: massive bleeding with stools; mostly in lower colon.
- *Crohn's disease*: skipping, "cobble-stone" lesions from mouth to anus.

Diagnosis: barium enema, ESR, CRP, colonoscopy

Treatment includes the following:

- Corticosteroids, mesalamine, azathioprine, folate supplements.
- Surgery: drain abscesses, fistula repair, and ostomy (severe.)
- Monitor the patient for ankylosing spondylitis, liver disease, carcinoma, infection, hemorrhage, perforated colon.
- Teaching: NSAIDs, stress, and certain dietary choices will aggravate IBS; report floating stools/limit fat, sitz baths and careful peri-care for comfort. Increase insoluble fiber in diet with diarrhea stools.

Celiac Disease

Celiac disease (gluten-sensitive enteropathy) occurs when the microvilli of the small intestine are damaged by gliadin, a protein of gluten found in wheat, rye, oats, and barley. Celiac disease is generally diagnosed in children, but can occur in adulthood. Atrophy and inflammatory processes in the small intestine are the result of celiac disease, leading to the impaired absorption of vitamins and minerals, causing malnutrition, anemia, and clotting disorders.

Signs and symptoms: loose stools, often diarrhea, fatty stools (steatorrhea), flatus, bloating, weakness, vitamin and nutrient deficiencies, anemia, failure to thrive, changes in personality such as lethargy or irritability.

Diagnosis: clinical symptoms, blood tests for antigens, scope of intestines.

Treatment includes the following:

- No cure: must remove products that contain gluten from the diet including wheat, rye, oat, and barley. Patients cannot digest even a small amount of these foods, nor can they eat food prepared in the same kitchen as foods with gluten.
- Monitor weight on a routine basis, document diet consumption, monitor growth patterns.

DIVERTICULITIS

Diverticulitis is inflammation of diverticula, which are bulging herniations in the intestinal wall, most commonly found in the sigmoid colon, although they can occur anywhere within the GI tract from pharynx to anus. Diverticulitis may result in bowel obstruction, infection, perforation, or hemorrhage as undigested food and bacteria accumulate in diverticula, forming a fecalith (hard mass) that can impair circulation.

Signs and symptoms: acute pain (usually LLQ), abdominal distention, nausea, flatus, fever, constipation, irregular bowel habits, and leukocytosis.

Diagnosis: upper GI, barium enema, and CBC. Colonoscopy is often avoided during acute diverticulitis because of the bowel prep needed.

Treatment: Mild to moderate cases are treated with bedrest, stool softeners, and liquid or bland diet followed by high residue diet and bulk-forming laxatives once symptoms subside. With severe diverticulitis, surgical resection of the bowel may be required, sometimes with a temporary colostomy.

HIATAL HERNIA

Hiatal hernia is an area of the stomach that has protruded upward into the chest via the esophageal hiatus. Hiatal hernias may occur due to weakness in the diaphragm, eructation (belching) on a routine basis, pregnancy, reduced motility of the esophagus (scleroderma), and gastric emptying delays. Disease processes such as Zollinger-Ellison syndrome, and Heller's myotomy are also known causes of hiatal hernia.

Signs and symptoms: heartburn, belching, chest/abdominal pain, GI bleed.

Diagnosis: blood work, x-ray/barium swallow, endoscopy (EGD.)

Treatment includes the following:

- Medications: H2 antagonists, such as ranitidine, famotidine, or cimetidine. Proton pump inhibitors (PPIs), such as esomeprazole or lansoprazole, are also used.
- Lifestyle modification: refraining from lying flat in bed/going to bed directly after consuming a meal, avoiding restrictive clothing, weight loss, avoiding caffeine and spicy foods.
- Clinical note: the H2 receptor agonists all have the suffix *-ine*, and PPIs all end in *-azole.*

INTUSSUSCEPTION

Intussusception is the inversion of one portion of the intestine into another resulting in intestinal obstruction, often called *telescoping* of the bowel. It is often found in infants and toddlers, but can occur in older adults as well. The cause is often unknown in children, but can be caused by tumors or adhesions in adults.

Signs and symptoms: severe intermittent or constant abdominal pain with drawing up of the lower extremities, abdominal distention, emesis with bile, diarrhea, or jelly-type stools (presence of blood and/or mucus), lethargy, palpable abdominal mass, fever and pallor.

Diagnosis: EGD, MRI with contrast, x-ray (shows "bullseye"), air/barium enema.

Treatment includes the following:

- NG tube and IV fluids for rehydration and gastric decompression.
- A barium/ air enema will diagnose as well as fix the problem for most children. Adults generally require surgical repair.
- Monitor for signs of peritonitis and dehydration.

Appendicitis

Appendicitis is an acute inflammation of the vermiform appendix. More commonly found in males than females, appendicitis can be deadly if not diagnosed and treated promptly.

Signs and symptoms: McBurney sign (rebound tenderness), Psoas sign (pain with right thigh extension), abdominal pain that starts near the umbilicus and moves to the right lower quadrant, guarding of the area, anorexia, nausea and vomiting, constipation or mild diarrhea, elevated temperature, rapid heart rate.

Diagnosis: blood work, rectal exam, CT scan, ultrasound

Treatment includes the following:

- Fluids for correction of any fluid or electrolyte imbalances.
- Broad-spectrum antibiotics.
- Surgical procedures to remove the appendix or drain any abscess that may have occurred.
- Teaching: full activity should return within 6 weeks post-op, resume diet as bowel function resumes (typically 24 to 48 hours post-op).
- Monitor for nausea, vomiting, pain, fever and chills; could be peritonitis.

Acute Pancreatitis

Acute pancreatitis is an inflammatory process of the pancreas caused by autodigestion of trypsin. Causes of pancreatitis include gallstones (microlithiasis), alcohol, and trauma, treatment for AIDS, antibiotics, diuretics, and treatments for inflammatory bowel disorders.

Signs and symptoms: epigastric pain that radiates to the back, nausea and vomiting, fever, shock, hypotension, jaundice; Grey Turner Sign is flank discoloration (bluish); Cullen sign - umbilical discoloration.

Diagnosis: blood work (amylase/lipase), C-reactive protein, CT/MRI, endoscopic ultrasound, stool studies; be aware that insulin and steroids have the potential to alter lab results in these patients.

Treatment: **PANCREAS**

- **P**: pain control: generally narcotics, pain is severe.
- **A**: arrest and shock will require intravenous (IV) fluids.
- **N**: nasogastric tube; clear liquids or NPO; possibly TPN.
- **C**: calcium monitoring.
- **R**: renal function evaluation (BUN/creatinine.)

- **E**: ensure adequate pulmonary function (risk of acidosis.)
- **A**: antimicrobial therapy.
- **S**: surgical or other procedures to assist with treatment.

Teaching: bedrest, position with pillows for comfort. Smoking and drinking cessation. Increase fluids, low-fat/high-protein diet; may take supplemental enzymes to aid digestion.

HEPATITIS CIRRHOSIS/PORTAL HYPERTENSION

Portal hypertension or *hepatitis cirrhosis* is a disruption in the normal configuration of hepatic lobules or obstruction of the portal vein leading to increased portal venous pressure and subsequent cell death. Portal hypertension occurs predominantly in older adult males. Risk factors for portal hypertension include cirrhosis, alcohol abuse, viral hepatitis B, hepatitis C, and hemochromatosis.

Signs and symptoms: Hepatosplenomegaly, caput medusa (varicose veins that radiate from the umbilicus), umbilical bruit, hemorrhoids, spider angiomata, gynecomastia, testicular atrophy, and digital clubbing.

Diagnosis: Blood work (AST/ALT), EGD, x-ray.

Treatment includes the following:

- Treat underlying cause: antivirals, drinking cessation, etc.
- Nutritional and metabolic support.
- Monitor for changes in level of consciousness (LOC) as this is the first sign of hepatic encephalopathy (buildup of ammonia causing damage to brain.)

NECROTIZING ENTEROCOLITIS

Necrotizing enterocolitis (NEC) is an acute inflammatory disease of the bowel in preterm and high-risk infants. While the cause is unknown, it leads to ischemia and death of the bowel tissue, often with fatal infection if not recognized and treated promptly. Risk factors include prematurity, formula feeding, and difficult delivery.

Signs and symptoms: swollen abdomen, nausea/vomiting, lethargy, refusal to eat, fever, tachycardia, constipation/bloody stools.

Diagnosis: x-ray, blood work, lab studies (stool, blood, urine cultures)

Treatment includes the following:

- IV antibiotics and fluids; TPN for nutrition.
- NG tube for gastric decompression.
- Bowel resection if perforation occurs; temporary or permanent ostomy.

Prevention: NPO for 24-48 h if suspected asphyxiation during birth or very low birth weight infant, human milk is preferred food for oral feeds.

UTIS

Urinary tract infections (UTIs) are bacterial infections that cause inflammation in one or more areas of the urinary tract. *Escherichia coli* is the most common causative organism with urinary tract infections, often transmitted from the GI tract. "Urinary tract infection" is an umbrella term used to discuss cystitis (bladder infection), pyelonephritis (kidney infection), and urethritis.

Types of UTIs are as follows:

- *Recurrent*—repeated episodes.
- *Persistent*—bacteriuria despite antibiotics.
- *Febrile*—typically indicates pyelonephritis.
- *Urosepsis*—bacterial illness; urinary pathogens in blood.

Signs and symptoms: fever, polyuria, and urgency with urination, dysuria, urinary retention, and enuresis (episodes of incontinence). Pain in low back, flank area, and lower abdominal area. *Elderly: only sign may be change in mental status; Pediatric - asymptomatic until septic.*

Diagnosis: urinalysis, blood tests, physical exam.

Treatment includes the following:

- Antibiotic therapy; may culture urine to use most effective medicine.
- Fluids: hydrate and flush out bacteria; cranberry juice may help.
- Teach: stay hydrated, avoid hot tubs and baths, Woman – urinate after sex, wipe front-to-back.

Acute Glomerulonephritis

Acute glomerulonephritis is characterized by inflammation of the glomeruli in the kidneys, most often caused by an antigen-antibody response to group A beta-hemolytic *Streptococcus*.

Signs and symptoms: cola-colored urine (hematuria), foamy urine, oliguria/anuria, edema, hypertension, protein, nitrates, cells, epithelial cells, and casts in urine.

Diagnosis: blood work (creatinine, BUN, ESR), urinalysis, x-ray/CT, renal biopsy

- Ask if patient has had a sore throat in the past 2 weeks, or history of heart valve replacement.

Treatment includes the following:

- Controlling blood pressure is priority: ACE inhibitors/angiotensin II blockers, diuretics.
- Usually will resolve on own without specific treatment.
- Teach: report and treat sore throat promptly to prevent systemic spread of strep infections.

BPH

Benign prostatic hypertrophy (BPH) is the enlargement of the prostate to the point that it begins to compress the urethra and cause some degree of urinary obstruction. BPH commences with changes in the periurethral glandular tissue. The enlarged tissue may obstruct the urethra or create a pouch within the bladder that results in urinary retention. BPH may result from hormonal changes, inflammation, or metabolic changes.

Signs and symptoms: Early indications include reduced urinary stream in both volume and force, difficulty initiating urination, urinary retention, and urgency. Later symptoms include frequent urination, nocturia, incontinence, and urinary obstruction.

Diagnosis: Urinalysis and culture positive for hematuria and/or pyuria, elevated BUN and creatinine (with impaired renal function), IVP, and cystourethroscopy. The prostate may be palpable on rectal exam.

Treatment: Conservative treatment includes sitz baths and prostatic massage. Definitive treatment is surgical prostatectomy. Transurethral resection of the prostate (TURP) is usually done if the prostate weighs less than 2 ounces. If patients are poor candidates for surgery, an indwelling Foley catheter (usually suprapubic) may be inserted.

GOUT

Gout is a disorder of altered purine metabolism characterized by elevated uric acid levels that cause inflammation. This results in a sudden onset of crystal deposits and sodium urate in the connective tissues and articular cartilage, usually affecting the joint of the big toe. Risk factors for gout include severe arthritis, family history, male sex, obesity, recent surgery/trauma, and alcohol abuse.

Signs and symptoms: acute onset of swelling, severe pain (even weight of sheet will seem unbearable), and erythema in 1 or more joints, soft tissue redness and warmth.

Diagnosis: blood work (uric acid, creatinine), joint fluid biopsy, physical exam, ultrasound.

Treatment includes the following:

- Medications: colchicine, NSAIDs, steroids for acute flareup.
- Fluids and rest; keep pressure off of affected area.

Prevention: allopurinol or febuxostat lowers uric acid in blood, and probenecid increases excretion of uric acid from the body.

Teaching: Take medications as directed to prevent flareups: gout is a recurring disorder; diet restrictions: low fat, low or no alcohol, decrease red meat/seafood, no sardines, anchovies, liver, or sweetbreads.

CUSHING SYNDROME

Cushing syndrome is an abnormal production of ACTH, which causes elevated cortisol levels. It can be caused by prolonged use of corticosteroids or tumor on adrenal cortex.

Signs and symptoms: Muscle weakness, central obesity distribution, hyperglycemia, hyperkalemia, bone and joint pain, hypertension, mood changes, headaches, frequent urination, moon-shaped facies, weight gain, acne, hirsutism, immunosuppression.

Diagnosis: dexamethasone suppression test, cortisol level check, MRI-check for tumors.

Treatment includes the following:

- Surgery to remove tumor.
- Monitor corticosteroid levels; avoid prolonged use of steroids.
- Symptom management; wash hands frequently to avoid infection, low-carb diet to manage blood sugar/weight gain, etc.
- Monitor the patient for kidney stones, HTN, diabetes, fractures.

Classifications of Diabetes

The National Institutes of Health (NIH) recognizes the following as **classifications of diabetes.**

- **Diabetes Mellitus (DM)**: an umbrella term that includes type I diabetes (insulin-dependent diabetes) and type II (non-insulin dependent diabetes). Type II divides into nonobese non-insulin dependent or obese non-insulin dependent diabetes.
- **Impaired Glucose Tolerance (IGT)**: Impaired glucose tolerance occurs when there is an increased amount of circulating blood glucose after consuming an increased amount of carbohydrates.
- **Gestational Diabetes Mellitus (GD)**: Gestational diabetes is a form of diabetes mellitus that occurs during pregnancy, characterized by the pregnant woman's intolerance of carbohydrates.

Type I Diabetes Mellitus

Type I diabetes mellitus or *insulin dependent diabetes mellitus (IDDM)* was formerly called childhood-onset diabetes because it typically surfaces early in life, before the age of 30. In these individuals, the beta cells of the islets of Langerhans have suffered damage, usually due to autoimmunity, childhood disease, exposure to toxins, or congenital damage. This results in the inability of the pancreas to produce insulin, and results in inability of the body to use glucose.

Signs and symptoms: polyuria, polydipsia, polyphagia, weight loss, weakness, fatigue, increased rates of infection, and increased healing time.

Diagnosis: fasting blood glucose, glucose tolerance test.

Treatment includes the following:

- Insulin replacement: use of short-acting and long-acting insulins to replace function of pancreas.
- Teaching: signs and symptoms of hypo/hyperglycemia, lifestyle modification (diabetic diet, sick-day rules, when and how to check blood sugar, etc.).
- *Ketoacidosis* from fat metabolism when insulin is under-administered; teach signs and symptoms as this complication can be life-threatening if not treated properly.

Treatment of Diabetes Mellitus Type I

People with **type I diabetes** produce no insulin of their own, so all insulin must be supplemented. Therefore, stabilization of blood glucose levels is the priority of care with the type I diabetic patient. Insulin therapy is the only course of medications that can be used with the type I diabetic patient; insulin injections serve to replace what is not being produced by the body. Clinical diabetic patients are educated on food exchanges to maintain the proper carbohydrate, protein, and fat ratios that promote normal blood glucose levels. Carbohydrates represent 50% of the diabetic diet, protein represents 20%, and fat represents the remaining 30% of the diabetic diet.

*Clinical note: Oral antidiabetic agents stimulate insulin production in the pancreas; in a patient with the type I diabetes, the pancreas is not capable of producing insulin. Therefore, oral antidiabetic agents are not effective for these individuals.

Review Video: Diabetes Type I
Visit mometrix.com/academy and enter code: 501396

Type II Diabetes Mellitus

Type II diabetes or *non-insulin dependent diabetes mellitus* (NIDDM) is characterized by insulin resistance in the peripheral tissues along with a decreased production of insulin by the beta cells of the pancreas. Obesity and increased age increase the risk of developing NIDDM. Diabetes mellitus type II causes the same systemic effects as type I diabetes, neuropathy, retinopathy, and increased rates of atherosclerosis leading to cardiovascular disease.

Signs and symptoms: polyuria, polydipsia, polyphagia, weight loss, weakness, fatigue, increased rates of infection, increased healing time.

Diagnosis: fasting blood sugar, glucose tolerance test.

Treatment includes the following:

- Oral hypoglycemics: desired glucose range is 70-110 mg/dL.
- Home glucose monitoring should be done before every meal and at bedtime and PRN.
- Diet education: 10%-20% protein, <10% fats, rest carbohydrates. Limit sugar.
- Lifestyle modification: regular exercise, weight loss can actually reverse disease process.

Review Video: Diabetes Complications
Visit mometrix.com/academy and enter code: 963669

Review Video: Diabetes: Diet and Exercise
Visit mometrix.com/academy and enter code: 861346

DKA

Diabetic ketoacidosis (DKA) is a condition that occurs in diabetic patients in which the body metabolizes fat instead of carbohydrates in the absence of insulin. As the body is utilizing fatty acids for energy, it begins producing an abnormal amount of ketones (ketosis). With ketoacidosis, the glucose level is elevated and the patient is suffering life-threatening hyperglycemia. Extreme physiological stress, illness, and poor blood glucose management are all potential causes of DKA.

Signs and symptoms: Kussmaul respirations; fruity odor to the breath, dehydration, anorexia or polyphagia, polydipsia, hypotension, hypothermia, confusion, tachycardia, tachypnea, hypothermia, weakness, malaise, lethargy, nausea, and/or vomiting.

Diagnosis: blood work (BMP/CBC), urinalysis (ketones), ABGs, chest x-ray, clinical picture, ECG.

Treatment includes the following:

- Fluid resuscitation -1000 mL the first hour is standard.
- Intravenous insulin.
- Monitor blood glucose and serum potassium closely, as both will drop dramatically with movement of glucose into cells.

Prevention: follow diabetes management plan, check sugar more often in times of illness and stress, report ketones in urine right away.

Thyroid Disorders

The **thyroid** is an important organ of the body that secretes hormones that stimulate growth and metabolism. The thyroid hormones are thyroxine (T4) and triiodothyronine (T3). Thyroid hormones contain iodine compounds that are crucial to normal development. Patients can either have hyperactive thyroid (Graves' disease) or hypothyroidism. Patients must be placed on life-long treatment to avoid ill effects.

Review Video: Thyroid and Antithyroid Drugs
Visit mometrix.com/academy and enter code: 816247

Signs and symptoms:

- *Hyperthyroidism:* hyperactive, hot, weight loss, fatigue.
- *Hypothyroidism*: depression, cold, weight gain, fatigue, constipation, goiter, myxedema, coma.
- *Congenital Hypothyroidism*: jaundice (>24 h), difficulty feeding, inactivity, constipation, umbilical hernia, wide-set eyes, broad, flat noses, tongue protrusion, and coarse, brittle hair, delayed dentition, anemia, developmental delays.

Diagnosis: blood work (TSH/T4 levels), physical exam

Treatment includes the following:

- Medication: will get regular blood work to assess efficacy
  - Hyperthyroidism: propylthiouracil (PTU), methimazole
  - Hypothyroidism: levothyroxine
- Surgical removal of thyroid (hyper); must then replace hormones with levothyroxine.

Review Video: Hyperthyroidism
Visit mometrix.com/academy and enter code: 374763

Review Video: Graves' Disease
Visit mometrix.com/academy and enter code: 543173

Acne

Acne is a disease that involves the sebaceous glands and hair follicles of the skin. Excessive sebum production causes the overgrowth of *Propionibacterium acnes* bacteria, causing the formation of pustules on the skin of the face, back, and chest. Acne is more common in boys than girls, and peak age is 16-17 years old for young women and 17-18 years for young men.

Treatment includes the following: (combined approach most effective)

- General - well-balanced diet, rest, decrease stress
- Cleansing - acne not caused by dirt or oil on the skin; however, gentle cleansing daily/ twice a day prevents spread of bacteria
- Medication
  - Topical: Retinoid and Benzoyl Peroxide: use 30 minutes after cleansing. Can cause photosensitivity; wear sunscreen outdoors.
  - Oral: Accutane (isotretinoin [13-cis-retinoic acid]); only in severe cases; *contraindicated in pregnancy* (causes severe birth defects.)
- Female only: Oral birth control is sometimes prescribed as it is found helpful in treating hormonal forms of acne.

Contusions and Hematomas

A **contusion (bruise)** is characterized by bleeding into the skin when it is crushed or squeezed and not broken. The progressive color changes of bruises or contusions reflect the time or duration of the bruise; initial contusions begin as red or deep purple, fade to blue or black, then yellow and/or green before fading back to normal skin tone. The discoloration relates to the extent of vascular injury.

A **hematoma** is characterized by blood that has collected or pooled into the soft tissue of an enclosed space. Hematomas may cause problems when they exert pressure on adjacent structures.

- *Subdural Hematoma:* A subdural hematoma is a pooling or collection of blood between the dura mater and the surface of the brain. Subdural hematomas result from shearing of small veins that connect the subdural space.
- *Epidermal Hematoma:* An epidermal hematoma is a collection or pooling of blood between the inner surface of the skull and the dura. Epidermal hematomas are the result of arterial tears.

Treatment includes the following:

- Document placement, size, and coloration—do not diagnose.
- Note: multiple bruises in different stages of healing/on the torso could indicate abuse.

Phases of Wound Healing

The four phases of wound healing are as follows:

- **Phase 1**: Inflammation

  Edema of the tissues as injured cells leak contents; angiogenesis - growth of new blood vessels in damaged tissue; phagocytosis – white blood cells destroy invading pathogens.

- **Phase 2**: Granulation/Proliferation

  Lasts 5-30 days; formation of granulation tissue, which helps rebuild lost cells in the base of the wound.

- **Phase 3**: Contraction

  Fibroblasts bring wound edges closer together to aid in closing the wound.

- **Phase 4**: Maturation

  Scab forms over wound, which eventually falls off and leaves scar tissue in some cases.

The following are **factors that influence healing**:

- Moist, crust-free environment enhances wound healing.
- Poor nutrition, stress, infection, diseases, and decreased circulation can all increase healing time.

Atopic Dermatitis

Atopic dermatitis is an inflammatory reaction that is traditionally caused by allergens that come in contact with the skin. The nurse will need to assess for secondary infection related to scratching.

Signs and symptoms: erythema, papules, vesicles and macules that may or may not produce exudates. The individual will experience itching (pruritus), and erythema to the affected areas. Lesions may appear on the face, trunk, limbs, or head.

Teaching:

- At the time of initial exam, the nurse should assess for exposure to chemicals, history of skin infections, climate exposure that includes excessive heat and cold, as well as determination of any changes taking place within the household.
- Instruct patient to limit or avoid stress as possible, minimize over exposure to heat or cold, take tepid baths, use oatmeal in the bath to help with pruritus, decrease or limit the use of perfumed soaps, decrease sun exposure, and avoid lotions that contain alcohol. Stress the use of emollient creams for symptom relief.

FRACTURES

A **fracture** is a full or partial break in a bone, and classified as open (compound) vs closed (simple) fractures. Open (compound) fractures are fractures in which the bone protrudes out of the skin. Types include:

- Pathological fractures: Breaks at the site of an abnormality/existing weakness (tumors, osteoporosis, infection, and metabolic disorders).
- Stress fractures: result from repeated stress placed on the bone.
- Oblique fractures: occur at a curve or slope.
- Greenstick: incomplete fracture caused by excessive bend (pediatric).
- Transverse: broken bone at right angle to axis.
- Comminuted: fractured into several pieces.
- Buckled/impacted: ends of bone are driven into each other (pediatric arm fractures).

Signs and symptoms: swelling/bruising, obvious deformity, pain with movement, loss of ROM.

Diagnosis: x-ray, physical exam

Treatment includes the following:

- Casting/immobilize bone.
- Surgery: may require pins/rods to help reconstruct bone.
- Teaching: do not stick anything into cast, cover during shower, may have to do PT/OT to regain strength in limb.

Note: If casted, watch for compartment syndrome (#1 symptom = pain unrelieved by narcotics).

SCLERODERMA

Scleroderma is a diffuse connective tissue disorder in which insoluble collagen forms and accumulates in the tissues, leading to fibrotic changes, loss of elasticity, and impaired movement. The disorder starts in the hands and spreads systemically to the heart, lungs, and digestive system.

Signs and symptoms: Scleroderma usually starts with Raynaud phenomenon in the hands. Symptoms are referred to as CREST syndrome:

- **(C)**alcium deposits in the skin
- **(R)**aynaud's phenomenon (spasm of blood vessel due to cold or emotional stress)

- **(E)**sophageal hardening (acid reflux)
- **(S)**clerodactyly (thickening of skin on fingers/hands)
- **(T)**elangiectasia (capillary dilation that forms vascular lesions)

Diagnosis: based on symptoms, skin biopsy, pulmonary studies, esophageal studies, echocardiography, and ANA (positive ANA indicates connective tissue disorder).

Treatment: There is no specific treatment for the disease but counseling and support should be offered to patients. Calcium channel blockers and antihypertensive may help alleviate Raynaud phenomenon, and NSAIDs may help relieve inflammation and pain. Careful skin care is indicated to prevent skin breakdown. Patient teaching must include protective measures to avoid cold, which will worsen Raynaud.

RSV

Respiratory syncytial virus (RSV) is a virus that attacks the respiratory system, usually of infants and young children; however, it can affect all age groups. It is highly contagious, and can spread throughout nurseries and day cares. It is a family of viruses, so there is no active immunity against the disease.

Signs and symptoms: fever, SOB, cyanosis, wheezing, nasal congestion, croupy cough.

Diagnosis: chest x-ray, ABGs, physical exam.

Treatment includes the following:

- Medications: ribavirin, bronchodilators.
- IV fluids for rehydration, thin secretions.
- May require ventilator in severe cases.
- Symptom management: Infants – sleep with head propped up (blocks under crib legs), frequent small feedings, suction nose and mouth (mouth first to prevent aspiration) with bulb suction, monitor for wheezing/respiratory distress (accessory muscle use, retractions, and cyanosis.)
- Monitor the patient for pneumonia, respiratory failure, and otitis media.

Opportunistic Infections Associated with AIDS

Opportunistic infections are infections that occur in AIDS patients. Due to the decreased immunity characterized by the disease, these infections now have the "opportunity" to infect the individual. Remember, AIDS patients do not die of AIDS, but of one of these diseases:

- Salmonellosis, syphilis, and neurosyphilis
- Tuberculosis (TB), bacillary angiomatosis ("cat-scratch disease")
- Aspergillosis, candidiasis (thrush, yeast infection)
- Coccidioidomycosis, cryptococcal meningitis
- Histoplasmosis, Kaposi sarcoma
- Lymphoma, systemic non-Hodgkin lymphoma (NHL)
- Primary CNS lymphoma, cryptosporidiosis
- Isosporiasis, microsporidiosis
- *Pneumocystis jiroveci* pneumonia (PCP), toxoplasmosis
- Cytomegalovirus (CMV), hepatitis
- Herpes simplex (HSV, genital herpes), herpes zoster (HZV, shingles)

- Human papilloma virus (HPV, genital warts, cervical cancer)
- AIDS dementia complex (ADC)

Review Video: AIDS Infections & Malignancies
Visit mometrix.com/academy and enter code: 217128

Hypothermia

Hypothermia is a condition that results when more heat is lost than the body can generate, and is defined as an internal body temperature less than 95 °F. Symptoms usually develop slowly; someone with hypothermia typically experiences gradual loss of mental acuity and physical ability; may be unaware of the need for emergency medical treatment. Older adults, infants, young children, and people who are underweight are at particular risk.

Signs and symptoms: shivering, bradycardia, slurred speech, abnormally slow breathing, cold/pale skin, loss of coordination, fatigue, lethargy, and coma.

Diagnosis: vital signs, clinical picture

Treatment includes the following:

- Emergency management: infusion of warmed IV fluids, Bair-Hugger (circulates continuously warmed air around patient), warm blankets, give warm fluids; use rectal temperature.

Prevention: community education about shelters during cold weather, avoid prolonged exposure to cold, layered clothing.

Note: Severe hypothermia can hide pulse and blood pressure—"They're not dead until they're warm and dead"

Heat Cramps, Heat Exhaustion, and Heat Stroke

Heat-related illnesses are a consequence of prolonged or intense exposure to elevated temperatures. There are three main types of heat-related illnesses:

1. **Heat cramps** are painful muscle spasms in the abdomen, arms, or legs following strenuous activity. The skin is usually moist and cool and the pulse is normal or slightly raised.
2. **Heat exhaustion** means the body is becoming overheated. The person may be thirsty, giddy, weak, uncoordinated, nauseous, and *sweating profusely*; the pulse is slowed and weak. The skin feels cold and clammy to the touch.
3. **Heat stroke** can be LIFE-THREATENING! Immediate medical attention is essential. Body temperature above 104 °F: may exhibit confusion/combativeness, lethargy/faintness, staggering, strong rapid or extremely slowed pulse, *dry flushed skin,* lack of sweating, possible delirium or coma.

Treatment: If a person is exhibiting signs of heat-related illness, immediately move him/her into a cool and shaded area. Remove any excess clothing, and offer fluids, preferably something with electrolytes. If symptoms do not immediately begin to improve, get immediate medical help.

Prevention: Stay hydrated when outdoors during hot weather, wear light-colored clothes, avoid hours of peak heat (2-5 PM).

Medical Emergencies

Advanced Cardiac Life Support Measures

Pulseless Electrical Activity (PEA)

Pulseless electrical activity is any rhythm without a palpable pulse (common after defibrillation). Identifying and correcting the underlying cause is critical for treatment. Common causes include:

5 Hs	5 Ts
Hypokalemia/Hyperkalemia	Toxins
Hypoxia	Tamponade (cardiac)
Hypothermia	Tension pneumothorax
Hypovolemia	Thrombosis (lungs)
Hydrogen ion (acidosis)	Thrombosis (heart)

Intervention: Begin CPR (100-120 per minute), IV access line, epinephrine1 mg/IV/IO every 3 to 5 minutes, intubation and ventilation (ventilate 10 times/minute), oxygen as indicated.

Asystole

Asystole ("flatlined") is absence of audible heartbeat, palpable pulse, and respirations. ECG may show some P waves initially, the QRS complex is absent although there may be an occasional QRS "escape beat." Intervention: Check leads, begin CPR, IV access line, epinephrine as for PEA every 3 to 5 minutes, intubation and ventilation (ventilate 10 times/minute), oxygen as indicated.

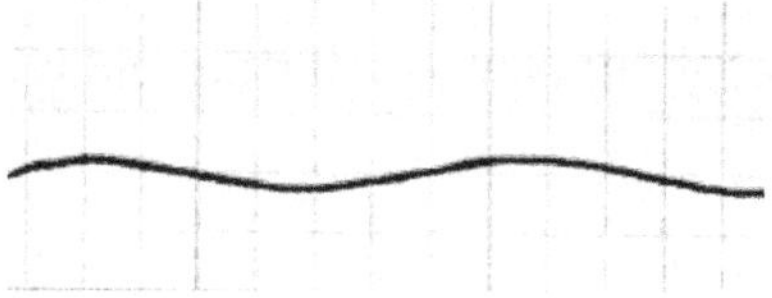

Ventricular Fibrillation/Pulseless Ventricular Tachycardia

Ventricular fibrillation/Pulseless ventricular tachycardia (VF) is a rapid, very irregular ventricular rate >300 beats per minute with no atrial activity observable on the ECG, caused by disorganized electrical activity in the ventricles. The QRS complex is not recognizable as ECG shows irregular undulations. The causes are the same as for ventricular tachycardia (VT) (alcohol, caffeine, nicotine, underlying coronary disease), and cardiac arrest may result if VF is not treated. VF may also result from an electrical shock or congenital disorder, such as Brugada syndrome. VF is accompanied by lack of palpable pulse, audible pulse, and respirations and is immediately life threatening without defibrillation. Emergent treatment includes initiating CPR (CAB protocol) and carrying out defibrillation as soon as possible. After emergency defibrillation, CPR should be continued for two minutes and then the rate and rhythm checked and cause considered. If VF persists, then epinephrine is given and repeated every 3-5 minutes. If ineffective, amiodarone 300 mg is given IV. Defibrillation and medication are given alternately with 2 minutes of CPR until the client recovers or recovery efforts are stopped. Mortality is high if VF occurs as part of a myocardial infarction.

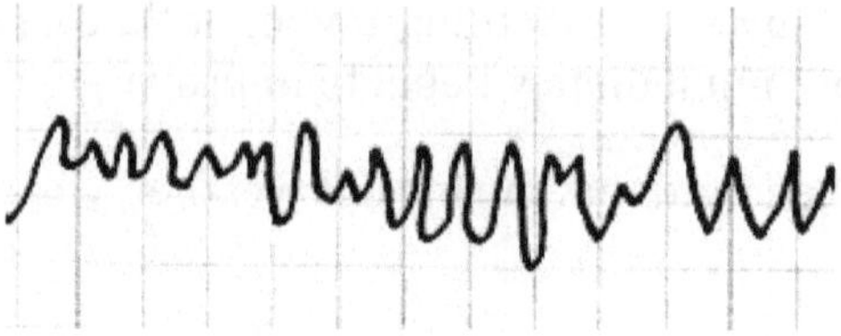

Symptomatic Bradycardia

Bradycardia (<60 bpm) may be benign in some clients but needs immediate intervention if the client has serious symptoms related to the slow heart rate (after other causes are ruled out). Symptoms may include: hypotension, pulmonary edema, chest pain, dyspnea, heart failure, fatigue, weakness, dizziness, altered mental status, and shock. The client's perfusion should be assessed and, if adequate, the client can be monitored, but if perfusion is inadequate, immediate interventions are needed, according to ACLS guidelines:

- Begin transcutaneous pacing if IV access is not yet available.
- If IV access available, begin with atropine 0.5 mg, repeated every 3-5 minutes to maximum 3 mg/6 doses while preparing for pacing.
- If bradycardia does not convert with atropine, begin transcutaneous pacing.
- If transcutaneous pacing is not effective (or while awaiting pacing instead of atropine in some cases), administer epinephrine 2-10 mcg/min or dopamine 2-20 mcg/kg/min.

Interventions should be carried out in rapid succession to prevent cardiac arrest.

Sustained and Symptomatic Atrial Fibrillation

Atrial fibrillation (Afib) is rapid, disorganized atrial beats that are ineffective in emptying the atria, so that blood pools and can lead to thrombus formation and emboli. The ventricular rate increases with a decreased stroke volume, and cardiac output decreases with increased myocardial ischemia, resulting in palpitations and fatigue. Afib is caused by coronary artery disease, valvular disease, pulmonary disease, heavy alcohol ingestion, and cardiac surgery. Afib in characterized by very irregular pulse with atrial rate of 300-600 and ventricular rate of 120-200, shape and duration (0.4 to 0.11 seconds) of QRS is usually normal. Fibrillatory (F) waves are seen instead of P waves. The PR interval cannot be measured and the P: QRS ratio is highly variable. Score as Afib during sleep with irregularly irregular ventricular rhythm and varying rapid oscillations replacing P waves. Treatment may include:

- Diltiazem or metoprolol to control heart rate. Amiodarone is sometimes used but is not FDA-approved for this condition. Digoxin may be used but is less effective.
- Anticoagulant: Heparin initially and then converted to warfarin if Afib persists >24 hours.
- Synchronized cardioversion (50-100 joules).
- Cardiac catheterization with ablation (more effective than cardioversion).

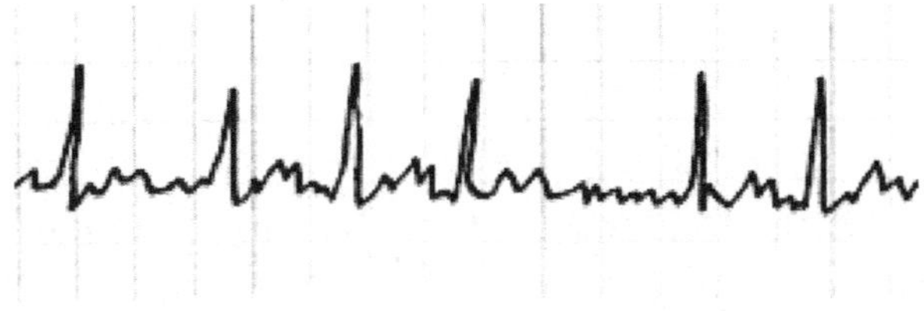

CVA

Cerebrovascular accident (CVA; stroke) is sudden impairment of circulation in one or more of the blood vessels supplying the brain because of thrombosis (most common), embolism, or hemorrhage, with strokes classified as ischemic or hemorrhagic. The lack of oxygen to the brain tissue can result in permanent brain damage. Risk factors include history of transient ischemic episodes (TIEs), atherosclerosis, hypertension, rheumatic heart disease, diabetes, gout, cardiomyopathy, oral contraceptives, cigarette smoking, and dysrhythmias.

Signs and symptoms: Varies depending on the site of the occlusion. If the stroke occurs on the left side, then right-sided paresis/paralysis occurs and *vice versa*, although damage to facial nerves results in nerve dysfunction on the same side.

Diagnosis: May include CT, MRI, EEG, and/or angiography.

Treatment includes the following:

- Ischemic strokes are treated with aspirin and tissue plasminogen activator (tPA) (within 4.5 hours) as well as supportive treatment.
- Hemorrhagic strokes may require supportive care and surgical repair (coil, clip, AVM repair, radiosurgery, intracranial bypass).
- Short-term or long-term physical and rehabilitative therapy.

Review Video: Strokes
Visit mometrix.com/academy and enter code: 148798

Development of Neurovascular Compromise

Compartment syndrome is excessively high pressure in a compartment of the body (most often the legs, arm, or abdomen) that usually results from blood or edema filling the area. This commonly happens after cast application or circumferential burns. *Acute arterial occlusions* happen when blood flow to an extremity (most often the leg) is suddenly stopped. It occurs most often in patients with a history of peripheral artery disease or in the postoperative period after many cardiovascular surgeries. These are both considered medical emergencies; if left untreated, they will result in tissue necrosis and death.

The following are the **key signs and symptoms of neurovascular compromise (6 P's)**:

- **P**araesthesia
- **P**ain out of proportion to injury; not relieved by narcotics (key)
- **P**aralysis
- **P**allor
- **P**ulselessness
- **P**oikilothermia (temperature difference between injured and uninjured limbs)

Phases of Burn Management

The three phases of burn management are:

1. The Emergent Phase (Resuscitative Phase)
   a. 24-48 h; begins with fluid loss/edema formation and continues until fluid motorization and diuresis begins.
   b. **Complications**: hypovolemic shock and obstructed airway (often delayed 24 h), pneumonia, arrhythmias, compartment syndrome (circumferential burns), acute tubular necrosis/ renal failure.
   c. **Interventions**: fluid resuscitation, vasopressors, artificial airway, escharotomy (restores circulation.)
2. The Acute Phase:
   a. Weeks/months: diuresis to complete wound healing.
   b. **Complications**: infection/sepsis (usually gram-negative); gastroparesis/intestinal ileus, ulcers, stress-induced diabetes mellitus, contractures.

c. **Interventions**: IV antibiotics – culture wounds/IV/Foley/etc. for bacteria/sensitivity, pain management, skin grafts, NG tube, PPIs for ulcer, wound care/debridement, passive/active ROM.

3. The Rehabilitative Phase:
   a. Weeks to months: from wound covered to optimal functioning.
   b. **Complications**: joint/skin contractures and scarring, permanent disability, regression/depression.
   c. **Interventions**: physical/occupational therapy, splints/pressure garments. May need psychiatric counseling for body image alterations and self-esteem issues, encourage support groups and counseling, protect grafts from sunlight for 1 year.

Burn Injuries

Burns occur when intense or prolonged heat causes injury to the cells.

The following are types of burn injury:

- *Thermal burns* - (common) flames, hot objects/water
  - Complications: massive skin loss – skin grafts
- *Chemical burns* - acids or alkaline; internal or external
  - Complications: tissue destruction may continue for 72 h
- *Electrical burns* - electrical current (coagulation necrosis)
  - Complications: fractures, cardiac arrest/arrhythmias (24-48 h), metabolic acidosis, renal failure (myoglobinuria)
- *Smoke & inhalation injury* -hot air or noxious chemicals
  - Complications: airway obstruction – look for singed nasal hairs/eyebrows, hoarse voice/cough, darkened membranes; obstruction can occur 24 h post burn

Treatment includes the following:

- Severity = Time of Exposure + Intensity of Heat
- BURNS
  - **B**reathing/**B**ody Image: watch for distress, counseling
  - **U**rine output: 30 mL/hr minimum (0.5mL/kg/hr most accurate)
  - **R**esuscitation (Fluid): first 24-48 h
  - **N**utrition: increase protein and calories
  - **S**hock/**S**ilvadene: Keep CVP ~12 cm water pressure, monitor U/O
- Tetanus if not up to date on vaccinations

Degrees of Burns and the Rule of Nines

The **degree** and **extent of burns** are ways to determine the severity of the injury. These are determined by the depth of the injury, as well as the total body surface area (TBSA) affected:

- Depth of injury
  - 1st degree—superficial: reddened skin, but intact.
  - 2nd degree—partial thickness; loss of skin, into dermis (most painful).
  - 3rd degree—full thickness; all skin is lost, can see fat/muscle.
  - 4th degree—full thickness + underlying tissue; can see to bone.

- Both 3rd and 4th degree burns are not painful since nerves are lost; however, they will not heal without skin grafting.
- TBSA - Rule of Nines (Adults)
  - Adults:
    - Head and neck - 9%
    - Anterior torso - 18%
    - Posterior torso - 18%
    - Each leg - 18%
    - Each arm - 9%
    - Genitalia/perineum - 1%
  - Children: Head/Neck increased to 18%, legs only 13.5% each. Note: 10% of total surface area burned in school-aged child or younger may be fatal.

Review Video: Rule of Nines: Burn Evaluation
Visit mometrix.com/academy and enter code: 988486

Common Reservoirs for Organisms That Infect Burns

Burn patients are at exceptional risk of infection because the barrier of protective skin is breached, and eschar provides a medium for microorganisms, along with the immunosuppression which occurs. There are a number of **reservoirs** of infection for organisms to grow, and many of these reservoirs can serve as sources for transmission on the hands of health care workers:

- **Burn wounds** are colonized within the first few hours by gram-positive organisms from sweat glands and hair follicles and within days by gram-negative organisms, so collectively the burn wounds of all patients on the unit may harbor organisms that can spread from one patient to another.
- **Gastrointestinal tract flora** can contaminate burn wounds directly if wounds are in proximity to fecal material or indirectly through cross-contamination.
- **Normal flora,** especially gram-positive cocci, on the skin are the cause of early burn infections, and an increasingly important reservoir, with nasal colonization often implicated in burn infections.
- **Environment** can harbor organisms on many inanimate surfaces. Hydrotherapy equipment has been a frequent cause of wound infection because contaminated equipment spreads the infection to subsequent patients being treated.

MODS

Multiple Organ Dysfunction Syndrome (MODS) results from a systemic inflammatory response syndrome (SIRS), and is progressive physiologic failure of two or more separate organ systems. MODS is the major cause of death of patients in the critical care units. Outcome is directly related to the number of organs that fail. The failure of three or more organs is associated with a 90% to 95% mortality rate. Organ failure may occur in a progressive pattern or organs may fail simultaneously. The lungs are generally the first organ and the most common organ to be affected.

Signs and symptoms: lethargy, altered level of consciousness, an elevated body temperature, lower than normal lymphocyte counts, lack energy, experience ascites, and may experience an alteration in bowel pattern or decreased peristalsis; Cardiovascular instability and central nervous system dysfunction may be present.

Diagnosis: blood work, clinical symptoms/examination, various testing.

Treatment includes the following:

- Intensive antibiotic therapy to treat underlying infection.
- Hypermetabolic states: requires increased calories; often placed on TPN or another alternate form of nutrition.
- Monitor in intensive care unit; anticipate need for intubation if respiratory system collapses.

Review Video: Multiple Organ Dysfunction Syndrome
Visit mometrix.com/academy and enter code: 394302

SIRS

Systemic inflammatory response syndrome (SIRS) is a generalized systemic inflammation in organs remote from the initial insult. The many causes of SIRS include infection (especially of heart and lungs), pancreatitis, trauma with massive tissue injury/ischemia, shock, massive transfusion, and autoimmune diseases.

Signs and symptoms: temperature <36 °C or >38 °C, heart rate >90 beats/min

Respiratory rate >20 breaths/min or $PaCO_2$ <32 mm Hg

WBC >12,000/mm^3 or <4000/mm^3, or ≥10% immature (bands) forms

Diagnosis: Blood work (CBC/BMP), physical exam/clinical picture

Treatment includes the following:

- Treat underlying cause (IV antibiotics, fluids, parenteral nutrition, supportive treatment).
- Be alert for progression to multiple organ dysfunction syndrome (MODS)!

Pathophysiology

Lobes of the Brain

The **brain** comprises three primary areas: cerebrum, cerebellum, and brain stem. The cerebrum is divided into two hemispheres (joined by the corpus callosum), thalamus, hypothalamus, and basal ganglia. The outer layer of the hemispheres is called the cerebral cortex and is comprised of gray matter while the innermost layer is comprised of white matter (myelinated nerve fibers and neuroglia cells). The cerebral hemispheres are further divided into pairs (right and left) of lobes:

- **Frontal**: controls information storage, memory, personality, problem solving, motor functions of speech, and judgment.
- **Parietal**: interprets sensory input, such as temperature, touch, pressure, and pain, as well as aids in understanding speech and using words to express ideas.
- **Temporal**: Responsible for hearing, remembering visual scenes, learning, music, and interprets sensory experiences.
- **Occipital**: Responsible for vision and associates visual images with other sensory experiences.

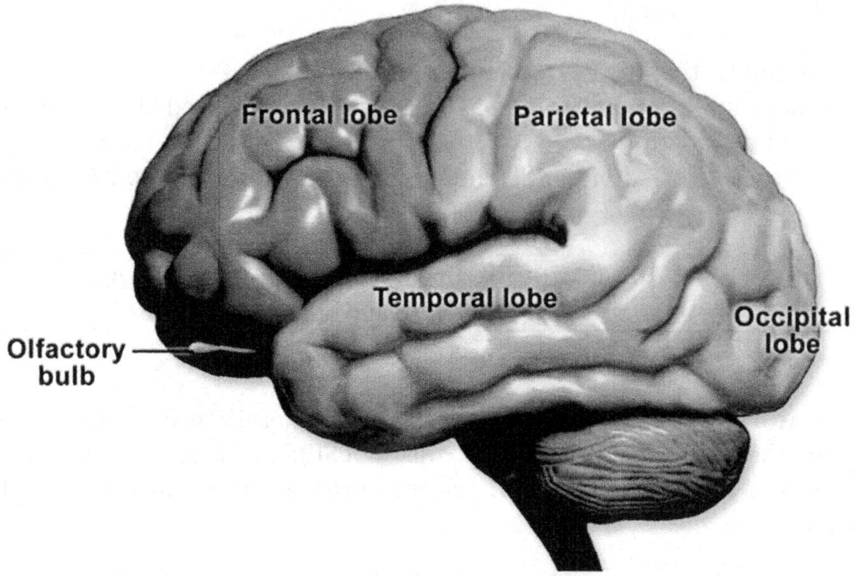

Adrenergic Receptors

The **sympathetic nervous system** is composed of adrenergic receptor sites, activated by epinephrine or norepinephrine. These sites are also where adrenergic drugs bind and produce their effect. They are divided into alpha-adrenergic and beta-adrenergic receptors, depending on whether they respond to norepinephrine or epinephrine. Both alpha- and beta-adrenergic receptors have subtypes designated 1 and 2. Medications classified as alpha-blockers and beta-blockers bind to the receptor sites for norepinephrine and epinephrine, blocking the stimulation of the sympathetic nervous system.

Location of Receptors:

- $Alpha_1$: muscles of veins and arteries.
- $Alpha_2$: central nervous system.
- $Beta_1$: primarily located in the heart.
- $Beta_2$: smooth muscle of bronchioles, arterioles, and visceral organs.

First Line of Defense Against Bacterial Infection

The body's **first line of defense** against microorganisms is the innate (primary) immune response, which is a *nonspecific* form of defense against infection. This includes the skin, mucous membranes, body fluids, and bacterial flora of the intestines:

- The skin provides a barrier to entry of bacteria. Fatty acids and lactic acids of sweat and sebaceous secretions also contribute to the first line of defense.
- The mucous lining of the respiratory and GI tracts traps bacteria and the trapped particles are removed by coughing and sneezing, aided by ciliated epithelial cells.
- Tears, saliva, and urine contain enzymes and acids that kill bacteria.
- Normal bacterial flora in humans defends against infectious bacteria by competitive inhibition—competing for nutrients, space to grow, etc.

TYPES OF IMMUNITY

Innate immunity is also called natural immunity. Innate immunity consists of all the immune defenses that lack immunologic memory. Innate immunity is acquired at birth and all humans have a resistance to certain types of organisms.

Acquired immunity includes active acquired immunity and passive acquired immunity. Acquired immunity is gained after birth as a result of an immune response. Active or passive immunity is related to the stimulation process and whether the response is activated by a donor or by the host. It can also be further classified as natural vs artificial.

- **Active acquired immunity**: Active acquired immunity is produced by a host after exposure from an antigen or immunization.
    - *Active natural*: immunity after sick from disease.
    - *Active artificial:* immunity after receiving immunization.
- **Passive acquired immunity**: Passive acquired immunity is when antibodies are given to the host.
    - *Passive natural:* breastfed infants receive antigens from milk.
    - *Passive artificial*: infusion of antigens to combat disease.

IMMUNOGLOBULINS

Immunoglobulins are antibodies that are produced from serum glycoprotein in plasma cells in response to pathogens. Immunoglobulins are receptors on the surfaces of mature B cells. Immunoglobulins have specific sensitivity to antigens. There are five molecular classes of immunoglobulin. The five classes of immunoglobulin are IgG, IgA, IgM, IgE, and IgD.

- **IgG** is responsible for most antibody functions, and can be found in all the fluids of the body. They fight most bacteria and viruses, and are responsible for activities such as precipitation, agglutination, and complement activation. IgG is also the only antibody that can pass from mother to baby through placenta.
- **IgA** is found in body secretions, such as those in the ear, nose, throat, digestive tract, vagina, etc. The IgA antibodies protect the body from infectious enzymes and secretions.
- **IgM** is the largest immunoglobulin and is the first antibody produced during the initial primary response to an antigen.
- **IgD** is found in low concentrations in the blood and peritoneal lining, and the function is unknown.
- **IgE** is the least concentrated immunoglobulin in circulation, primarily found in the respiratory system. IgE is the primary antibody with allergic reactions, and also responds to parasitic infections.

ANTIGENS AND IMMUNOGENS

Antigens are molecules or molecular complexes that react with preformed components of the immune system such as lymphocytes and antibodies. *Antigenicity* is the molecules' innate capacity to react with those preformed components. Self-antigens are produced within the body and nonself antigens are foreign to the body or not formed by the body. *Immunogens* are antigens that have the capacity to initiate an immune response.

Immunogens and antigens result in stimulation of an immune response by the body. The body responds with antibodies or immune cells when activated to protect the body from invasion of bacteria, viruses, and/or any other inflammatory process, illness, or injury.

Humoral vs. Cell-Mediated Immunity

Humoral immunity is associated with circulating antibodies, and B cells are the primary source of humoral immunity. The primary immunocyte of the immune response is the lymphocyte. The process of humoral immunity involves the lymphocyte migration through lymphatic system and blood vessels. As lymphocytes make their way through the lymph, they become B cells. B cells that encounter antigens are stimulated to mature into plasma cells that produce antibodies.

Platelets

Platelets, also called thrombocytes, are the smallest cell-like component of human blood, originating in the bone marrow where they are fragments of a large cell, the megakaryocyte. Because platelets are fragments of a cell, they have no nucleus. In the blood, the platelets are disk-shaped but change into a globular form with pseudopodia (false feet) when activated. These pseudopodia help to form a clot in a two-step process that involves first **adhesion**, where the platelets bind to a wound site, and then **activation**, where the platelets change shape and release agents to attract other platelets. Fibrin forms from fibrinogen (a protein produced in the liver), creating a stabilizing mesh over the platelet plug to control bleeding. Normal platelet counts range from 150,000 to 400,000 per mm^3. Platelet counts may increase with infections, cirrhosis, heart disease, malignancies, pancreatitis, and polycythemia. Platelet counts may decrease with alcohol toxicity, aplastic anemia, iron-deficiency anemia, megaloblastic anemia drug toxicity, prolonged hypoxia, viral infection, and immune thrombocytopenic purpura.

White Blood Cells

Types and functions of white blood cells are described below:

- **Lymphocytes**: Work closely with macrophages. Subtypes include B cells, which produce specific antibodies to destroy foreign substances; T cells, which help regulate immune response and attack virus-infected cells, foreign tissue, and cancer cells; natural killer (NK) cells, which utilize phagocytosis and destroy cancer cells and virus-infected cells.
- **Monocytes**: Production increases during an immune response. Mature into macrophages, which engage in phagocytosis and help activate T cells and B cells.
- **Eosinophils (granulocyte)**: Become active in parasitic infections and allergic responses. Contain granules that are toxic to many organisms as well as tissue.
- **Basophils (granulocyte)**: Involved in type 1 hypersensitivity (IgE-mediated) and may result in anaphylaxis.
- **Neutrophils** (polymorphonuclear granulocytes): Primary role is in fighting inflammation and arrive first at site of inflammation by leaving the blood and entering tissue where they act as phagocytes, ingesting and killing microorganisms.

Lipids

Lipids are fats, which combine with plasma proteins to form lipoproteins (e.g., LDL, HDL), which are carried throughout the body. The primary lipids include:

- **Triglycerides**: This is "neutral" fat composed of glycerol and fatty acids. It is found in adipose tissue throughout the body, and its primary role is to store energy. Levels tend to elevate with obesity, alcohol use, and diabetes.
- **Steroids (Cholesterol)**: Cholesterol is required for formation of the cell membrane and serves as a precursor for hormone synthesis of other steroids (such as estrogen, testosterone, and bile salts). Cholesterol is found in the cell membranes and the digestive and endocrine systems.

- **Phospholipids**: These lipids are derived from triglycerides and are important constituents of all cell membranes, forming lipid bilayers that form barriers around cells but allow passage of small molecules, such as oxygen.

Anterior Pituitary Gland Hormones

Anterior pituitary gland (adenohypophysis) hormones include:

- **Growth hormone (somatotropin)**: Protein that stimulates cells to enlarge and divide, increases rate of protein synthesis, decreases rate cells utilize carbohydrates, increases rate cells utilize fats, and stimulates elongation of bones. Peak secretion is during the night.
- **Prolactin**: Protein that promotes production of milk after labor and delivery. May help maintain sperm production in males.
- **Thyroid-stimulating hormone (thyrotropin)**: Glycoprotein that controls secretions of thyroid hormones and may stimulate excess growth (goiter) if levels are high.
- **Adrenocorticotropic hormone**: Peptide that controls the manufacture and secretion of adrenal hormones.
- **Follicle-stimulating hormone**: Glycoprotein that controls growth and development of follicles that contain eggs in the female ovaries. Stimulates the follicles to secrete estrogens. In males, stimulates production of sperm cells in testes.
- **Luteinizing hormone**: Glycoprotein that stimulates secretion of sex hormones in both males and females and controls release of egg cells from ovaries.

Digestion

The **digestive system** is a sequence of organs that function together to breakdown ingested nutrients for *digestion* and *absorption*. Digestion is a method of altering foods into smaller and smaller particles until the nutrients are absorbed into the body. The digestive system is also considered a protective mechanism for the body as it relates to absorption of microorganisms and/or noxious substances.

The **process of digestion** takes place as follows: first, the *oral cavity (mouth)* facilitates chewing to break down ingested materials. The *salivary glands* are located in the oral cavity, which produce saliva rich in *amylase* that lubricates the ingested materials and begins the initial phase of carbohydrate breakdown. Swallowing is facilitated by the *pharynx*. Food is moved from the oral cavity into the stomach via the *esophagus*. The *stomach* secretes acid and maintains motion to break down foods. The *liver* produces digestive bile, which the *gallbladder* concentrates and stores. *Bile* is then secreted into the small intestine to break down fats. The *pancreas* produces *bicarbonate* (a base) that assists in the regulation of stomach acid and the production of *insulin* (a hormone) to regulate blood glucose levels. The *small intestine* is responsible for the absorption nutrients once food has been broken into particles small enough to cross the cell membrane of the digestive mucosa. The *large intestine* is responsible to absorb mostly water; by the time food reaches the large intestine, it is a mass that is known as *feces*. The *rectum* is the distal portion of the large intestine and stores feces. The *anus* serves as the outlet for fecal material.

Absorption

Absorption is the body's process of assimilating the nutrients from digested food. Absorption takes place when microscopic digested food particles diffuse through the walls of the mucosa of the small intestine into the bloodstream or lymph fluid. There are several types of diffusion that must occur depending on which nutrient the body is absorbing.

- **Passive diffusion** is the simplest type, where molecules travel from an area of high concentration to low concentration.
- **Facilitated diffusion** is used when nutrient molecules being transported through the cell membrane must use transporter proteins to get inside, though still moving from high to low concentration.
- **Active transport** takes place when cellular energy is used to transfer molecules into areas of high pressure via transporter proteins.

Effects of Malnourishment on the Immune System

When the body is deprived of adequate nutrients, the functioning of the immune system is altered, leaving the body vulnerable to disease. The immune system activates a response to infectious organisms as a measure of protection for the body. If the immune system is compromised, its defense mechanisms will become altered. With malnutrition, the skin becomes less elastic and healing is delayed, giving a point of entry for bacteria. Under-nourishment causes the microvilli of the mucous membranes in the intestines to flatten, further decreasing the amount of nutrient absorption and antibody excretion. At the cellular level, the different white blood cells and antibodies may be slow to respond and/or may not have enough energy to mount a cell-mediated immune response if not properly supplied with nutrients to create adenosine triphosphate (ATP). This could allow the invasion of harmful viruses/bacteria and the growth of organisms.

Iatrogenic Malnutrition

The term "iatrogenic" means "related to health care/health treatment." **Iatrogenic malnutrition** is malnutrition that occurs with prolonged hospitalization, surgical procedures, and/or prescribed treatments. Monitoring diet, hydration status, level of consciousness, fatigue, and overall health are some ways nurses can prevent iatrogenic malnutrition in hospitalized patients. Some populations at an increased risk of iatrogenic malnutrition include patients with cancer, pulmonary disorders, or Alzheimer disease, and elderly patients with fractures.

Metabolism

Metabolism occurs when absorbed nutrients are utilized by the body to maintain proper function, energy levels, and maintenance. Metabolism occurs in two forms: catabolism and anabolism. **Catabolism** is when food particles are broken down into molecular particles. The body mainly uses catabolism to produce chemical and heat energy. **Anabolism**, however, is the formation of new substances using the catabolized nutrients to build larger molecules. Anabolism is responsible for the production of new tissue.

To maintain proper metabolic function, the patient's nutritional intake must be in balance with their body's requirements for daily functional needs. Maintaining this balance is critical in preventing and treating obesity, cachexia, and other forms of malnourishment.

Nurses' Role in Dealing with Unexpected Responses to Therapies

While treatments and therapies often follow an expected and reliable course, there are times when a patient can have an **adverse or unexpected reaction.** This can be a fearful time for the patient as well as the nurse. When the patient has an unexpected response to a therapy, here are some actions that the nurse should take:

1. First, immediately cease whatever therapy is causing the reaction if possible (stop the blood or IV medication, remove that patient from the area, etc.).
2. Remember ABC – airway, breathing, circulation. If the patient stops breathing or loses a pulse, call for help and begin CPR immediately.
3. If the patient is having an allergic reaction to a medication, notify the physician immediately and administer an antihistamine or reversal agent (often Benadryl or epinephrine for anaphylaxis).
4. After resolution of the event, regardless of the outcome, be sure to thoroughly document what happened, including all the steps taken before and after the incident to ensure patient safety.

NCLEX Test Question Strategies

Sometimes when you are testing, you may know an answer immediately on reading the choices. Other times, you may need to choose an answer without being certain. In those situations, here are some tips to help you eliminate the answer choices most likely to be incorrect. Use these strategies to dissect complex nursing questions and improve your NCLEX test taking skills.

Do NOT select an answer choice that:

- Asks "**Why**?"
- You have never heard of or are **unfamiliar** with.
- Requires you to **speculate** or read extra information into the question that isn't there.
- Is based on a scenario you may have seen at **work** or in **clinicals**; instead focus only on the information you are given.
- **Degrades** the patient or a member of the health care team.
- Involves bringing up potentially **controversial** material.
- Goes against a **general rule**.
- Involves **leaving** the patient, unless absolutely necessary.
- Tries to **persuade** the patient to make a choice or agree with something; instead look for answers that are associated with **caring** about the client's feelings.
- Tells the patient not to **worry**; this minimizes the patient's concerns and feelings.
- Tries to avoid **responsibility** or passes it to someone else.
- Is **unreasonable** or under normal circumstances could/should not be done.
- Involves "**doing nothing**" or "waiting" for an unspecified period of time unless you are absolutely certain it is the best option.
- Makes **absolute** statements involving words like always, never, or must.
- Only cites a **hospital rule** for its rationale. If the hospital has a rule about something, there will be an **underlying reason**, usually patient **safety** or hospital **liability**, which you should be aware of.

If you are asked to pick which nursing action to take first or next, remember that every answer choice listed could be a correct action to take, but the question is asking for the **highest priority action**.

NCLEX Practice Test #1

1. A client is to receive 1,000 mL of 0.15% potassium chloride in 5% dextrose injection (D5W) intravenously over 3 hours and 20 minutes using a drop factor of 15 drops/mL. What is the required flow rate (drops) per minute? *Record your answer using a whole number.*

2. A client develops mastitis in the postpartum period. Which of the following instructions does the nurse anticipate when notifying the physician? *Select all that apply.*

1. antibiotics for 7 to 14 days
2. opioid analgesia
3. alternating hot and cold compresses to relieve the pain
4. discontinuation of breastfeeding
5. continuation of breastfeeding

3. The nurse is teaching a new parent about the use of car seats for infants. Which of the following information should the nurse include? *Select all that apply.*

1. the shoulder straps should be fed through slots at or below the infant's shoulders
2. infants should always be in rear-facing car seats
3. the mother should place padding on the car seat underneath the infant
4. the harness clip should be positioned at the infant's abdomen
5. the car seat should be positioned so that the infant's head does not fall forward

4. A client is to wear a Holter monitor for continuous cardiac monitoring for 48 hours. The nurse should advise the client to avoid which of the following activities during the monitoring period? *Select all that apply.*

1. watching television
2. using a remote control
3. using an iPad or other wireless device
4. showering and bathing
5. drinking caffeinated beverages
6. exercising

5. A client requires insertion of a nasogastric tube. When preparing the client for the procedure, the nurse should place the client in which of the following positions?

1. high Fowler's position with the head tilted forward
2. high Fowler's position with the head tilted backward
3. semi-Fowler's position with the head in a neutral position
4. semi-Fowler's position with the head tilted backward

6. A client returns to his room after a liver biopsy. The nurse should place the client in which of the following positions?

1. left side-lying with a folded towel under the biopsy site
2. right side-lying with a folded towel under the biopsy site
3. supine with a pressure dressing over the biopsy site
4. prone with a small pillow under the biopsy site

7. Following insertion of a nasogastric (NG) tube, the nurse aspirates the gastric contents to check the pH to determine if the NG tube is correctly placed. Which of the following pH values is consistent with gastric secretions?

1. 9
2. 8
3. 6
4. 4

8. A client with a tracheostomy is exhibiting difficulty breathing, and respirations are increasingly noisy. Secretions are very thick. Which of the following initial interventions is <u>most</u> indicated?

1. increase humidification, and suction the tracheostomy tube
2. notify the physician
3. sit the client upright, and encourage the client to breathe deeply and cough
4. gently irrigate and suction the tracheostomy tube

9. A client has a chest tube in place with a three-chamber chest drainage system. The nurse notes continuous bubbling in the water seal chamber. This indicates which of the following?

1. pneumothorax
2. suction is adequate
3. system air leak
4. the tube is positioned incorrectly

10. An elderly client with moderate Alzheimer's disease lives with her daughter and appears dirty and disheveled and has lost five pounds over the previous month. Which of the following does the nurse suspect?

1. physical abuse
2. caregiver neglect
3. self-neglect
4. psychological abuse

11. The nurse is reviewing medications with a client who is to be scheduled for outpatient rotator cuff repair. Which of the following medications does the nurse anticipate the client will be advised to avoid on the morning of the surgery?

1. metoprolol.
2. levothyroxine.
3. aspirin.
4. fluoxetine.

12. A patient with hypothyroidism states that she takes levothyroxine 0.112 mg daily, but the pharmacy has issued the drug labeled in micrograms. How many micrograms of levothyroxine is equivalent to 0.112 mg? *Record your answer using a whole number.*

13. The nurse is caring for an unvaccinated child who developed complications related to German measles (rubella). Which of the following infection control protocols is appropriate?

1. standard only
2. standard and contact
3. standard and droplet
4. standard and airborne

14. A client is scheduled for knee replacement surgery, and the nurse is reviewing preoperative laboratory results. The nurse should notify the physician about which of the following abnormal laboratory results?

1. platelets 119,000
2. glucose 83
3. hemoglobin 13.7
4. sodium 141

15. The nurse is caring for a client with diabetes mellitus, type 1. Which of the following signs and symptoms are indicative of diabetic ketoacidosis? *Select all that apply.*

1. dehydration
2. polyuria
3. hyperventilation
4. polydipsia
5. blurred vision
6. abdominal pain

16. A 15-year-old client was involved in an auto accident and requires emergency surgery to control bleeding, but both parents are out of town and unable to sign the consent form. Which of the following is the <u>most</u> appropriate action?

1. the client signs the consent form
2. the parents give telephone consent with two witnesses listening
3. the parents give email consent
4. the physician operates without consent because of the emergency situation

17. The nurse is administering an intermittent tube feeding to a client through a nasogastric tube. Which of the following positions is optimal for tube feedings?

1. the head of the bed is elevated to at least 45°
2. the head of the bed is elevated to at least 90°
3. the head of the bed is elevated to at least 30°
4. the head of the bed is flat with the client supine

18. When considering fluid balance, if 60% of an adult's body is composed of water, approximately what percentage of this is found in intracellular fluid?

1. 33%
2. 25%
3. 67%
4. 8%

19. Whole blood is primarily indicated for which of the following purposes?

1. to treat extreme loss of blood volume
2. to increase clotting factors
3. to increase oxygen-carrying capacity for those with anemia
4. to control acute bleeding

20. A client who has undergone a thyroidectomy complains of numbness, tingling, and stiffness in her hands, feet, and face as well as muscle tremors, spasmodic muscle contractions, and anxiety during the postoperative period. Which laboratory tests does the nurse anticipate that the physician will request?

1. hemoglobin
2. sodium
3. thyroid-stimulating hormone (TSH)
4. calcium

21. A client receiving chemotherapy and opioids for renal cancer has had no bowel movement for five days and no results from two doses of laxatives in the past 48 hours. The client is passing no flatus and complains of increasing abdominal pain and nausea. Which of the following does the nurse anticipate?

1. abdominal examination and abdominal x-ray
2. oil retention enema and manual removal of impaction
3. oil retention enema followed by a soapsuds enema
4. another dose of laxative followed by a soapsuds enema if there are no results in 24 hours

22. An 82-year-old female complains of generalized fatigue and has new onset of urinary incontinence as well as anorexia, hyperventilation, and low-grade fever. The nurse anticipates that the client will be evaluated for which of the following?

1. diabetes mellitus
2. bladder cancer
3. urinary tract infection
4. influenza

23. The nurse administers a dose of acetaminophen to the wrong client. Which of the following actions is the most appropriate after notifying the physician?

1. notify her supervisor and complete an incident report
2. ask the physician for an order of acetaminophen to cover the inadvertent administration
3. take no further action because acetaminophen is relatively benign
4. document in the client's record that an error in drug administration occurred

24. The nurse is aware that African-Americans are at higher risk than Caucasians for which of the following conditions? *Select all that apply.*

1. hypertension
2. diabetes mellitus
3. asthma
4. skin cancer
5. osteoporosis

25. The nurse is instructing a client who has had an eye removed in the proper procedure for inserting a prosthetic eye. Place the following steps of prosthetic-eye insertion (in Roman numerals) in the correct sequence from the first to the last.

i. Raise the upper eyelid.
ii. Pull the lower eyelid down.
iii. Slide the prosthesis under and behind the upper eyelid.
iv. Identify landmarks on the prosthetic eye for the inner and outer areas and the superior and inferior aspects.
v. Check the positioning.
vi. Cleanse the prosthetic eye according to the manufacturer's directions.

1.
2.
3.
4.
5.
6.

26. A client's wife states that her elderly husband has begun to slightly slur his words and drop word endings, he has become increasingly withdrawn socially, and he is irritable, accusing her of talking behind his back and whispering at him. The nurse suspects that the client should be <u>initially</u> evaluated for which of the following?

1. depression
2. Alzheimer's disease
3. hearing loss
4. stroke

27. Which of the following tasks are appropriate for the nurse to delegate to unlicensed assistive personnel? *Select all that apply.*

1. checking temperature and vital signs for a client acutely ill with sepsis
2. checking routine temperature and vital signs for clients at the beginning of the shift
3. emptying catheter bags and measuring the urinary output from Foley catheters
4. monitoring the transfusion of red blood cells
5. assisting an ambulatory client to walk to the bathroom

28. Two days' postpartum, a nursing mother develops swollen, taut, and very painful breasts. Which of the following is the <u>most</u> likely cause?

1. engorgement
2. insufficient milk
3. blocked milk ducts
4. mastitis

29. Following surgical repair of a fractured femur, a client's hemoglobin falls to 7.4 and the physician orders one unit of packed red blood cells (250 mL) to be administered over two hours with a drop factor of 10 drops/mL. What flow rate (drops per minute) is needed? *Record your answer using a whole number.*

30. Place the following metric capacity measures (in Roman numerals) in the correct position in the table below.

i. Deciliter
ii. Milliliter
iii. Dekaliter
iv. Kiloliter.
v. Hectoliter.

(1)	Centiliter	(2)	Liter	(3)	(4)	(5)

1.
2.
3.
4.
5.

31. A client with recurrent episodes of gout has been advised to eat a low-purine diet. Which of the following foods should the nurse advise him to limit or avoid? *Select all that apply.*

1. liver
2. sardines
3. wine
4. low-fat yogurt
5. beef broth
6. potatoes

32. A client develops anaphylaxis syndrome and loses consciousness after eating fruit salad containing kiwi fruit, to which the client is severely allergic. The nurse is aware that the <u>initial</u> concern is which of the following?

1. establish a patent airway
2. administer intravenous fluids
3. administer oxygen at 100% high flow
4. administer epinephrine

33. An infant is to receive 250 mL of 5% dextrose/0.45 normal saline (D5/0.45 NS) in five hours. The pediatric IV system has a drop factor of 60 drops per mL. What is the flow rate (in drops per minute)? *Record your answer using a whole number.*

34. A client states that he takes five grains of aspirin daily, but the hospital issues aspirin in milligrams. How many milligrams are approximately equivalent to five grains of aspirin?

1. 81 mg
2. 120 mg
3. 325 mg
4. 500 mg

35. A child who weighs 40 kg is prescribed clarithromycin 15 mg/kg per day for 10 days in two divided doses for acute strep throat. If the medication is provided in suspension with 250 mg/5 mL, how many total milliliters of medication are required to complete the treatment? ***Record your answer using a whole number.***

36. The physician had prescribed 10 mL of oral suspension twice daily for a child, but the mother is confused about the metric system and wants to know how many teaspoons of medication to give the child. How many teaspoons are equivalent to 10 mL of oral suspension? ***Record your answer using a whole number.***

37. An electrical fire occurs in a client's room shortly after the client returns from the recovery room after repair of a hip fracture with insertion of a prosthesis. What is the best method of removing the client from the room?

1. place the client in a wheelchair
2. transfer the client to a gurney
3. move the bed with the client on it
4. do a two-person carry

38. A client is confused after receiving morphine for analgesia and repeatedly tries to pull out the intravenous (IV) line in her left arm. Which of the following actions is the best initial solution?

1. attempt to camouflage the IV and tie a piece of tubing to the bedrail so the client can pull on that safely
2. apply wrist restraints
3. apply wrist and vest restraints
4. discontinue the IV line and reinsert at a more distant site

39. A nurse must teach a client how to do wound care and dressing changes prior to discharge. Which of the following are barriers to learning? ***Select all that apply.***

1. the client is 55 years old
2. the client is fearful
3. the client is illiterate
4. the client is weak and frail
5. the client has many questions about the procedures
6. the client is hard of hearing

40. A client is prescribed 0.25 mg terbutaline subcutaneously, but the medication is provided as 1 mg/mL. How much medication is needed to provide the correct dosage? ***Record your answer using a decimal to two places.***

41. A client has returned from surgery after removal of a tumor of the colon and creation of a temporary colostomy. She refuses to take a deep breath and cough then refuses to turn. Which of the following should the nurse assess first in trying to understand her lack of cooperation?

1. delirium status
2. vital signs
3. oxygen saturation.
4. level of pain

42. When assisting a client with range-of-motion exercises, which movements should be carried out on the client's elbows? *Select all that apply.*

1. supination
2. flexion
3. circumduction
4. pronation
5. rotation
6. hyperextension

43. A client has had a long leg cast removed after eight weeks. Which of the following actions is the correct method of cleansing the skin after cast removal?

1. advise the client to use a bath brush on his skin during a shower
2. advise the client to soak in a tub of water and wash his leg with a washcloth
3. apply a cold-water enzyme wash to the client's skin, leave it in place for 20 minutes, and then rinse it off with warm water
4. wash the skin with hot, soapy water and then rinse with warm water

44. The nurse has documented a treatment on the wrong client's record. Which of the following methods of indicating the error is correct?

1. the nurse draws a straight line through the incorrect entry and writes "error" above it and initials the correction
2. the nurse uses correction fluid to cover the incorrect entry
3. the nurse draws multiple lines through the incorrect entry so it is unreadable, writes "error" above it, and initials the correction
4. the nurse leaves the incorrect entry in place, writes "error" in the margin, and initials and dates the notation

45. A client in Dunlop traction experiences numbness of the thumb and index finger and cannot move the thumb to touch the tips of the other fingers. The capillary refill time is four seconds. Which of the following actions is indicated?

1. remove and reapply the forearm elastic bandage more loosely
2. decrease the weights on the traction
3. release the countertraction
4. increase the weights on the traction

46. For which of the following reasons would the nurse use the Braden Scale to assess a client?

1. to determine if the client is suffering from delirium
2. to determine if the client is at risk for developing pressure sores
3. to determine if the client is at risk for falls
4. to determine if the client is at risk for substance abuse

47. Following a disaster with multiple victims and danger to those present, which group should have <u>priority</u> for protection from injury?

1. The clients/victims.
2. The firefighters and police officers.
3. The bystanders and news reporters.
4. The healthcare providers.

48. Which of the following statements by the client suggests that the client has not made informed consent for a craniotomy?

1. "I know that surgery could cause a stroke, and I'm scared."
2. "I told the doctor I didn't want to know anything about the surgery, and she agreed."
3. "I have one more question before I sign the consent form."
4. "This is a really complicated procedure. So many things could go wrong."

49. The computers for documenting client care and treatment are located at the nursing station. Which of the following is the <u>most</u> important consideration regarding the computers?

1. height of the computer stations
2. ratio of computers to staff
3. positioning of the computer screens away from the line of sight of unauthorized persons
4. brand of computer and operating system

50. The physician has ordered that a serum trough level be drawn for a medication. Which of the following is the correct time to draw blood for a trough level?

1. at the midpoint in time between two scheduled doses of the drug
2. at the time the drug peaks
3. immediately after a scheduled dose is administered
4. immediately before a scheduled dose is due

51. A client tells the nurse that she is on a high-protein diet and averages 75 g of protein daily, 120 g of carbohydrates, and 40 g of fat. If fat is equal to 9 calories per gram and protein and carbohydrates are equal to 4 calories per gram, how many total calories is the client averaging each day? *Record your answer using a whole number.*

52. An elderly preoperative client seems very anxious but denies concerns when the nurse asks; however, the client's son confides that the client is very superstitious and believes it is bad luck that he is in room 113. Which of the following actions is the <u>best</u> response?

1. reassure the client that the room number will not affect his surgery outcome
2. contact the admissions department and request that the client be reassigned to a different room
3. ask the physician for medication to relax the client
4. ask the son to stay with the client to reassure him

53. A transient homeless client with a history of mental illness and substance abuse is to be discharged. Which of the following support systems are most likely to provide social support for the client? *Select all that apply.*

1. self-help programs
2. internet-based programs
3. community agencies
4. governmental agencies
5. friends
6. family

54. A client is receiving oxygen therapy at 3 L/min per nasal cannula. Which of the following fraction of inspired oxygen (FiO_2) measurements does the nurse expect that the client is receiving?

1. 24%
2. 60%
3. 32%
4. 100%

55. A 43-year-old client has developed progressive frontotemporal dementia and is exhibiting inappropriate and compulsive behaviors, difficulty with language, and impaired judgment. Which statement by the client's wife suggests that she has not accepted a permanent role change in their relationship?

1. "I need my husband to take care of financial matters."
2. "It's so frustrating that my husband refuses to bathe."
3. "My husband doesn't pay attention to anything I try to tell him."
4. "I want my husband to do the things that he can still manage independently."

56. A client undergoing "cold-turkey" withdrawal from years of substance abuse is most at risk of serious life-threatening complications with which of the following substances?

1. heroin
2. cocaine
3. alcohol
4. marijuana

57. The nurse finds a client smoking marijuana in the hospital and tells her that no smoking or use of drugs is allowed in the facility. The client responds by shouting, "What business is it of yours? Leave me alone!" Which of the following <u>initial</u> responses is the best for the nurse to use to defuse the situation?

1. "It's my business because I'm your nurse."
2. "If you don't put that out immediately, I will call security."
3. "You are violating the facility policies and the law!"
4. "I'm sorry, but I have to ask you again to put out your marijuana cigarette."

58. A client who served three tours of duty in Afghanistan has been diagnosed with posttraumatic stress disorder (PTSD). Which of the following signs and symptoms does the nurse expect the client to exhibit? *Select all that apply.*

1. recurring flashbacks
2. detachment from others
3. anger
4. hyperacute memory regarding the events associated with the trauma
5. nightmares
6. excessive sleeping

59. A diabetic client self-administers insulin four times daily. Which of the following statements by the client indicates the need for further education?

1. "I flush the used needles down the toilet."
2. "I carry glucose tablets with me at all times."
3. "I eat a little dessert occasionally."
4. "I avoid wearing sandals."

60. A hospice client is to receive 4 mg of morphine sulfate (MS) subcutaneously from a vial that contains 10 mg/mL. How many milliliters of MS should the patient receive to equal a dose of 4 mg? ***Record your answer using one decimal place.***

61. Which of the following findings are indicative of peripheral arterial insufficiency? ***Select all that apply.***

1. throbbing, cramping pain that increases with exercise
2. aching pain that increases with dependency
3. capillary refill time of less than two seconds
4. shiny skin with decreased hair
5. brown pigment about the ankles and lower legs
6. pale color on elevation and redness on dependency

62. The nurse is assisting a client with a colostomy irrigation. The client is positioned on the toilet and has removed the colostomy pouch, and the irrigation bag is filled with 1000 mL of warm water. Place the following actions (in Roman numerals) in the correct order from first to last.

i. Allow 15 to 20 minutes for evacuation and then fold the sleeve, secure it, and leave it in place for 30 to 45 minutes before removing it.
ii. Allow the solution to flow in for 5 to 10 minutes and then clamp the tubing and close the top of the irrigation sleeve.
iii. Apply gloves, lubricate the cone tip, and insert it into the stoma, holding it securely.
iv. Apply the irrigation sleeve over the stoma.
v. Hang the irrigation solution with the bottom of the bag being 20 inches above the stoma.

1.
2.
3.
4.
5.

63. A client complains of sleeping poorly, arousing many times during the night, awakening with a headache, and feeling tired and sluggish in the morning and throughout the day. For which of the following tests does the nurse anticipate that the client will be scheduled?

1. electroencephalogram
2. electrocardiogram
3. nocturnal polysomnogram
4. magnetic resonance imaging (MRI) of the brain

64. A pregnant woman undergoes a 40-minute nonstress test for evaluation of fetal heart rate (FHR) accelerations. Which of the following test results is <u>normal</u> (reactive)?

1. one acceleration of the FHR of 10 beats per minute (bpm) above the baseline for 10 seconds
2. two accelerations of the FHR of 10 bpm above the baseline for 15 seconds
3. no accelerations of the FHR.
4. three accelerations of the FHR of 15 bpm above the baseline for 20 seconds

65. The nurse is conducting an aphasia assessment of a client who has suffered a stroke. Which of the following observations should the nurse include in the assessment? *Select all that apply.*

1. spontaneous speech
2. comprehension of the spoken and written word
3. ability to name objects
4. ability to describe objects
5. ability to write
6. ability to recall four named items after five minutes

66. The nurse must obtain wound cultures for anaerobic and aerobic bacteria from the traumatic leg wound of a three-year-old child, but the wound is quite painful even with analgesia. Which is the best approach?

1. do the cultures in the child's room with the child in bed and the mother assisting
2. do the cultures in the child's room with the child in bed with a nurse assisting and the mother comforting the child
3. do the cultures in a separate treatment room with the mother holding the child and a nurse assisting
4. do the cultures in a separate treatment room with a nurse assisting and the mother comforting the child

67. A nurse is at a local swimming pool, and a man collapses with a cardiac arrest after exiting the pool. The man is still wet when the nurse begins cardiopulmonary resuscitation (CPR), and another person brings the automated external defibrillator (AED). Which of the following should the nurse do next?

1. apply the AED pads and deliver a shock
2. wipe the chest dry with an available cloth or towel
3. continue CPR because a client who is wet cannot receive a shock
4. wipe the chest with an alcohol hand wipe to speed the evaporation of the water

68. The client's intravenous (IV) line has a gauze pad wrapped around the IV catheter at the insertion site and a transparent dressing over the gauze dressing. How long after application should the nurse change the dressing?

1. at the normal rotation time for the IV
2. when the transparent dressing loosens
3. in 48 hours
4. in 24 hours

69. Which of the following groups of neonates should be screened for hearing loss?

1. premature neonates
2. neonates with risk factors for hearing loss
3. neonates with abnormal Apgar scores
4. all neonates

70. A child weighing 20 kg is to receive 45 mg/kg of amoxicillin per day in a divided dose every 12 hours. The oral suspension contains 250 mg/5 mL. How many milliliters should the child receive in each dose? *Record your answer using a whole number.*

71. A client has a rate-responsive permanent pacemaker in his upper chest. The nurse understands rate-responsive to mean which of the following?

1. a pacemaker function prevents excessive changes in the pacing rate
2. the pacing rate increases above the normal pacing rate with sudden bradycardia
3. the pacemaker switches from atrial tracking mode to nontracking mode with atrial fibrillation
4. the pacing rate increases when the sensors note increased activity

72. The "5 A's" of smoking cessation intervention begin with which of the following?

1. advise all clients who smoke to stop smoking
2. ask all clients about tobacco use at every visit
3. assess clients' willingness to stop smoking
4. assist the client to stop smoking

73. The nurse is educating a client about lifestyle modifications to manage hypertension. Which of the following modifications should the nurse recommend? *Select all that apply.*

1. limit fluid intake to 2000 mL daily
2. engage in regular aerobic exercise (30 minutes most days)
3. adopt the dietary approaches to stop hypertension (DASH) eating plan
4. lose weight
5. eliminate all alcoholic beverages
6. stop smoking

74. The nurse is caring for a Muslim client who is recovering from an automobile accident and is unable to cleanse herself after a bowel movement. Which of the following should the nurse do to show respect for the woman's cultural and religious beliefs?

1. use the left hand to cleanse the client's rectal area
2. ask a female family member to assist the client
3. wear gloves when cleansing the client's rectal area
4. ask the client's husband to assist the client

75. A client with multiple sclerosis tires easily, so the nurse is instructing the client in energy-conservation techniques. Which of the following techniques may help the client conserve energy? *Select all that apply.*

1. sit down to perform activities instead of standing
2. keep frequently used items close at hand on the floor or on a high shelf
3. rest 10 minutes out of every hour
4. plan ahead to avoid extra movements
5. watch for stress signals, such as dyspnea or fatigue
6. pull objects instead of pushing them

76. The mother of a 24-month-old child tells the nurse that she is concerned that her child's language abilities are delayed. Which of the following language milestones does the nurse expect the child to exhibit?

1. understands 300 words and uses two- and three-word sentences
2. says and understands a few words, such as "Mama" and "Dada," and can imitate animal sounds, such as "moo" and "woof"
3. says and understands four to six words but understands more and can point to items he wants
4. says and understands up to 20 words and can point to his body parts

77. A client who experienced a cardiac arrest and resuscitation is exhibiting characteristics of mild anoxic brain injury. Which of the following characteristics does the nurse expect her to exhibit? *Select all that apply.*

1. decreased ability to concentrate
2. seizures
3. memory impairment
4. semicomatose state
5. decreased balance
6. restlessness

78. A client has developed osteomyelitis of the bones of the left foot following the infection of a diabetic ulcer. The nurse anticipates which of the following treatments to be the primary focus?

1. warm wet soaks
2. analgesia
3. surgical debridement.
4. intravenous (IV) antibiotic therapy

79. During the second stage of labor, the baby's head becomes compressed because the mother has a narrow, bony pelvis. Which of the following is the most common result for the infant from this type of compression?

1. cerebral palsy
2. Intracranial hemorrhage
3. cranial molding
4. epilepsy

80. A client with rheumatoid arthritis tells the nurse that she is having increasing difficulty cooking, cleaning, and attending to activities of daily living. Which of the following referrals is the most appropriate?

1. occupational therapist
2. physical therapist
3. home health agency
4. assisted-living facility

81. If the nurse is teaching a group of clients about risk factors for diabetes mellitus, type 2, the nurse should include which of the following? *Select all that apply.*

1. obesity
2. hypertension and/or heart disease
3. 45 years or older
4. caucasian race
5. family history of diabetes mellitus, type 2

82. The nurse is assessing an older adult. The client does not appear to always understand the questions, sometimes answering incorrectly, and stares at the nurse's mouth rather than the nurse's eyes when the nurse is speaking. The client answers in an unusually loud voice. Which of the following impairments should the nurse suspect?

1. hearing impairment
2. cognitive impairment
3. vision impairment
4. anxiety

83. A client is to be discharged 48 hours after a normal vaginal delivery of an infant with no laceration or episiotomy. Which of the following danger signs should the client be advised to report to her physician? *Select all that apply.*

1. temperature higher than 38 °C (100.4 °F)
2. difficulty urinating
3. swelling, redness, or pain in one or both legs
4. fatigue
5. foul-smelling vaginal discharge

84. When assessing a client's skin, the nurse notes a scattered red rash on the trunk. The individual lesions are about 0.5 cm in diameter and are flat, nonpalpable, and circumscribed. How would this type of lesion be classified?

1. papule
2. nodule
3. macule
4. patch

85. An older client says that she frequently experiences stress incontinence and may have to stop playing golf because swinging the golf club often results in small amounts of urinary incontinence. Which of the following suggestions may be <u>most</u> effective?

1. take a deep breath while swinging the golf club
2. utilize the "knack" (precisely timed muscle contractions)
3. wear incontinence pads
4. urinate immediately before playing golf

86. A client has had a recent below-knee (BK) amputation of the right leg because of a traumatic injury. After removing the elastic wrap, which the client had applied, the nurse notes an unusual pattern of swelling. Which of the following is the <u>most</u> likely reason for this observation?

1. wound infection
2. impaired circulation to the stump
3. incorrect wrap technique
4. bleeding into the tissues

87. A client has recurrent episodes of constipation and fecal impaction. The nurse is assisting the client with a bowel-training regimen. Which of the following interventions should be included? *Select all that apply.*

1. scheduled toileting
2. stool softeners
3. high-fiber diet
4. daily laxatives
5. periodic enemas
6. routine exercise

88. Which of the following descriptions is typical of a Parkinsonian gait?

1. uncoordinated and unsteady, wide-based, staggering, high stepping, flat footed step
2. short, slow, stiff steps with thighs crossing while moving forward
3. decreased speed and balance, slight flexion of hips and knees, stooped posture, and decreased stride length
4. slight flexion of hips and knees, short shuffling steps, trunk leaning forward, and no arm swing

89. A client has increasing pain in both hands. On examination, the nurse notes that the metacarpophalangeal and proximal interphalangeal joints are enlarged and swollen, swan-neck deformity is evident, and the fingers on both hands show ulnar deviation. These findings are consistent with which of the following disorders?

1. osteoarthritis
2. rheumatoid arthritis
3. gouty arthritis
4. psoriatic arthritis

90. A client with pelvic skin traction for low back pain is at risk of which of the following problems associated with decreased mobility? *Select all that apply.*

1. orthostatic hypotension
2. muscle weakness
3. venous stasis
4. dysuria
5. confusion

91. If a client weighs 132 lb and has a caloric requirement of 28 calories per kg of body weight per day, what is the number of calories that the client needs each day to maintain body weight? *Record your answer using a whole number.*

________ calories

92. If a client has had repair of a right fractured hip and has an overhead trapeze on the bed to assist with movement, which of the following instructions should the client receive about use of the assistive device? *Select all that apply.*

1. the client should always grasp the bar with both hands before moving
2. the client should grasp the bar with the left hand and place the right hand flat on the bed to assist movement
3. the client should flex the left hip and knee and place the foot flat on the bed before moving
4. the client should keep the left hip and knee extended when moving

93. If a 6-year-old child has influenza with a fever and cough, which statements by the child's caregiver suggest a need for education? *Select all that apply.*

1. "If his fever gets too high, I'll give him a bath in cold water."
2. "I try to offer him plenty of liquids."
3. "Sipping hot lemonade seems to help relieve his cough."
4. "I've been giving him baby aspirin to lower his fever."
5. "I alternate giving him acetaminophen and ibuprofen for this fever."

94. Nutrients per serving:

Nutrients	Lunch meat	Peanuts	Cheese	Apple
Fat	6 grams	14 grams	9 grams	0.3 grams
Carbs	1 gram	5 grams	1 gram	25 grams
Insol. Fiber	0	1 gram	0	5 grams
Protein	7 grams	7 grams	7 grams	0.5 grams

Which of the snacks—lunch meat, peanuts, cheese, or apple—has the lowest number of calories per serving?

1. lunch meat
2. peanuts
3. cheese
4. apple

95. The nurse must administer in one syringe a combined dose of two different insulins from two vials. The procedure includes:

i. Cleanse tops of vials.
ii. Inject air into vial 1.
iii. Withdraw medication from vial 1.
iv. Change needles.
v. Withdraw medication from vial 2.
vi. Inject air into vial 2.

Place the steps (Roman numerals) in the correct order in the chart below.

Step	Procedure
1	
2	
3	
4	
5	
6	

96. If teaching a client to use a metered-dose inhaler (MDI) without a spacer, how far away from the mouth should the nurse advise the client that the inhaler be positioned when administering a dose of inhaled medication?

1. the inhaler should be enclosed within the client's lips
2. the inhaler should be immediately outside of the client's lips
3. the inhaler should be 1 to 2 inches away from the client's lips
4. the inhaler should be 3 to 4 inches away from the client's lips

97. A client is receiving an opioid per patient-controlled analgesia (PCA) pump to control postoperative pain; however, when the nurse assesses the client, she finds the client is pale and hypotensive, and has a respiratory rate of 6 breaths per minute. The PCA pump record shows that the limit for maximum dosage was set far too high, resulting in an overdose. The client is very somnolent and barely responsive. What interventions does the nurse anticipate? *Select all that apply.*

1. immediately stop the infusion
2. discontinue the PCA pump
3. administer naloxone per standing orders
4. administer supplementary oxygen
5. file an incident report

98. A client is hospitalized in a long-term care facility because of Alzheimer's disease. The client is incontinent of urine and feces. The nurse has delegated incontinent care to unlicensed assistive personnel (UAP). How frequently should the nurse advise that the UAP check the client for dryness?

1. every 2 hours
2. every hour
3. when the client appears restless
4. before meals and at bedtime

99. A client with epilepsy is taking phenytoin. What long-term effects should the nurse advise the client can occur with prolonged administration of phenytoin? *Select all that apply.*

1. gingival hypertrophy
2. hirsutism
3. hypertrophy of facial subcutaneous tissue
4. dementia
5. anemia

100. A 60-year-old client has undergone a nerve-sparing prostatectomy and has been advised by his physician that he may not recover normal sexual functioning. The client is very concerned about this and asks the nurse for more information. Which of the following information should the nurse include? *Select all that apply.*

1. retrograde ejaculation may occur
2. recovery rates vary but can take up to a year or more
3. if sexual functioning is going to return, it will do so within a month
4. attempts at sexual intercourse are usually avoided for 1 month after surgery
5. anxiety can interfere with sexual functioning
6. other forms of sexual intimacy are more important than sexual intercourse

101. A client is receiving end-of-life care and tells the nurse that he has not always lived the way he should have or treated his children well. Which of the following responses is the <u>most</u> appropriate?

1. "What kinds of things have you done?"
2. "There are things that you regret."
3. "I'm sure those things don't matter anymore."
4. "It's not too late to ask for forgiveness."

102. A client who was prescribed increasing dosages of baclofen to relieve muscle spasms should have taken 80 mg daily in 4 divided doses but misunderstood and took 80 mg four times a day, resulting in an overdose and pronounced CNS depression. Which of the following treatments does the nurse anticipate?

1. administration of naloxone
2. administration of atropine
3. supportive care only
4. administration of flumazenil

103. A client has been diagnosed with Parkinson disease and has been prescribed levodopa. Which of the following are contraindications to levodopa? *Select all that apply.*

1. narrow-angle glaucoma
2. macular degeneration
3. pregnancy
4. melanoma
5. cataracts

104. A 78-year-old client with a history of diabetes mellitus type 2, GERD, and hypertension is hospitalized with pneumonia and rings the call bell at 11 PM, complaining of being unable to sleep and having "indigestion" and "heartburn." Which of the following initial interventions is <u>most</u> indicated?

1. administer antacid per prn order
2. administer acetaminophen per prn order
3. administer hypnotic per prn order
4. assess cardiac and respiratory status

105. A client is upset that the physician has refused to order a stronger pain medication for the client and berates the nurse, calling the nurse "worthless and stupid" when the nurse brings the prescribed medication. Which of the following ego defense mechanisms is the client exhibiting?

1. compensation
2. reaction formation
3. displacement
4. regression

106. When determining whether or not a client is a candidate for restraints, which of the following would be considered an appropriate reason for a restraint?

1. current dangerous behavior
2. history of falls
3. recent violent attack on a staff member
4. refusal to cooperate with treatment

107. A 52-year-old client is undergoing menopause. Which of the following physical sign or symptom is often attributed to decreased estrogen production associated with menopause?

1. weight loss
2. excessive sleeping
3. increased fat deposits on hips and abdomen
4. increased metabolic rate

108. An older client has been sleeping poorly at night, and her daughter states that the client has always loved music and suggests that listening to music might relax the client. Which type of music is <u>most</u> likely to help the client relax?

1. classical music
2. jazz
3. single instrument music (guitar, piano)
4. client's favorite music

109. If a client's waist measurement is 38 inches and the hip measurement is 45 inches, what is the client's waist-to-hip ratio. *Record your answer rounded to two decimal places.*

________ waist-to-hip ratio

110. If a client is to have a nasogastric (NG) tube inserted for intermittent feedings, which of the following is an appropriate task to delegate to unlicensed assistive personnel?

1. inserting the NG tube
2. verifying tube position
3. administer tube feedings
4. reposition a displaced NG tube

111. A client received a unit of packed red blood cells; 2 hours after the transfusion had been initiated, the client developed severe chills and a 2 °C elevation of temperature. The client had no dyspnea, swelling, or urticaria. Which of the following is the <u>most</u> likely cause of the client's symptoms?

1. circulatory overload
2. acute hemolytic reaction
3. febrile nonhemolytic reaction
4. allergic reaction

112. A client with prostate cancer has been given the option of various treatments and asks the nurse for advice. Which of the following is the <u>most</u> appropriate response?

1. "Let's discuss the different options and how you feel about them."
2. "I can't help you to make a decision about your treatment."
3. "You need to discuss this decision with your physician."
4. "I would choose surgery if I were in your position."

113. If a client with psoriasis is to begin NB-UVB phototherapy, how long should the initial treatment be?

1. 30 seconds to 1 minute
2. 1 to 2 minutes
3. 5 to 10 minutes
4. 15 to 20 minutes

114. A neonate has severe congenital abnormalities that make death imminent, and the NICU team believes that further attempts at treatment or feeding are not warranted and that palliative care only should be provided. When speaking with the parents about this, which of the following is the best approach?

1. tell the parents that the team suggests that all food and treatment will be withheld
2. tell the parents that the team suggests a change in care plan to focus on comfort measures
3. tell the parents that any further efforts at treatment are futile as the infant is dying
4. tell the parents that the best thing is to let nature take its course

115. A client has an open draining wound infected with MRSA and is on contact precautions. If the nurse is entering the room to care for the client, when are gloving and gowning necessary?

1. when the nurse has direct contact with the wound or drainage
2. when the nurse has direct contact with the client's body, wound, or drainage
3. when the nurse enters the room for any type of patient or environmental contact
4. when drainage is not contained by a dressing

116. Clients taking anticholinergic drugs, such as benztropine mesylate (Cogentin), to relieve muscle tremors and muscle rigidity associated with Parkinson disease should be advised to avoid which of the following?

1. overheating
2. overeating
3. excessive fluid intake
4. skipping meals

117. Following procurement of organs from a standard criteria donor (donor younger than 50 years who suffered brain death), within what time period should the heart and lungs be transplanted?

1. 4-6 hours
2. 8-12 hours
3. 24 hours
4. 36 hours

118. A nurse who is a friend on a social media site with a coworker finds that the coworker has written on the media site confidential information about a well-known client's health history (information obtained from the client's EHR). What is the most appropriate response?

1. tell the coworker that the information must be deleted from the site
2. advise the client that the security of the EHR has been breached
3. do nothing as this is not a serious problem
4. report the incident to an appropriate supervisor/administrator

119. In order to ensure adequate protein intake during pregnancy, how many additional grams of protein should the woman ingest daily during the second half of the pregnancy? *Report your answer using a whole number.*

________ grams

120. Following application of a right BK prosthesis for an amputated limb, the client returns for evaluation, and the nurse notes that the client has an unstable gait and the right hip and knee are showing signs of slight flexion contractures. The client admits to infrequent use of the prosthesis. Which of the following interventions are <u>most</u> indicated? *Select all that apply.*

1. providing sympathetic encouragement
2. arranging for retraining
3. chastising the client for failure to use the prosthesis
4. suggesting the client meet with a counselor

Answer Key and Explanations for Test #1

1. 75 drops per minute. Calculation:

$$\text{Volume (mL)} \times \text{drop factor/total minutes} = \text{flow rate.}$$

$$\text{3 hours and 20 minutes} = \text{200 minutes.}$$

$$1{,}000 \times 15/200 = 75 \text{ drops/min.}$$

2. 1, 3, and 5: Mastitis is a bacterial infection of the breast, most often caused by *Staphylococcus aureus* from the infant, so the mother can continue to breastfeed. The usual treatment includes antibiotics (such as penicillin G or erythromycin). Pain control is achieved with ibuprofen or acetaminophen and alternating hot and cold compresses. The mother should be encouraged to massage her breasts in a hot shower and to pump or express milk on the infected side to prevent an abscess from forming.

3. 1, 2, and 5: Parents should be advised to follow the manufacturer's directions for securing a car seat. Infants should be placed in rear-facing car seats with no padding underneath the infant. The shoulder straps should be fed through slots at or below the infant's shoulders and the harness positioned with the clasp at midchest. The car seat should be positioned so that the infant's head does not fall forward. For neonates, bolsters (such as a rolled infant blanket or diaper) should be placed beside the infant's head to maintain it in a neutral position.

4. 2, 3, and 4: Clients with a Holter monitor (usually in place for 24 to 48 hours) should avoid using wireless electronic devices, such as remote controls, iPads, and laptops, because these may interfere with the monitor. They may use desktop computers but should stay at least 10 feet away from routers. Although microwaves and other equipment may be used in the home, the client should avoid direct or close contact. The client may not shower or bathe until the monitor is removed. Clients may be asked to exercise and drink caffeinated beverages so the effects can be monitored.

5. 1: For insertion of a nasogastric tube, the client should be placed in the high Fowler's position with the head tilted forward because this position helps to close the trachea and open the esophagus, facilitating correct insertion. The nurse should examine the nasal passages by occluding one naris and then the other while the client is breathing through the nose and should use the side with the best airflow. The length of the tube should be estimated by measuring the distance from the tip of the nose, around the ear, and down to just below the left coastal margin. The end of the tube is lubricated, and then the tube is inserted slowly. The client may suck on ice cubes or swallow small sips of water during the procedure.

6. 2: Because the liver is located on the right side, the client should be positioned in the right side-lying position with a folded towel or small pillow under the biopsy site to apply pressure for at least three hours after the procedure is completed. The client should avoid straining or coughing. If this procedure is done on an outpatient basis, upon discharge the client should be advised to avoid any heavy lifting, strenuous exercise, or straining for one week.

7. 4: Gastric secretions are usually acidic with gastric tube aspirate having a pH of 5.5 or less. However, medications may alter the acidity, so depending on the pH alone is not adequate. Additionally, tube feedings usually have a pH of about 6.6, so aspirating with continuous feedings to check the pH is not effective. Intestinal fluid is less acidic than gastric secretions, usually 6 or higher. A pH of greater than 7 often indicates that the end of the tube is located in the respiratory system rather than the gastrointestinal system. Note that some nasogastric tubes contain built-in pH sensors.

8. 1: The client is exhibiting signs of obstruction. Because the secretions are very thick, the best action is to increase the humidification to help loosen the secretions and suction the tracheostomy tube. Suction should not be used during insertion of the suction catheter because this removes oxygen and may traumatize the tracheal tissue, but suction should be used for 5 to 10 seconds while the catheter is removed. Suctioning for longer periods should be avoided because it may result in hypoxia.

9. 3: Continuous bubbling in the water seal chamber indicates a system air leak. Intermittent bubbling occurs with pneumothorax as the air flows from the chest cavity into the chamber. The water level in the water seal chamber should fluctuate. If the fluctuation stops, this is generally an indication of a problem, such as obstruction of the chest tube or inadequate suction. However, it may also indicate reexpansion of the lung. The collection chamber is monitored for drainage. The suction control chamber should exhibit gentle bubbling.

10. 2: The client is exhibiting signs of caregiver neglect: her dirty, disheveled appearance and her loss of weight, which may indicate that she is not receiving sufficient food or sufficient assistance with eating. A client with moderate Alzheimer's disease is not usually able to manage self-care without assistance. For example, clients may forget where their clothing is or believe they have already bathed, changed clothes, and eaten when they haven't done so.

11. 3: Medications with antithrombotic properties, such as aspirin or nonsteroidal anti-inflammatory drugs (NSAIDs), are usually avoided the morning of a surgery, although other routine medications may generally be taken with a sip of water a few hours before scheduled surgery. Some medications, such as warfarin, may be discontinued for a few days prior to surgery because of the increased risk of bleeding. All medications (prescription and over the counter [OTC]) should be reviewed with the client, and instructions about use of the medication in relation to the surgery should be provided.

12. 112 micrograms: One milligram contains 1,000 micrograms, and 1 gram contains one million micrograms. Although the symbol μg is used to represent micrograms, the Food and Drug Administration (FDA) and the Institute for Safe Medication Practices (ISMP) recommend against using this symbol because it may easily be confused with the abbreviation for milligrams (mg). The abbreviation mcg is sometimes used. Calculation:

0.112 mg × 1,000 = 112 micrograms.

13. 3: Clients with rubella (German measles) must be maintained on droplet precautions. Standard precautions apply to all clients regardless of other precautions.

Contact	Use personal protective equipment (PPE), including gown and gloves, for all contact with the client or the client's immediate environment. Clients should be in private rooms or >3 feet from other clients.
Droplet	Use a mask while caring for the client. Clients should be in a private room or >3 feet away from other clients with a curtain separating them. The patient must be masked for transport.

Airborne	Place the client in an airborne infection isolation room, and use ≥N95 respirators (or masks) for client care.

14. 1: All of the laboratory results are within the normal range except for the platelet count. The normal range for platelets is 150,000 to 450,000, so 119,000 is low, indicating thrombocytopenia, which may increase the risk of bleeding and bruising. A decrease in platelets may indicate aplastic anemia, alcohol toxicity, prolonged hypoxia, iron-deficiency anemia, megaloblastic anemia, or viral infection. Severe infection may also suppress platelets. The risk of bleeding with invasive procedures is usually minimal until the count drops below 50,000, and the risk is most severe with counts below 20,000.

15. 1, 2, 3, 4, 5 and 6: Diabetic ketoacidosis (DKA) occurs when the amount of insulin is insufficient, resulting in hyperglycemia. Indications include polyuria and polydipsia, hyperventilation (Kussmaul respirations), blurred vision, weakness, headache, abdominal pain, orthostatic hypotension, and mental status changes. Clinically, the primary indications are hyperglycemia, dehydration, electrolyte imbalance, and acidosis. The primary causes of DKA are missing a dose of insulin, illness/infection, and untreated diabetes mellitus. Illness and infection can increase the need for insulin even if food intake is decreased.

16. 2: A minor cannot sign a surgical consent unless she is emancipated. Although a surgeon may, in an emergency, perform surgery on a minor without parental or legal guardian consent, every effort should be made to locate a parent or guardian. If reached by telephone, the parent or guardian can give consent verbally, but two witnesses should listen to the conversation and document that consent was given for the procedure, noting the name of the person granting consent.

17. 3: For intermittent tube feedings, the client should be positioned with the head of the bed elevated to 30° to prevent aspiration. The client should remain in this position for at least an hour after each feeding, and the head of the bed should stay elevated to at least 30° at all times if he is receiving continuous feedings. Placement of the tube should be verified through aspiration and assessing the pH of aspirant prior to every intermittent feeding and at least every 12 hours for continuous feeding.

18. 3: Although 60% of the adult's body is composed of water, 67% of this amount is intracellular fluid (ICF), 25% is interstitial fluid (ISF) (found in the spaces between cells, tissues, and organs), and 8% is plasma volume (PV). ISF and PV are classified as extracellular fluids. Fluid balance is extremely important for life because death usually occurs when 20% to 25% of the total body water is lost, such as through dehydration.

19. 1: Whole blood is rarely administered nowadays, although it may be given for extreme loss of blood volume when the red blood cells and the plasma need replacement. The most commonly used blood products are packed red blood cells and fresh frozen plasma, so whole blood is usually separated into these components. Red blood cells are preferred for most indications because the extra plasma found in whole blood may result in transfusion-associated circulatory overload.

20. 4: These symptoms are consistent with hypoparathyroidism and hypocalcemia, so the physician is likely to monitor the calcium level. One complication of thyroidectomy is trauma to or inadvertent removal of the parathyroid glands, resulting in hyperphosphatemia and hypocalcemia because of decreased intestinal absorption of dietary calcium as well as decreased resorption from bone related to inadequate parathyroid hormone. Hypocalcemia causes tetany, which may manifest as numbness, tingling, and stiffness in the hands, feet, and face and muscle spasms and contractions. Clients may experience anxiety, depression, and hypotension.

21. 1: Constipation and fecal impaction are common with chemotherapy and opioids. Chemotherapeutic agents may cause dysfunction of the autonomic nerves, resulting in abdominal discomfort, and rectal emptying may be slowed. Opioids slow the intestinal motility, so the combination increases the risk of obstruction. The client should have an abdominal examination and abdominal x-ray to evaluate for obstruction before further treatments because the client has not been passing flatus and has increasing pain and nausea.

22. 3: Although difficulty with urination, frequency, and urgency are the usual signs of urinary tract infection (UTI), these may be absent in elderly clients, who frequently exhibit nonspecific symptoms, such as anorexia, hyperventilation, low-grade fever, and new onset of urinary incontinence. General fatigue/malaise is the most common presenting symptom in older adults. Cognitive function may also be impaired, and those with dementia may show a sudden cognitive decline. The most common causative agent for UTI in elderly clients is *Escherichia coli.*

23. 1: Although protocols for dealing with medication errors may vary from one institution to another, in most cases, the correct response is to notify the physician, notify the supervisor, and complete an incident report. The nurse should not attempt to cover the mistake by obtaining a physician's order after the fact. Usually, documenting an error on the client's record consists only of documenting the actual treatment given—in this case the acetaminophen—but omitting further information about the error and documenting that only in the incident report.

24. 1, 2, and 3: Although African-Americans have a lower risk than Caucasians for skin cancer and osteoporosis; they have a higher risk for a number of other diseases:

- Hypertension: Forty-one percent have hypertension compared to 27% of Caucasians.
- Diabetes mellitus: The incidence is 60% higher than for Caucasians with about two-and-a-half times as many amputations and more than five times as much kidney disease.
- Asthma: The rate of death is three times that of Caucasians.
- Lung cancer: African-American males have twice the incidence of lung cancer than do Caucasian males.
- Heart disease.
- Stroke: The risk is twice that of Caucasians, and resulting deaths are four times higher.

25. Correct order:

1. vi: Cleanse the prosthetic eye according to the manufacturer's directions.
2. iv: Identify landmarks on the prosthetic eye for the inner and outer areas and superior and inferior aspects.
3. i: Raise the upper eyelid.
4. iii: Slide the prosthesis under and behind the upper eyelid.
5. ii: Pull the lower eyelid down.
6. v: Check the positioning.

26. 3: These are indications that the client may be experiencing hearing loss. Hearing loss may be insidious, with the client not being fully aware that his hearing is impaired. Because hearing loss may impair the person's ability to hear his own voice as well as others' voices, he may begin slurring his words or dropping word endings. Clients may react to hearing loss by becoming depressed, withdrawn, and irritable, and they may believe that people are whispering or talking behind their backs because they cannot hear what people are saying.

27. 2, 3, and 5: Although unlicensed assistive personnel (UAP) can check routine temperatures and vital signs, they should not be responsible for assessing the condition of a client who is acutely ill. UAP may empty catheter bags and measure urinary output as long as they have been trained in the proper techniques, and they may assist ambulatory clients to walk to the bathroom or help clients with a bedpan. The nurse who delegates the task is always responsible for supervising the UAP and ensuring that the task is completed appropriately.

28. 1: Engorgement often occurs in the first two to three days after delivery as the mother begins to produce milk and nurse the infant. Because the infant's intake the first few days is usually very small, the production of milk may exceed demand, resulting in breasts that are swollen, taut, and painful. The mother should be encouraged to continue to nurse and gently massage the breast toward the nipple. Application of cold compresses for 15-20 minutes in between feedings may relieve swelling and discomfort. The mother may take acetaminophen for pain. Engorgement usually lasts only 24 to 48 hours.

29. 21 drops per minute. Calculation:

Volume (mL) × drop factor/total minutes = flow rate.
250 × 10 = 2,500.
2 hours = 120 minutes.
2,500/120 = 20.83 = 21 drops per minute.

30. Correct order:

Milliliter	Centiliter	Deciliter	Liter	Dekaliter	Hectoliter	Kiloliter

1: ii. Milliliter
2: i. Deciliter.
3: iii. Dekaliter.
4: v. Hectoliter.
5: iv. Kiloliter.

31. 1, 2, 3, and 5: Organ meats, such as liver, and some seafood, such as sardines, mackerels, and scallops, are high in purines and should be avoided. All meats contain purines, so their intake should be limited to 4 to 6 ounces per day. Broth made from meats should be avoided. Because alcohol impairs the elimination of uric acid, wine intake should not exceed 10 ounces daily. Foods high in fat also impair elimination, so high-fat foods, such as avocados and ice cream, should be limited.

32. 1: Although all of these are important, histamine is released in response to the antigen, causing erythema and edema, which can result in airway obstruction, so the primary concern is to ensure patency of the airway. This may require intubation. Epinephrine should be administered as soon as possible, and oxygen is provided at 100% high flow. Intravenous fluids are provided to combat hypotension. Albuterol may be given to relieve bronchospasm. If shock continues, diphenhydramine and methylprednisolone may be required.

33. 50 drops/minute. Calculation:

$$\text{Volume (mL)} \times \text{drop factor/total minutes} = \text{flow rate.}$$
$$250 \times 60/5 \times 60 = 15{,}000/300.$$
$$15{,}000/300 = 50 \text{ drops per minute.}$$

34. 3: One grain is equal to 60 to 65 mg (the calculation depends on the manufacturer), so 325 mg is approximately equivalent to five grains of aspirin. Grains are used in the apothecary method of measurement, but only a few medications are still provided using this measurement because most are now provided using metric measurements, such as milligrams. Household measurements, such as ounces and teaspoons, are also used for medications, so nurses should be familiar with conversions among the different measurement systems.

35. 120 mL. Calculation:

$$\begin{aligned} 40\text{ (kg)} \times 15\text{ (mg per kg)} &= 600\text{ mg per day} \\ 600\text{ (mg per day)} \times 10\text{ (total days)} &= 6{,}000\text{ mg total} \\ 250/5 &= 6{,}000/x \\ 250 \times x &= 250x \\ 5 \times 6{,}000 &= 30{,}000 \\ 250x &= 30{,}000 \\ 30{,}000/250 &= 120\text{ mL} \end{aligned}$$

36. Two teaspoons: Milliliters are metric measurements, and teaspoons are household measurements. Five milliliters is approximately equivalent to one teaspoon, so the child will require two teaspoons for 10 mL of oral suspension. Oral suspensions are often prescribed in household measurements to reduce the chance of medication errors for those unfamiliar with the metric system.

37. 3: In the event of a fire, the client must be evacuated as quickly as possible. Because the client has not yet ambulated and the repaired hip must remain abducted, transferring the client to a wheelchair or attempting to carry the client is precluded. Transferring the client to a gurney is too time-consuming. The best solution to moving a client to a safe area as quickly as possible is to move the client in the bed.

38. 1: Restraints cannot be applied as the first intervention, so the nurse must attempt other interventions first, such as trying to camouflage the IV with clothing or dressings. Tying a length of IV tubing to the bedrail and allowing the client to pull on it may distract the client. Restraints may result in injuries and should be avoided whenever possible. Vest restraints have resulted in a number of deaths, so many facilities no longer allow their use.

39. 2, 3, 4, and 6: Although advanced age may be a barrier to learning, age should not be a concern for a 55-year-old unless she has cognitive impairment. However, fear and lack of literacy may impact the client's ability to learn. Clients who are weak and frail may not be able to concentrate fully, and those who are hard of hearing may miss important points, especially if the nurse is unaware of the hearing deficit. Asking questions is usually a good sign that the client is alert and attentive.

40. 0.25 mL. Calculation:

$$\begin{aligned} 1\text{ (mg)}/1\text{ (mL)} &= 0.25\text{ (mg)}/x\text{ (mL)} \\ 1 \times x &= 1x \\ 1 \times 0.25 &= 0.25 \\ 1x &= 0.25 \\ x &= 0.25\text{ mL} \end{aligned}$$

41. 4: The nurse should assess the client's level of pain. Deep breathing, coughing, and turning may be very painful in the first 24 to 48 hours after major surgery, but they are necessary to prevent atelectasis and other complications. Clients who are in pain are often very reluctant to cooperate, so the nurse should ensure that the client has received adequate analgesia prior to the first time she is asked to deep breathe, cough, and turn.

42. 2: The elbow comprises the simplest type of joint: the hinge. The only movements a hinge joint can perform are flexion and extension. Flexion involves the biceps brachii, brachialis, and brachioradialis muscles, and extension uses the triceps brachii. Three bones (the humerus, ulna, and radius) come together at the elbow but in two different joints—the hinged elbow joint and the pivot proximal radioulnar joint, which allows the forearm to supinate and pronate.

43. 3: After a cast is removed, the skin is covered with fatty deposits and dead skin. The nurse should apply a cold-water enzyme wash to the skin, leave it in place for about 20 minutes, and then rinse or soak the leg in warm water to remove the enzyme wash. The skin can then be gently washed with warm water and mild soap, but it should not be rubbed vigorously or scrubbed. The skin should be gently patted dry, and an emollient is applied.

44. 1: The correct method of indicating that information has been documented on the wrong record is to draw a straight line (one only) through the incorrect documentation, write "error" above it, and initial the correction. No attempt should be made to obliterate the entry with correction fluid, erasure, or drawing multiple lines through it because the entry must remain readable for legal reasons so that it does not appear that the client's record has been altered.

45. 1: Numbness of the thumb and index finger, inability move the thumb to touch the tips of the other fingers, and capillary refill time greater than three seconds are all indications that the radial nerve is compressed. While the arm is supported, the elastic bandage on the forearm should be removed and reapplied more loosely, and then the circulation is reevaluated to determine if this alleviates the problem. If the numbness, impaired movement, and slow capillary refill persist, then further evaluation is indicated.

46. 2: The Braden Scale is used to determine if the client is at risk for developing pressure sores. The scale assesses six different areas with scores of 1 to 4 or 1 to 3. The lower the total score, the higher the risk. The six areas are sensory perception, moisture, activity, mobility, usual nutrition pattern, and friction and sheer. The Braden Scale is used to help identify the need for a support surface and the type of support surface appropriate for the client's needs.

47. 4: Healthcare providers should have priority for protection from injury because if they are injured, then no one will be available to provide care to the others who are injured. Police officers and firefighters are usually the first responders in a disaster, and they must determine when it is safe for healthcare providers to enter the area and provide care. In some cases, this may mean that care for the injured is delayed because of unsafe conditions.

48. 2: The statement that indicates the client has not made informed consent is "I told the doctor I didn't want to know anything about the surgery, and she agreed." The physician has a responsibility to inform the client of the risks and benefits of the treatment and any alternative treatment options even if the client does not want this information. A client who refuses to receive the information may be in denial or may not yet be emotionally prepared to deal with the reality of the treatment.

49. 3: Although these are all important considerations, the installed height, the ratio of computers to staff, and the brand of computer are focused on the needs of the staff. However, the positioning of the computer screens away from the line of sight of clients and visitors is essential for maintaining client confidentiality. The screens must be positioned so that others cannot read what is being documented about a client. Computers must be kept in a secure area. In some cases, privacy screens or filters may be used.

50. 4: The trough time is when the blood level is at its lowest (in the trough), so the serum trough level should be drawn immediately before a scheduled dose of the medication is due. Blood levels of a drug may also be measured at the peak time, and this will vary from drug to drug and should always be checked and the time prescribed. When drawing blood for trough and peak levels, it's important that the medication doses be administered on time.

51. 1,140 calories. Calculation:

$$75 \text{ (g protein)} \times 4 = 300 \text{ (calories)}.$$
$$120 \text{ (g carbohydrate)} \times 4 = 480 \text{ (calories)}.$$
$$40 \text{ (g fat)} \times 9 = 360 \text{ (calories)}.$$
$$300 + 480 + 360 = 1{,}140.$$

52. 2: The nurse should contact the admissions department and ask that the client be reassigned to a different room. Although superstitions may seem irrational at times, fear and anxiety can negatively impact recovery. Anxiety before surgery is common, and severe anxiety can result in increased time necessary for induction and an increased need for analgesia in the postoperative period. Superstitions can compound the fear because the client may feel that the negative outcomes he fears (pain, disability) are more likely to occur.

53. 1, 3, and 4: Because this client is transient and homeless, he probably does not have easy access to a computer or friends and family who can help, so he will most likely have to rely on public agencies and services, such as self-help programs, community agencies (including mental health outreach services), and government agencies (such as Medicaid or Social Security). Although the nurse can provide homeless clients with information, follow-up can be poor among homeless and transient populations.

54. 3: At 3 L/min per nasal cannula, the client should receive about 32% FiO_2. Nasal cannulas deliver low concentrations of oxygen, but they are relatively safe and easily tolerated, although they may cause drying and irritation of nasal passages. The FiO_2 measurement may be affected by nasal obstruction and breathing patterns. FiO_2 per L/min:

1 L/min: 24%.
2 L/min: 28%.
3 L/min: 32%.
4 L/min: 36%.
5 L/min: 40%.
6 L/min: 44%.

55. 1: The statement "I need my husband to take care of financial matters" suggests that the client's wife has not accepted that her husband's condition will continue to deteriorate and, because of behavioral and language difficulties, he will not be able to manage their financial affairs. She will need to assume responsibilities that were previously handled by her husband, who will become increasingly dependent. This change in roles can be very difficult for a spouse, especially as the behaviors worsen and profound personality changes occur.

56. 3: Alcohol, benzodiazepines, and barbiturates pose the greatest risk to life if clients attempt to undergo "cold-turkey" withdrawal. Patients may experience seizures, heart attacks, or strokes. Withdrawal from alcohol may result in delirium tremens (DTs). Clients undergoing withdrawal from opiates, such as heroin, may experience severe physical symptoms (nausea, vomiting, pain, muscle cramping, dyspnea, tremors, palpitations, and sweating) but they are rarely life threatening. Those withdrawing from cocaine and marijuana have milder withdrawal symptoms (anxiety, insomnia, headaches, and depression).

57. 4: In a crisis situation, such as a client shouting at the nurse and refusing to stop smoking marijuana, the best initial response is to remain calm and simply repeat the request. Challenges and threats often cause the client who is angry and belligerent to escalate her behavior. The nurse should not intrude on the client's personal space and should be aware of body language and nonverbal communication so as not to appear to be challenging. If possible, the nurse should try to identify the cause of the client's behavior by asking, "Are you feeling nervous about your upcoming tests?" so the nurse can better understand the whole situation.

58. 1, 2, 3, and 5: The diagnostic criteria for PTSD includes exposure to actual or threatened death, serious injury or sexual violation. The disturbance causes clinically significant distress or impairment and diagnosis is based on behavioral symptoms which include (1) *re-experiencing* (flashbacks, spontaneous memories of the traumatic event, nightmares, or other intense psychological distress), (2) *avoidance* (estrangement from others or diminished interest in activities, to an inability to remember key aspects of the event), (3) *negative cognitions and mood* (wide range of feelings from a persistent and distorted sense of blame of self or others, to distressing memories, feelings, thoughts or external reminders of the event), and (4) *arousal* (aggressive, reckless or self-destructive behavior, insomnia, hypervigilance or related problems). Symptoms usually present within three months of a traumatic event, although the reaction may be delayed for many months or years in some individuals.

59. 1: Clients should never flush needles or sharps down the toilet but should instead store and dispose of them in accordance with state or local regulations. In some places, needles and sharps must be placed in special sharps containers, but in other places, they may be placed in any secure, puncture-proof container with a lid. People who must dispose of needles and sharps in the community should contact their local refuse disposal service for information about disposal.

60. 0.4 mL. Calculation:

$$\begin{aligned} 10\text{ (mg)}/1\text{ (mL)} &= 4\text{ (mg)}/x\text{ (mL)} \\ 10 \times x &= 10x \\ 4 \times 1 &= 4 \\ 10x &= 4 \\ 4/10 &= 0.4\text{ mL} \end{aligned}$$

61. 1, 4, and 6: Peripheral arterial insufficiency is characterized by throbbing, cramping pain that increases with exercise; shiny skin with decreased hair; pale color on elevation; and redness on dependency. The skin is cool to the touch because of impaired circulation. Clients may complain of numbness and tingling and reduced sensation. Capillary refill is greater than two seconds. Ulcerations tend to occur on the tips of the toes or at the sites of trauma and are deep and well delineated.

62. Order of actions:

1. v: Hang the irrigation solution bag with the bottom being 20 inches above the stoma.
2. iv: Apply the irrigation sleeve over the stoma.
3. iii: Apply gloves, lubricate the cone tip, and insert it into the stoma, holding it securely.
4. ii: Allow the solution to flow in for 5 to 10 minutes and then clamp the tubing and close the top of the irrigation sleeve.
5. i: Allow 15 to 20 minutes for evacuation and then fold the sleeve, secure it, and leave it in place for 30 to 45 minutes before removing it.

63. 3: Because these signs and symptoms are indicative of obstructive sleep apnea, the client will likely be scheduled for a nocturnal polysomnogram. For the test, which is generally conducted in a sleep center, electrodes are placed on the head, face, and body as well as sensors to evaluate respiratory effort, snore, airflow, and oxygen saturation. The client spends the night in the sleep center so the different stages of sleep can be observed.

64. 4: A nonstress test measures the fetus's heart rate and accelerations during a 20- to 40-minute period. The mother is in the semi-Fowler's position with support placed beneath the right hip so the uterus is displaced to the left. An ultrasound transducer is placed on the abdomen to measure the FHR, and a tocodynamometer is placed over the fundus area of the uterus to monitor uterine contractions and fetal movement. A normal (reactive) result is 2 or more accelerations of the FHR of 15 bpm above baseline for ≥15 seconds. An abnormal (nonreactive) result is 0 to 1 acceleration of the FHR in a 40-minute period.

65. 1, 2, 3, and 5: An aphasia assessment includes observations of spontaneous speech (fluent, nonfluent, grammatical errors, and slow or hesitant speech), comprehension of spoken language (ability to follow simple and then more complex commands), comprehension of written language (ability to read and follow written commands), ability to name items (but not describe), ability to recall four named items (immediately, not after five minutes), and the ability to write. The nurse should observe the client carefully during the assessment for signs of frustration or fatigue.

66. 3: The nurse should take the child to a separate treatment area for unpleasant or painful procedures so the child can consider her own room as a safe place. Because the nurse must obtain two specimens (aerobic and anaerobic) from the leg wound, the best position for the child is in the mother's arms (facing the mother in a comfort hold), and a nurse assists to keep the leg from moving because the child will likely react by kicking.

67. 2: The area of contact for the automated external defibrillator (AED) pads must be dry, so the nurse should wipe the chest dry with an available dry cloth or ask someone else to do it while she continues cardiopulmonary resuscitation (CPR). The chest should not be wiped with alcohol because this could cause a spark and a fire when the AED shocks the heart. The pads should also not be placed over medicine patches, pacemakers, or implanted defibrillators. Different models of AEDs have slightly different directions, but most have audible directions and pictures that are easy to follow.

68. 3: Dressings over intravenous (IV) insertion sites are usually left undisturbed if they are transparent and allow clear visibility and if there is no tenderness until the rotation time for the IV. However, gauze dressings must be changed every 48 hours. If a gauze dressing is under a transparent dressing, then the dressing change schedule remains at 48 hours. In any case, the dressing should be changed if it loosens or is compromised or if signs of infection are evident.

69. 4: All neonates should be screened for hearing loss, according to the U.S. Preventive Services Task Force. Although those with identifiable risk factors, such as family history, admission to a neonatal intensive care, and craniofacial abnormalities, have up to 20 times the risk of other infants of having hearing loss, about half of infants with hearing loss have no identifiable risk factors. Testing is recommended for all neonates within one month of birth. Those who fail the hearing test should undergo a complete evaluation by three months.

70. 9 mL. Calculation:

$$
\begin{aligned}
20\text{ (kg)} \times 45\text{ (mg)} &= 900\text{ mg in 24 hours} \\
900/2 &= 450\text{ mg each dose (every 12 hours)} \\
250\text{ (mg)}/5\text{ (mL)} &= 450\text{ (mg)}/x\text{ (mL)} \\
250 \times x &= 250x \\
5 \times 450 &= 2{,}250 \\
250x &= 2{,}250 \\
25x &= 225 \\
225/25 &= 9\text{ mL}
\end{aligned}
$$

71. 4: Rate response: The pacing rate increases when the sensors note increased activity. Rate smoothing: A pacemaker function prevents excessive changes in the pacing rate. Rate drop response: The pacing rate increases above the normal pacing rate with sudden bradycardia. Mode switching: The pacemaker switches from atrial tracking mode to nontracking mode with atrial fibrillation. Pacemakers may be permanent or temporary and may include single-chamber, dual-chamber, and biventricular pacing. Pacemakers are classified with a five-letter pacemaker code indicating the chamber paced, chamber sensed, response to sensing, programmability, and pacing functions.

72. 2: The "5 A's" of the smoking cessation intervention include the following:

Step 1: Ask all clients about tobacco use at every visit. Questions about smoking should be included in all history and physical assessments.
Step 2: Advise all clients who smoke to stop smoking, advising them that smoking is harming their health.
Step 3: Assess clients' willingness to stop smoking. If they are unwilling, ask questions about why.
Step 4: Assist the client to stop smoking. Establish a quit plan with a quit date and a plan for intervention.
Step 5: Arrange for follow-up.

73. 2, 3, 4, and 6: Those with hypertension should engage in regular aerobic exercise, such as walking, for 30 minutes most days and should switch to the dietary approaches to stop hypertension (DASH) diet, which is high in fruits and vegetables and low in saturated fat and should limit alcohol to no more than one drink per day for females and two for males, but they need not completely eliminate alcohol. Smoking cessation is essential as is losing weight for those who are overweight.

74. 1: Muslims use the left hand, which is considered unclean, for toileting, so the nurse should use the left hand to cleanse the client's rectal area. For the same reason, the nurse should be careful to always pass food, medications, and other items to the client using the right hand and not the left. Wearing gloves to provide rectal cleansing is required by standard precautions and is unrelated to the woman's cultural and religious beliefs.

75. 1, 3, 4 and 5: Energy-conservation techniques include sitting down to perform activities instead of standing and keeping frequently used items close at hand but at arm level, so the person does not have to reach up or bend down because these activities require increased energy. The client should plan ahead to avoid extra movements; ask for help when needed; and use correct body mechanics, including pushing items instead of pulling them. The client should be advised to watch for stress signals, such as dyspnea or fatigue.

76. 1: 24 months: Although children develop at different rates, generally, by age 24 months a child is able to understand about 300 words and is beginning to use two- and three-word sentences ("want candy"). 16 to 18 months: Says and understands 7 to 20 words and can point to body parts. 13 to 15 months: Says and understand 4 to 6 words but understands more and can point to items he wants. 12 months: Says and understands a few words, such as "Mama" and "Dada," and can imitate animal sounds, such as "moo" and "woof."

77. 1, 3, 5, and 6: Anoxic brain injuries result from insufficient blood flow and oxygen to the brain, resulting from trauma, near-drowning, choking, cardiac arrest, trauma, drug overdose, and operative complications. Mild anoxic brain injury: Decreased ability to concentrate, memory impairment, decreased balance, and restlessness. Severe anoxic brain injury: Same as mild anoxic brain injury as well as unclear mumbled speech, dysphasia, seizures, and spasticity. Critical anoxic brain injury: Impaired ability to communicate, semicomatose state but able to open eyes; however, she has inconsistent response to environmental stimuli.

78. 4: The primary focus of treatment for osteomyelitis is intravenous (IV) antibiotic therapy, based on the results of a wound culture. IV antibiotics are administered continuously for three to six weeks, and then oral antibiotics are administered for up to three months. If the wound does not respond adequately to antibiotic therapy, then surgical debridement is indicated, during which time antibiotic-impregnated beads may be inserted into the wound. The infected area is immobilized to reduce pain and to reduce the risk of pathological fractures. Warm, wet soaks may be used to increase circulation, and analgesia may be used to reduce pain.

79. 3: Although brain damage can occur during labor and delivery, it is more often caused by a lack of oxygen than from compression. In most cases, compression results in cranial molding, which is a relatively benign condition that resolves within a few days of birth. Compression occurs during the second stage of labor, with molding being more pronounced if there is a disparity between the size of the fetal head and the maternal bony pelvis. The bones of the baby's skull are soft and flexible with sutures that allow the plates of the skull to overlap if necessary.

80. 1: Because this client faces many challenges in the home environment, the most appropriate referral is to an occupational therapist. The occupational therapist can meet with the client to determine her goals and may observe her carrying out activities of daily living (ADLs) to evaluate her abilities and deficits and can then advise her about modifications needed in the home environment and assistive devices so she can remain independent for as long as possible.

81. 1, 2, 3, and 5: If the nurse is teaching a group of clients about risk factors for diabetes mellitus, type 2, the nurse should include the following:

- Obesity
- Hypertension and/or heart disease
- 45 years and older (risk increases with age)
- Non-Caucasian race: African American, Asian, Hispanic, Pacific Islander
- History of diabetes mellitus in family

- High level of LDL cholesterol or low level of HDL cholesterol and high level of triglycerides
- History of polycystic ovarian syndrome

82. 1: Clients who are hearing impaired often are reluctant to say so but may try to compensate by reading lips. Because their hearing of their own voice may also be impaired, they may speak more loudly than usual. Even clients who are quite adept at lip reading may misunderstand some words, resulting in answering incorrectly. If a client appears to have hearing impairment, the nurse should ask the client directly if he or she is having trouble hearing the nurse and ask how to best communicate.

83. 1, 2, 3, and 5: When a client is discharged 48 hours after delivery of an infant, the client should be apprised of danger signs that could indicate infection or other complications. Constant fatigue, although debilitating, is usually normal so soon after delivery. Danger signs include:

- Temperature higher than 38 °C (100.4 °F)
- Difficulty urinating
- Swelling, redness, or pain in one or both legs
- Increased vaginal bleeding or foul vaginal discharge
- Swelling, masses, or red streaks in the breasts or bleeding nipples
- Blurred vision, persistent headache
- Depression, overwhelming feeling of sadness

84. 3: If the nurse notes a scattered red rash on a client's trunk, and the individual lesions are about 0.5 cm in diameter and are flat, nonpalpable, and circumscribed, this type of lesion would be classified as a macule. Macular lesions include those associated with petechiae, measles, and scarlet fever. Freckles are benign macules. A patch is similar to a macule but larger than 1 cm. Papules are solid, elevated, and less than 1 cm in diameter. Nodules are similar to papules but larger than 1 cm.

85. 2: If the client has stress incontinence while playing golf, she should certainly be encouraged to urinate immediately before playing golf and to wear incontinence pads for security, but the most effect technique is likely the "knack," which is the use of precisely timed muscle contractions (Kegel exercises). The client should contract the pelvic muscles immediately before stressful events, such as the golf swing, and maintain the contraction until the event is over. This maneuver provides support to the proximal urethra, preventing incontinence.

86. 3: If a client has had a recent BK amputation of the right leg and the nurse notes an unusual pattern of swelling after removing the elastic wrap, which the client had applied, the most likely reason for this observation is incorrect wrap technique in which the pressure from the wrap is uneven. The nurse should point out the swelling and discuss the reasons, demonstrating the correct wrap procedure and then observing the client rewrap the stump.

87. 1, 2, 3, and 6: If a client has recurrent episodes of constipation and fecal impaction, interventions that should be part of bowel training include scheduled toileting, such as attempting to defecate at the same time each day. The client should be advised to increase fluid intake and eat high-fiber foods. Stool softeners may be taken but not daily laxatives, which may in time make constipation worse. Stimulants, such as a suppository or a hot cup of coffee, may help to promote defecation. Routine exercise may help to stimulate intestinal contractions.

88. 4: Gait disturbances:

- Parkinsonian gait: slight flexion of hips and knees, short shuffling steps, trunk leaning forward, and no arm swing
- Ataxic gait: uncoordinated and unsteady, wide-based, staggering, high stepping, flat-footed step
- Geriatric gait: decreased speed and balance, slight flexion of hips and knees, stooped posture, and short or decreased stride length
- Scissors gait: short, slow, stiff steps with thighs crossing while moving forward

89. 2: If a client has bilateral pain, enlarged and swollen metacarpophalangeal and proximal interphalangeal joints, swan-neck deformity, and ulnar deviation, these signs and symptoms are consistent with rheumatoid arthritis (RA), an autoimmune disorder that results in inflammation and damage to the joints. RA may also affect other organs of the body. Clients typically experience periods when the disease exacerbates and symptoms worsen. Treatment includes NSAIDs, analgesics, disease-modifying antirheumatic drugs (DMARDs), and biologics.

90. 1, 2, and 3: A client with pelvic skin traction for low back pain (as well as any client on bedrest with decreased mobility) is at risk of the development of the following:

- Orthostatic hypotension: Vessels in the lower extremities lose tone and then dilate when the person stands, resulting in decreased blood flow to the brain and other parts of the body.
- Muscle weakness: Lack of movement results in weakness of muscles.
- Venous stasis: Blood flow slows when vessels lose their tone, resulting in increased risk of thrombus formation.

91. 1680 calories: In order to calculate a client's necessary caloric intake to maintain body weight, the first step is to convert the client's weight in pounds in kilograms:

- 132/2.2 = 60

Then, the caloric requirement (usually between 25 and 30 calories per kg) is multiplied by the number of kilograms:

- 60 × 28 = 1680 calories

Clients who are exceptionally active, such as athletes, may need to have a higher number of calories, so caloric requirements must be individualized.

92. 1 and 3: If a client has had repair of a right fractured hip and has an overhead trapeze on the bed to assist with movement, the client should receive instructions on the proper use of the assistive device:

- The client should always grasp the bar with both hands before moving in order to move smoothly and prevent straining the muscles.
- After grasping the bar, the client should flex the unaffected (in this case left) knee and hip and place the foot flat on the bed.
- In one movement, the client should pull on the trapeze while pushing down on the left foot and moving the body.

93. 1 and 4: If a 6-year-old child has influenza with a fever and cough, the statements by the child's caregiver that suggest a need for information include:

- "If his fever gets too high, I'll give him a bath in cold water": This could lower the child's fever too quickly. If the child's fever is high (>102 °F/39 °C), then the child may be bathed with lukewarm water.
- "I've been giving him baby aspirin to lower his fever": Children should not be administered any salicylate for viral infections because this places the child at risk for developing Reye syndrome, which can cause progressive encephalopathy, liver failure, and death.

94. 4: The snack with the lowest number of calories per serving is the apple; however, it has very little protein. When calculating calories, each gram of fat is equal to 9 calories and each gram of carbohydrate and protein is equal to 4 calories. Insoluble fiber grams are not absorbed and can be subtracted from the carbohydrate total:

- Lunch meat: $(6 \times 9) + (1 \times 4) + (7 \times 4) = 86$ calories
- Peanuts: $(14 \times 9) + (5 \times 4) - (1 \times 4) + (7 \times 4) = 170$ calories
- Cheese: $(9 \times 9) + (1 \times 4) + (7 \times 4) = 113$ calories
- Apple: $(0.3 \times 9) + (25 \times 4) - (5 \times 4) + (0.5 \times 4) = 84.7$ calories

95. The steps to combining doses of two different insulins from two vials in one syringe include:

Step	Procedure
1	i. Cleanse top of vials.
2	ii. Inject air into vial 1.
3	vi. Inject air into vial 2.
4	v. Withdraw medication from vial 2.
5	iv. Change needles.
6	iii. Withdraw medication from vial 1.

96. 3: If teaching a client to use a metered-dose inhaler without a spacer, the inhaler should be positioned 1 to 2 inches away from the client's lips for administration of a dose of inhaled medication. The client should be advised to exhale and then to deliver a dose while breathing in slowly for about 5 seconds, followed by holding the breath for 10 seconds before exhaling. If an adult has difficulty with coordinating breathing and delivering of a dosage or holding the inhaler at the correct distance, then a spacer should be used. Children should also use a spacer.

97. 1, 3, 4, and 5: If a client has received an overdose of opioid per PCA pump because the limit for maximum dosage was set far too high, resulting in the client's being pale, hypotensive, somnolent, and barely responsive with a respiratory rate of 6 breaths per minute, the nurse should immediately stop the infusion. The nurse should also administer naloxone per standing order (or immediately consult the physician to obtain the order). Because the respirations are so slow, supplementary oxygen will generally be administered. Because an error occurred in setting the parameters of dosage on the PCA, an incident report must be filed.

98. 1: If a client with Alzheimer's disease is incontinent of urine and feces and incontinent care has been delegated to UAP, then the UAP should be advised to check the client for dryness on a regular schedule of every 2 hours. Eating and drinking often trigger urination and/or bowel movements, so scheduling checks after meals is advisable. However, if the client appears restless or pulls at clothing at other times, the UAP should check for dryness then as well.

99. 1, 2, and 3: The long-term effects of prolonged use of phenytoin include a condition referred to as "Dilantin facies," which is characterized by gingival hypertrophy, hirsutism, and hypertrophy of facial subcutaneous tissue. Clients must be advised to maintain good dental care. Additionally, clients may develop osteoporosis, so supplementary vitamin D is usually advised. Clients with low levels of albumin (usually associated with renal disease or malnutrition) may have more severe effects.

100. 1, 2, 4, and 5: If a 60-year-old client has undergone a nerve-sparing prostatectomy and has been advised that he may not recover normal sexual functioning and the client is concerned and asks the nurse for more information, the nurse should include the following:

- Retrograde ejaculation may occur.
- Recovery rates vary but can take up to a year or more.
- Attempts at sexual intercourse are usually avoided for 1 month.
- Anxiety can interfere with sexual functioning.
- The client may want to explore other forms of sexual intimacy even though these are not likely as important to the client as sexual intercourse at this time.

101. 2: If a client receiving end-of-life care tells the nurse that he has not always lived the way he should have or treated his children well, the most appropriate response is: "There are things that you regret," which is stating the point that the client is making without being judgmental or questioning. At the end of life, clients often think back over their lives and consider both positive and negative aspects. They often are not seeking advice but rather an opportunity to verbalize feelings.

102. 3: There is no antidote for an overdose of muscle relaxants, such as baclofen. Therefore, treatment consists of supportive care. The client should receive large volumes of intravenous fluids to prevent the development of crystalluria, and may require mechanical ventilation if respirations are severely depressed. The client should be placed on cardiac monitoring. If other CNS depressant drugs are taken along with the overdose of muscle relaxant, the client is more at risk.

103. 1, 3, and 4: Contraindications to levodopa include narrow-angle glaucoma, pregnancy, and melanoma (or suspicious skin lesions that may be melanoma). Additionally, levodopa should not be given to clients with psychoses and must be monitored carefully if administered to clients with a history of cardiac problems. Levodopa interacts with numerous drugs, so the client's list of medications should be reviewed by a pharmacist.

104. 4: If a 78-year-old client with a history of diabetes mellitus, type 2, GERD, and hypertension is hospitalized with pneumonia and rings the call bell at 11 PM, complaining of being unable to sleep and having "indigestion" and "heartburn," the initial intervention should be to assess the client's cardiac and respiratory status before deciding how to proceed. The nurse should never assume to know the reason for a client's symptoms without conducting an assessment.

105. 3: If a client is upset that the physician has refused to order a stronger pain medication for the client and berates the nurse, calling the nurse "worthless and stupid" when the nurse brings the prescribed medication, the ego defense mechanisms that the client is exhibiting is displacement, which is the transference of feelings from one target to another. Compensation is compensating for a perceived weakness by emphasizing a strength. Reaction formation is covering up unacceptable thoughts/behaviors by emphasizing the opposite. Regression is reverting to an earlier level of development.

106. 1: When determining whether or not a client is a candidate for restraints, only current behavior should be considered. If the client currently poses a danger to others or to self and no other reasonable alternative exists, then restraints may be considered. Restraints cannot be applied as a preventive measure for such things as history of violent attack against a staff member or a history of falls. There must be evidence of current risk.

107. 3: Physical signs and symptoms often attributed to decreased estrogen production associated with menopause include increased fat deposits on hips and abdomen, often associated with weight gain and decreased metabolic rate. Clients may have difficulty sleeping and develop restless leg syndrome and heart palpitations. Hot flashes are common. Clients lose subcutaneous fat in the labia and are more at risk for problems with the lower urinary tract, such as stress incontinence and bladder and vaginal infections.

108. 4: If an older client has been sleeping poorly at night, and the daughter states that the mother has always loved music and suggests listening to music might relax the client, the nurse should ask about the client's favorite music. Tastes in music are very individual. For example, while classical music may seem relaxing to some, others may find it boring or irritating. If the client is not in a private room, then the client should use earphones.

109. 0.84: If a client's waist measurement is 38 inches and the hip measurement is 45 inches, then the calculations are:

- Waist measurement/Hip measurement = waist-to-hip (WTH) ratio.
- 38/45 = 0.8444 = 0.84.

According to the National Institute of Diabetes and Digestive and Kidney Diseases (NIDDK), a female is considered obese if the WTH ratio is greater than 0.8, and a male is considered obese if the WTH ratio is greater than 1.

110. 3: If a client is to have a nasogastric tube inserted for intermittent feedings, an appropriate task to delegate to unlicensed assistive personnel (UAP) is to administer the tube feedings if the person has been trained in doing so. However, an RN or LVN/LPN must verify the tube position first because this cannot be delegated to UAP. UAP cannot insert or reposition a displaced NG tube. UAP can be advised to monitor the client's condition and to report any changes in condition, such as dyspnea or nausea.

111. 3: If a client who received a unit of packed red blood cells developed severe chills and a 2 °C elevation of temperature 2 hours after initiation of the transfusion and the client had no dyspnea, swelling, or urticaria, the most likely cause of the client's symptoms is febrile nonhemolytic reaction. This reaction results from antibodies against the leukocytes that remain in the PRBCs. This is the most common transfusion reaction and is generally treated with nonaspirin antipyretics, such as acetaminophen and ibuprofen. The transfusion is usually resumed after acute hemolytic reaction is excluded.

112. 1: If a client with prostate cancer has been given the option of various treatments and asks the nurse for advice, the most appropriate response is: "Let's discuss the different options and how you feel about them." The nurse must avoid trying to directly influence the client's choice; however, since the client asked for advice, this is a good opportunity for the client to express feelings and concerns about the diagnosis and treatment. Additionally, talking through the options may help the client reach an independent decision.

113. 2: If a client with psoriasis is to begin NB-UVB phototherapy, the initial treatment is 1 to 2 minutes long with the time increased gradually by 10% to 15% until the optimal duration is reached. Treatments are usually done 3 times weekly to a maximum of 20 to 30 treatments. The phototherapy dosage is adjusted so that only slight erythema occurs during treatment. If the dose is too high, the client may experience marked erythema or burns.

114. 2: If a neonate has severe congenital abnormalities, death is imminent, and the NICU team feels that no further attempts at treatment or feeding are warranted, the best approach is to tell the parents that the team suggests a change in care plan to focus on comfort measures. The nurse should avoid such phrases as "stopping" or "withdrawing" treatment or feeding because these terms may make the parents feel as though they are starving or killing their infant, although the exact plan for care should be explained.

115. 3: If a client is on contact precautions because of a MRSA infection and has an open, draining wound, the nurse should glove and gown whenever entering the room for any type of patient or environmental contact. MRSA can be spread from the client to surfaces, such as the bedrails or bedside table. Upon leaving the room, the gloves and gown should be removed and placed into a receptacle near the door and inside of the client's room.

116. 1: Clients taking anticholinergic drugs to relieve muscle tremors and muscle rigidity associated with Parkinson disease should be advised to avoid overheating. Clients taking anticholinergics should be advised to avoid high environmental temperatures or activities, which may increase internal temperature, such as excessive exercise during warm weather. Because anticholinergics interfere with the body's ability to perspire, the body cannot adequately cool if overheated. Anticholinergics are often used as adjuncts to primary Parkinson drugs.

117. 1: Following procurement of organs from a standard criteria donor (donor younger than 50 years who suffered brain death), the heart and lungs should be transplanted within 4 to 6 hours, liver and pancreas within 12 hours, and the kidney within 24 hours. Organ and tissue recovery is carried out in the operating room with members of the recovery team present and transportation to the recipient available. The corneas and skin can be harvested for up to 2 hours after death and bone up to 36 hours. Heart valves can be harvested up to 72 hours after death.

118. 4: If a nurse who is a friend on a social media site with a coworker finds that the coworker has written on the media site confidential information about a well-known client's health history (information obtained from the client's EHR), the most appropriate response is to report the incident to an appropriate supervisor/administrator as soon as possible because breaching the security of the EHR is illegal and unethical. In most cases, this type of breach will result in the guilty person being fired.

119. 25 grams: While the average woman should have approximately 46 grams of protein daily, pregnancy increases the demand for protein in order to expand the blood volume and support fetal growth and maternal nutrition. By halfway through the pregnancy, the average woman should have increased the intake of protein by 25 grams. If mothers are vegetarian or vegan, they should especially seek guidance about their diet from a dietitian to ensure that their protein intake is adequate.

120. 1 and 2: Flexion contractures and impaired gait can occur if the client fails to routinely use the prosthesis, but clients may find it easier at times to use a wheelchair, and then this can become a habit. The interventions that are most indicated are to provide sympathetic encouragement without chastising the client, but pointing out the problems that are arising and arranging for a period of retraining, as retraining may be essential to ensuring the client understands and follows instructions for use of the prosthesis.

NCLEX Practice Test #2

1. A client has received 10 mg of morphine sulfate subcutaneously. When does the nurse anticipate the maximal period of respiratory depression will occur?

1. 7 minutes
2. 30 minutes
3. 60 minutes
4. 90 minutes

2. How many hours of activity per day are necessary to prevent disuse syndrome with muscle atrophy and joint contracture?

1. 6 hours
2. 4 hours
3. 2 hours
4. 1 hour

3. The nurse is one of the first on the scene of a bus accident and is triaging injured riders. Place the following injured clients (Roman numerals) into the correct triage classification.

i. 40-year-old woman with arterial bleed
ii. 20-year-old male with sprained wrist, small cuts, and bruises
iii. 14-year-old female with severe crush injuries to the head and chest and dilated, non-responsive pupils
iv. 56-year-old male with fractured femur

Minor injury (Ambulatory injured)	Immediate care	Delayed care	Unsalvageable
1.	2.	3.	4.

4. A client nearing death has an Advance Directive in his records indicating that he does not want intravenous fluids or other invasive procedures, but the client's physician has ordered IV fluids. Which of the following initial actions by the nurse is <u>most</u> appropriate?

1. notify the bioethics committee
2. inform the physician of the Advance Directive regarding intravenous fluids
3. administer intravenous fluids
4. contact a supervisor to resolve the issue

5. A client has been instructed in the application and use of anti-embolic compression stockings. Which of the following statements by the client indicates a need for more teaching? *Select all that apply.*

1. "After I apply the stocking, I roll the top back down about 2 inches to hold the stockings in place."
2. "I remove the stocking and reapply about every day or two."
3. "To apply, I turn the stocking inside out while holding onto the toe."
4. "I apply a small amount of baby powder to my legs before applying the stockings."
5. "These stockings help prevent blood clots."

6. A client with a demand pacemaker complains that he has developed persistent chronic hiccupping and is experiencing mild discomfort in the chest. Which of the following causes does the nurse suspect?

1. pacemaker syndrome
2. dislocation of a lead
3. esophageal reflux
4. myocardial infarction

7. Which of the following are common neurological changes are <u>not</u> associated with aging? *Select all that apply.*

1. dementia occurs
2. threshold for sensory input increases
3. perspiration is reduced
4. short-term memory is impaired
5. muscles atrophy

8. When examining an 80-year-old client with chronic COPD receiving home health care, the nurse notes that over the previous 48 hours the client has developed scattered painful pustular lesions on the right arm near the elbow (see photo), on the back of the neck, the face, and on both legs.

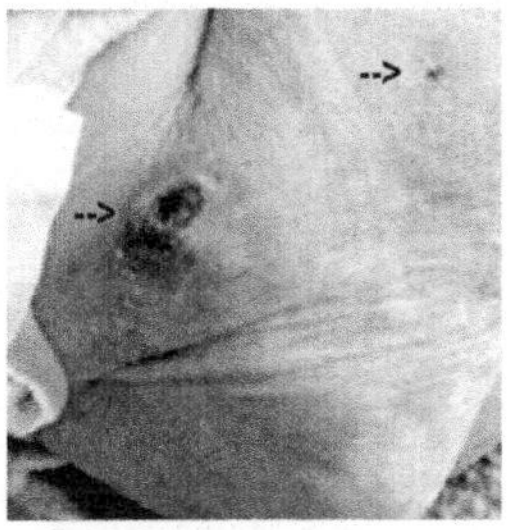

Which of the following does the nurse suspect is the <u>most</u> likely cause of the lesions?

1. psoriasis
2. herpes zoster
3. MRSA
4. contact dermatitis

9. A Turkish-speaking client is scheduled for a colonoscopy, and the nurse must provide printed directions to the client, but directions are not available in Turkish. Which of the following is <u>most</u> appropriate?

1. the nurse contacts a medical translator to translate
2. the client's 10-year-old daughter translates the directions
3. the nurse draws pictures and pantomimes directions
4. client's daughter is advised to tell her parent to seek a translator

10. While a dosage of oral morphine has approximately 25% bioavailability, what percentage is the bioavailability of an intravenous dose of morphine? *Record your answer using a whole number.*

11. The nurse is teaching the mother of a newborn to care for the umbilical cord. What should the nurse advise the mother to do if the cord becomes soiled with urine or feces?

1. swab with alcohol
2. wipe with a dry cloth
3. wash with mild soap and water, rinse and dry
4. swab with povidone-iodine

12. A client is in acute postoperative pain, and the physician orders 85 mg of meperidine (Demerol®) stat. The vial contains 100 mg in 2 mL. How many milliliters should the nurse administer? *Record your answer using a decimal number.*

13. The physician has ordered that a client recovering from back surgery be logrolled. The client has a draw sheet in place, and the nurse and an assistant are positioned with one on each side of the bed. Place the steps to logrolling (Roman numerals) in the correct sequence from first to last.

i. grasping draw sheet at shoulder and lower hips, roll patient on count of three
ii. place a small pillow between client's knees
iii. place pillows along length of client's back
iv. cross client's arms across chest

1.
2.
3.
4.

14. The physician has ordered that a 132-pound client with increased intracranial pressure receive 0.5 g of mannitol per kg in an IV solution. How many grams should be in the total mannitol dose? *Record your answer using a whole number.*

15. When applying the leads for a 12-lead electrocardiogram, the nurse places V1 and V2 at the fourth intercostal space to the right and left of the sternum. Which of the remaining leads is placed at the fifth intercostal space on the left midclavicular line?

1. lead V3
2. lead V4
3. lead V5
4. lead V6

16. A client is recovering from a stroke and the nurse is doing range-of-motion exercises. Which movements should be included for ROM of the elbow on the weak side? *Select all that apply.*

1. abduction and adduction
2. hyperextension
3. supination and pronation
4. flexion and extension
5. rotation

17. The nurse is assisting a client to adjust crutches to the proper measurement. With the client in standing position, where should the tips of the crutches be placed?

1. 2 to 3 inches directly to the side of the client's legs
2. 4 to 6 inches to the side of the client's legs and 4 to 6 inches in front of feet
3. 2 to 3 inches to the side of the client's legs and 4 to 6 inches in front of feet
4. 4 to 6 inches directly to the side of the client's legs

18. A client who is very confused removed a diamond ring and threw it on the floor. Which of the following is the <u>most</u> appropriate action?

1. give the ring to a visiting granddaughter for safekeeping
2. place the ring in the client's bedside stand in an envelope clearly marked "Valuables"
3. replace the ring on the client's finger
4. place the ring in a secured container, according to organizational policy

19. If the first day of a pregnant woman's last menstrual period fell on May 1, 2013, what is the expected delivery month and year? *Record your answer using the month (word) and year (whole number).*

20. Twenty micrograms (mcg) are equal to how many milligrams? *Record your answer using a decimal number.*

21. A physician orders chest physiotherapy for a 4-year-old child with cystic fibrosis, but the respiratory therapists are off duty, so the physician tells the nurse to do the therapy. The nurse, however, rarely works in pediatrics, has never done chest physiotherapy, and does not know the procedure. Which of the following is the <u>most</u> appropriate response by the nurse?

1. ask the child's mother to explain the procedure
2. check the procedure manual and attempt to do the therapy
3. refuse to do the procedure
4. advise the physician that the nurse will try to locate another staff person knowledgeable about chest physiotherapy

22. A pregnant woman has experienced repeated vaginal monilial infections. When educating the client about the infection, which information should the nurse include? *Select all that apply.*

1. advise client to bathe daily
2. explain the effects of increased estrogen production
3. advise client to wear cotton panties and avoid nylon or pantyhose
4. suggest client use panty liners to protect clothing
5. advise the client to avoid wearing any panties

23. When drawing up a dosage of subcutaneous heparin, how much air should be drawn into the syringe after the correct dosage is obtained?

1. 1 mL
2. 0.6 mL
3. 0.2 to 0.3 mL
4. 0.01 mL

24. Lochia serosa usually is evident on days 4 to 10 postpartum. When teaching the client about postpartum care, how should the nurse describe lochia serosa?

1. dark red discharge with small clots
2. yellowish discharge
3. pinkish to brownish discharge
4. clear watery discharge

25. The Z-track injection technique should be used with which of the following? *Select all that apply.*

1. iron
2. haloperidol
3. heparin
4. hydroxyzine (Vistaril®)
5. insulin

26. A Mexican-American client states that she and her family live next door to her brother and his family and that they share goods, services, and childcare. How is this type of family classified?

1. nuclear
2. dual career/dual earner
3. extended
4. extended kin network

27. The physician has ordered sublingual nitroglycerin for a client. Which of the following are contraindications for administration of sublingual or buccal medications? *Select all that apply.*

1. client is edentulous
2. client has mild dementia
3. mucous membranes are red and irritated
4. client is dehydrated
5. client has productive aphasia

28. The nurse is teaching a new breastfeeding mother about breast care, but the mother has engorgement and asks if she should quit breastfeeding. Which information should the nurse include? *Select all that apply.*

1. "Continue to nurse every 2 to 3 hours."
2. "Gently massage the breast toward the nipple while breastfeeding."
3. "Apply hot compresses to the breast."
4. "Acetaminophen or ibuprofen is safe to use to relieve pain."
5. "Engorgement usually recedes in 24 to 48 hours."

29. When administering a capsule that is individually wrapped to a client, when should the wrapping be removed?

1. when initially obtained from the medicine cart
2. when placed in the medicine cup
3. prior to entering the client's room
4. at bedside in the client's presence

30. Which of the following are important factors in facilitating attachment between a newborn and mother?

1. rooming in
2. swaddling and holding the infant
3. knowledge of childcare
4. beginning breastfeeding within 24 hours of birth

31. Which of the following are controlled substances (Schedules I through V) regulated by the Drug Enforcement Agency (DEA)? *Select all that apply.*

1. codeine
2. ibuprofen
3. diphenhydramine (Benadryl®)
4. hydrocodone

32. Which of the following ethnic groups has the highest risk of developing diabetes mellitus type 2 and should be routinely screened for diabetes?

1. Hispanics
2. Asians
3. Caucasians
4. African-Americans

33. A hospice client is receiving high doses of opioid analgesia and is exhibiting nocturnal myoclonus with restless leg movement and involuntary jerking. Which of the following responses would the nurse expect?

1. discontinue opioids
2. reduce dosage by half and administer a benzodiazepine
3. administer naloxone
4. administer flumazenil

34. A 16-year-old female has been sexually active for two years but was recently treated for a gonorrhea infection. The nurse is teaching the adolescent about safe sex practices. Which of the following statements by the adolescent indicate a need for more information? *Select all that apply.*

1. "I'm never going to have sex again until I'm married, so I don't need to know about safe sex!"
2. "I should never have any kind of sex unless my partner wears a condom."
3. "We don't need to use a condom for oral sex."
4. "I'm confused about different birth control methods."
5. "Birth control pills are more effective than diaphragms."

35. A client receiving high doses of hydromorphone (Dilaudid®) develops acute respiratory depression with a drop in blood pressure. Which of the following treatments is most indicated?

1. naloxone
2. naproxen
3. fumazenil
4. nortriptyline

36. A 20-year-old client has taken forty 500-mg tablets of acetaminophen with 4 ounces of alcohol in a suicide attempt. The client is <u>most</u> at risk for which of the following?

1. gastrointestinal hemorrhage
2. respiratory depression
3. liver failure
4. brain damage

37. A client with bipolar disorder is taking lithium to control symptoms. Which of the following statements indicates the need for further education?

1. "I need to have regular tests for thyroid function."
2. "Once I'm stabilized, I won't need further testing."
3. "I should avoid taking ibuprofen."
4. "It's important for me to avoid dehydration."

38. Which of the following antibiotics is contraindicated in children younger than 8 years?

1. tetracycline
2. amoxicillin/clavulanic acid
3. azithromycin
4. amoxicillin

39. A nurse notes that clients of one surgeon have developed at least twice as many infections as clients of other surgeons on the unit. Which of the following is the <u>most</u> appropriate action?

1. report the physician to the hospital administration
2. ask the physician why his rate of infections is so high
3. report the observations to the infection control nurse
4. say nothing as infection rates vary from time to time

40. Which type of laxative agent is usually the safest for most people?

1. bulk laxatives
2. stool softeners
3. stimulants
4. osmotics/saline

41. Prior to drawing blood for blood gas analysis, the nurse conducts the modified Allen test to ensure there is adequate collateral circulation. The nurse asks the client to extend the wrist over a rolled towel and make a fist. Place the following steps (Roman numerals) in order from first to last.

i. ask the client to open and close the hand until the skin blanches
ii. palpate the ulnar and radial pulses and apply pressure to both arteries
iii. observe the hand for color
iv. release the ulnar artery while maintaining pressure on the radial artery

1. (Step 1)
2. (Step 2)
3. (Step 3)
4. (Step 4)

42. What is the critical point for PO2 (the "ICU" point), the percentage point at which there is marked decrease in oxygen saturation? ***Record your answer using a whole number.***

43. A client with heart failure has been prescribed the DASH diet (dietary approaches to stop hypertension) and must limit sodium intake to 2300 mg per day. Which of the following statements by the client indicates a need for further education?

1. "All I really have to do for this diet is stop adding salt to foods."
2. "I can have 2 or 3 servings of nonfat or low-fat dairy products each day."
3. "I should have 4 or 5 servings of both vegetables and fruits daily."
4. "I should limit lean meat, poultry, and fish to 6 ounces per day."

44. A client has immune thrombocytopenic purpura. The client's platelet count is 19,000. Which initial treatment does the nurse expect?

1. splenectomy
2. immunosuppressive therapy
3. observation only
4. platelet administration

45. A client is being assessed for neutropenia. The client's total white blood cell count is 5200 with 45% neutrophils and 5% bands. What is the absolute neutrophil count (ANC)? ***Record your answer using a whole number.***

46. Each staff person has an individual password that allows access to electronic health records. Under which of the following circumstances should a nurse allow another staff person to use his/her password?

1. a physician asks to use the password to access records of a former client.
2. another nurse asks to use the password because he has forgotten his own.
3. the nurse's supervisor asks to use the password to access client records.
4. the nurse should not allow anyone else to use the password, regardless of circumstances.

47. The nurse is part of an interdisciplinary team in a rehabilitation unit. Which of the following statements by a client is <u>most</u> important to be communicated to the social worker on the team?

1. "I can't afford to hire anyone to help me when I am discharged."
2. "I'm worried about falling when I go home."
3. "I need to learn how to get in and out of the shower."
4. "I'm not sure what kinds of adaptive equipment I will need."

48. An 84-year-old female with COPD in an extended-care facility is alert and responsive and has been maintained on low-flow oxygen and nebulizer treatments, but the client, who is bedridden, has removed the oxygen and refused nebulizer treatments, telling the nurse that she is ready to die and only wants comfort measures. Which of the following actions by the nurse is <u>most</u> appropriate?

1. insist the client take treatments as ordered by the physician
2. notify the physician of the client's refusal
3. ask family members to intervene
4. remind the client that committing suicide is contrary to her religious beliefs

49. If a client's LDL cholesterol is 100, HDL cholesterol is 50, and triglycerides are 150, what is the client's total cholesterol? ***Record your answer using a whole number.***

50. The nurse is conducting a physical examination of a client's abdomen. Place the examination techniques listed below (Roman numerals) in the correct sequence, from first to last.

i. percussion
ii. palpation
iii. inspection
iv. auscultation

1. (First)
2. (Second)
3. (Third)
4. (Fourth)

51. The nurse is conducting an examination of the abdomen and auscultating for bruits. Label the lettered points on the diagram with Roman numerals identifying the position of the arteries.

i. Femoral
ii. Aorta
iii. Iliac
iv. Renal

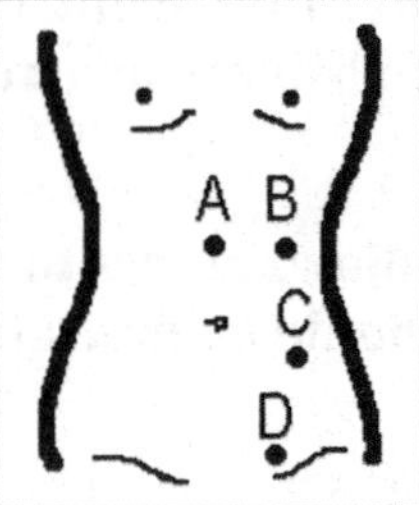

1. (A)
2. (B)
3. (C)
4. (D)

52. A female client is scheduled for a routine pelvic exam. Which of the following should the nurse ask the client to do prior to the exam?

1. refrain from drinking
2. urinate
3. wash perineal area
4. perform relaxation exercises

53. The nurse is inserting an intravenous line into the right arm and has identified a potential insertion site. Place the steps (indicated in Roman numerals) of venipuncture in the proper sequential order.

i. palpate vein.
ii. cleanse skin.
iii. apply tourniquet.
iv. perform venipuncture.

1.
2.
3.
4.

54. A client is receiving oxygen per nasal cannula at 3L/minute. Which of the following is the approximate inspired oxygen concentration (FiO_2)?

1. 60%
2. 50%
3. 40–42%
4. 28–32%

55. A client is taking nebulizer treatments for asthma, and the nurse is instructing the client in the correct method for measuring peak expiratory flow rates (PEFR) after treatment. The nurse prepares the meter with the indicator at the base of the scale. Place the following steps (Roman numerals) in the correct order from first to last.

i. client sits upright or stands
ii. client places the meter in the mouth and seals lips
iii. client expels air through the meter as forcefully as possible
iv. client takes a deep breath

1.
2.
3.
4.

56. Following a lumbar puncture, a client develops a severe headache that persists 24 hours and is unrelieved by bedrest or oral fluids. Which of the following interventions does the nurse anticipate?

1. bedrest for 3 days
2. opioid analgesia
3. epidural blood patch
4. intravenous fluids

57. The nurse is assisting a client who is to undergo a thoracentesis. Which of the following is the optimal position for the procedure?

1. lying prone with arms above head
2. side lying on the unaffected side
3. side lying on the affected side
4. upright position, leaning forward over an over-bed tray table

58. A client has experienced 48 hours of severe repeated bouts of vomiting. Which acid-base imbalance is of most concern?

1. respiratory acidosis
2. respiratory alkalosis
3. metabolic acidosis
4. metabolic alkalosis

59. A client is scheduled for hemodialysis twice weekly through an arteriovenous fistula in the left arm. Following each hemodialysis treatment, the nurse should evaluate the client for which of the following because of risks associated with hemodialysis? *Select all that apply.*

1. fluid volume deficit
2. fluid volume excess
3. bleeding
4. metabolic acidosis
5. pulmonary edema

60. A client with liver failure and ascites is having a paracentesis to relieve severe dyspnea resulting from abdominal fluid accumulation. Prior to the procedure, the nurse assists the client to urinate. Which of the following is the <u>most</u> important reason to have the patient urinate?

1. patient comfort
2. prevention of incontinence
3. prevention of bladder puncture
4. fluid displacement

61. A client is to be discharged with a tracheostomy. Which of the following should the nurse most stress when educating the client about home management? *Select all that apply.*

1. bowel care
2. pulmonary hygiene
3. dietary supplements
4. tracheostomy care
5. exercise program

62. A 72-year-old client with Parkinson disease is recovering from pneumonia and is to be discharged, but he remains weak and has poor control of his hands because of tremors. A home health aide will visit three times weekly to assist the client to bathe, and his daughter will visit every evening after work to help with laundry and housework. Which of the following referrals is <u>most</u> indicated to allow the client to remain independent in his home?

1. home meal delivery program (Meals on Wheels)
2. friendly Visitors program
3. hospice
4. occupational therapist

63. A client is receiving hospice and palliative care, including analgesia and other comfort measures. Which of the following indicates the client is undergoing life review? *Select all that apply.*

1. the client looks through old photo albums.
2. the client states that her analgesia is not adequate.
3. the client reminisces about her children when they were young and her parenting skills.
4. the client states that she is ready to die.
5. the client states she does not want her children to have a funeral for her.

64. A mother brings her child to the clinic because of repeated bouts of head lice. Which of the following statements by the mother suggests a need for education? *Select all that apply.*

1. "I've repeatedly used mayonnaise and olive oil treatments."
2. "I spent hours combing nits from my child's hair."
3. "I washed her clothing and bedding in hot water and dried in a hot dryer for 20 minutes."
4. "I warned my child not to use anyone else's comb or brush."
5. "I treated the dogs for lice as well."

65. A client comes to the emergency department with scalding burns covering his entire left arm, anterior and posterior surfaces. Using the rule of nines, how much total body surface area (TBSA) has been burned? *Record your answer using a whole number.*

66. A client has been on prolonged bedrest following surgery. The nurse notes that the patient has pain in the right calf on palpation with dorsiflexion of the ankle. Which of the following causes does the nurse suspect?

1. arthritis
2. muscle strain
3. compartment syndrome
4. deep vein thrombosis

67. A client had a craniotomy for a basal meningioma and is being monitored postoperatively. The client's baseline blood pressure and pulse were BP 138/72 and P 82. Temperature was 97.5°F/36.4°C. The client is awake and responding. Which of the following findings <u>most</u> indicates possible increasing intracranial pressure?

1. patient restless, BP 146/80 and P 90. Temperature 98.2°F/36.7°C
2. patient restless and complaining of headache. BP 160/64 and P 70. Temperature 99.4°F/37.4°C
3. patient sleeping. BP 142/76 and P 86. Temperature 97.8°F/36.6°C
4. patient complaining of headache, BP 160/110, P 92. Temperature 98°F/36.7°C

68. A client is being discharged with an implantable cardioverter-defibrillator (ICD), and the nurse is educating the client about home management. The client asks what he should do if the ICD fires one time but he has no other symptoms. Which of the following is the <u>best</u> advice?

1. "Call 9-1-1."
2. "Go to the emergency department when recovered from the firing."
3. "Resume normal activities."
4. "Lie down and rest and report the event to the physician by telephone."

69. The nurse is monitoring a client's cardiac rhythm when an abnormal rhythm occurs. Which of the following cardiac rhythms does the ECG strip (see image) indicate?

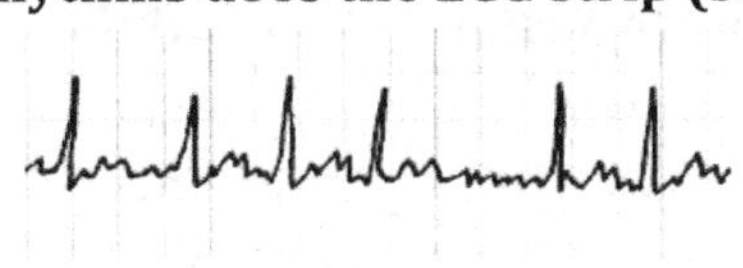

1. ventricular fibrillation
2. ventricular tachycardia
3. atrial fibrillation
4. atrial flutter

70. A client is to be discharged on warfarin (Coumadin®) therapy, and the nurse is teaching the client about the medication. Which of the following statements by the client indicates that the client's education has been effective? *Select all that apply.*

1. "I should use a soft toothbrush."
2. "My stools will routinely be black."
3. "Swimming is a good choice for exercise."
4. "I should wear a Medical Alert bracelet."
5. "I should avoid all green, leafy vegetables."

71. A client has had a central catheter inserted for administration of parenteral nutrition. An X-ray was taken to ensure correct positioning prior to commencing infusions. The X-ray report indicates that the catheter tip is in the right atrium. Which of the following actions by the nurse is correct?

1. hold the infusion and notify the MD
2. gently withdraw the catheter 2 to 3 inches
3. begin the infusion as the catheter is placed correctly
4. gently insert the catheter 2 to 3 inches further

72. A client was to receive 1 g of vancomycin intravenously in 200 mL of iso-osmotic solution over 60 minutes per infusion pump. However, the IV administration was discontinued after 45 minutes because the client developed nausea and chills. How many milligrams of vancomycin did the client receive? *Record your answer using a whole number.*

73. A client is receiving enteral feedings through a nasogastric tube, and the nurse is administering the client's medications. Which of the following can be administered through the NG tube? *Select all that apply.*

1. hard extended-release capsules (opened, crushed, and dissolved)
2. pills (crushed and dissolved)
3. enteric-coated tablets (crushed and dissolved)
4. liquid suspension
5. soft-gel capsules (dissolved)
6. sublingual wafer (dissolved)

74. The nurse is monitoring a client following postoperative cardiac catheterization and is checking the client's oxygen saturation (SPO2) per pulse oximetry. The nurse recognizes that the SPO2 should be maintained above what percentage in most clients to ensure adequate oxygenation? *Record your answer using a whole number.*

75. An older adult has become very confused after surgery for repair of a hip fracture. The client has repeatedly tried to climb over the bedrails and the nurse is considering placing the client in a Posey vest that is secured to the bed. Which of the following must the nurse consider when applying restraints to a client? *Select all that apply.*

1. an alternate method should be tried prior to applying a restraint
2. confused clients are almost always safer in restraints
3. restraints must be removed and the client reassessed at least every 2 hours
4. a written policy for application of restraints must be in place
5. the most restrictive restraint should be applied
6. the nurse does not need an order for a restraint if the client is in danger

76. The nurse is working with mothers and newborns. When educating a new mother about security measures to protect her infant, which of the following should the nurse include?

1. "Never leave your infant unattended for more than 5 minutes."
2. "Only allow people in hospital attire to remove the infant from the mother's room."
3. "Notify your assigned nurse if anyone attempts to carry the child from the room in his/her arms."
4. "Anyone with a hospital ID can be considered safe."

77. The nurse must administer 120 mg of amoxicillin oral suspension to a child. However, the only dosage available in the pharmacy is 200 mg per 5 mL. How many milliliters of suspension should the nurse administer? *Record your answer using a whole number only.*

78. Based on clinical findings, the physician suspects that a 65-year-old client has kidney disease and has ordered a blood-urea-nitrogen (BUN) test. Which of the following results is within normal limits?

1. 5 mg/dL
2. 15 mg/dL
3. 40 mg/dL
4. 100 mg/dL

79. A physician has ordered the HbA1c test for a client who complains of increased thirst and urination. Which of the following results (on two separate testings) is the lowest value considered diagnostic for diabetes mellitus?

1. 3.5 to 4.5%
2. 4.5 to 6%
3. 5.7 to 6.4%
4. ≥6.5%

80. A client with an artificial eye is too ill to remove the eye, but the lids are crusted and irritated, so the nurse must remove the prosthesis for cleaning and to inspect the eye socket. The nurse has washed hands and applied disposable gloves. Place the remaining steps to removing the prosthesis (Roman numerals) in the correct order.

i. gently retract the upper lid
ii. exert slight pressure below the eyelid and slip index finger under prosthesis
iii. break suction and slide prosthesis out of eye
iv. gently retract the lower eyelid against the orbital ridge with the thumb

1. (First)
2. (Second)
3. (Third)
4. (Fourth)

81. If a nurse accidentally punctures a finger with a needle after withdrawing blood from a client, which of the following actions should be carried out first?

1. notify a supervisor
2. wash the puncture area with soap and water
3. apply pressure to the wound
4. file an incident/injury report

82. When withdrawing blood from a peripheral vein in the arm and using a tourniquet, what is the maximum duration of time in minutes that the tourniquet should be left in place? *Record your answer using a whole number.*

_________ minute(s)

83. Which of the following factors increase the risk of developing deep vein thrombosis (DVT)? *Select all that apply.*

1. being underweight
2. smoking
3. having surgery
4. taking oral contraceptives
5. high-protein diet
6. immobility

84. A client with COPD must have the arterial blood gas (ABG) test and asks the nurse to explain the purpose of the test. Which of the following information should the nurse include? *Select all that apply.*

1. ABGs measure the levels of carbon dioxide, oxygen, and acidity in the blood
2. ABGs help to evaluate the effectiveness of treatment
3. ABGs measure the degree of anemia that has developed
4. ABGs can help to determine the need for supplemental oxygen

85. The nurse is doing a digital removal of stool for a client with a large fecal impaction resulting from opioid use when the client feels faint, and assessment of vital signs shows a marked decrease in pulse. Which of the following is the <u>most</u> likely reason for the change in pulse rate?

1. stimulation of the vagus nerve
2. onset of shock
3. internal bleeding
4. anxiety

86. A 15-year-old client took a full bottle of extra-strength acetaminophen in a suicide attempt 5 hours prior to admission to the emergency department for treatment, and the serum level of the drug is 180 mcg/mL. Which of the following interventions does the nurse anticipate? *Select all that apply.*

1. antidote: 72-hour N-acetylcysteine (NAC) protocol
2. supportive care
3. GI decontamination with activated charcoal
4. monitoring of hepatic function
5. psychiatric consultation

87. The nurse has inserted a nasogastric tube and aspirated gastric contents to check the pH with color-coded pH paper. The aspirate is dark brown, and pH measures slightly less than 5 according to the color chart. What does this pH usually indicate?

1. gastric aspirate
2. intestinal aspirate
3. respiratory aspirate
4. inconclusive results

88. A client who is to undergo electroconvulsive therapy for severe depression is quite anxious about the treatment and asks the nurse what to expect after treatment. Which of the following information should the nurse include? *Select all that apply.*

1. the client will experience confusion for a short time
2. headache and muscle soreness are common
3. some degree of memory loss, usually transient, may occur
4. possible urinary incontinence may occur for 12 hours
5. the client may experience hallucinations for 2 to 3 weeks

89. A 40-year-old male client has been diagnosed with Huntington disease and his spouse asks the nurse if their 3-year-old son should be tested to determine if the son inherited the genetic disorder. Which of the following is the <u>most</u> appropriate response?

1. "It's best to go ahead and have testing completed so that you don't have to worry about it."
2. "You should discuss the pros and cons about this with a genetic counselor."
3. "That's a bad idea. Your son may not want to know if he has the disease."
4. "Most authorities recommended letting your child decide when he is older and can make an informed decision about testing."

90. Following femoral catheterization for percutaneous coronary intervention (PCI), the client has increasing pain in the catheterization site, and the nurse notes visible edema and induration surrounding the site. The nurse suspects a hematoma and notifies the physician. Which of the following interventions does the nurse anticipate? *Select all that apply.*

1. apply pressure to the site
2. mark margins of edematous, indurated area
3. monitor hemoglobin and hematocrit
4. maintain bedrest
5. administration of clotting factors

91. If both parents are carriers of the defective gene for a disease with an autosomal recessive inheritance, what percentage chance does each child have of inheriting the gene from both parents and developing the disorder? *Report your answer using a whole number.*

________ %

92. A client has been diagnosed with immune thrombocytic purpura (ITP). Which of the following signs and symptoms indicate increased thrombocytopenia? *Select all that apply.*

1. frequent nosebleeds
2. petechiae and increased bruising
3. temporary changes in vision
4. numbness and tingling in distal limbs
5. confusion

93. A client seen in the emergency department for influenza asks for an antibiotic prescription. Which of the following guidelines are important in helping the client decrease the risk of developing an antibiotic-resistant infection? *Select all that apply.*

1. stop taking antibiotics as soon as symptoms subside
2. do not take antibiotics for viral infections, as they do no good
3. do not take preventive antibiotics to avoid infection
4. follow prescription directions when taking antibiotics
5. take the same antibiotic for every infection

94. A client who received an IV antibiotic mistakenly believed she was receiving opioid analgesia and reported a few minutes later that the medication had relieved her pain. Which of the following is the <u>most</u> likely reason for the client's response?

1. the client was lying about having pain
2. the antibiotic actually relieved the pain
3. the client experienced a placebo effect
4. the client's pain subsided coincidentally

95. A client has suffered a severe traumatic brain injury and is being treated in the ICU. Which of the following interventions does the nurse anticipate to control intracranial pressure? *Select all that apply.*

1. elevate the head of the bed
2. administer oxygen to maintain a PaO_2 >85 mm Hg
3. maintain neutral alignment of the head
4. administer sedation to prevent or reduce agitation
5. maintain body temperature below normal limits

96. A pregnant client is keeping a "kick count" log during the last trimester. Which of the following may indicate fetal distress?

1. fewer than 5 movements within 2 hours
2. fewer than 5 movements within 1 hour
3. fewer than 10 movements within 2 hours
4. fewer than 10 movements within 1 hour

97. Which of the following are intrinsic factors that increase risk of falls in older adults? *Select all that apply.*

1. sensory impairment
2. steep and unlit stairs
3. throw rugs and loose carpet
4. chronic illness
5. medications

98. During which stage of injury repair does the wound show evidence of erythema and edema, and phagocytosis begins?

1. proliferation
2. inflammation
3. hemostasis
4. maturation

99. A client with heart failure has a left ventricular ejection fraction of 38%. When educating the client about managing the condition, which of the follow advice should the nurse include? *Select all that apply.*

1. the client should take frequent rest periods
2. the client should avoid strenuous activities
3. the client should stop all exercises
4. the client should stop smoking
5. the client should limit alcohol intake to 2 to 3 drinks daily

100. Which type of behavior modification is most likely to benefit a client who has a severe phobia regarding spiders?

1. positive reinforcement
2. negative reinforcement
3. desensitization
4. aversion therapy

101. A pregnant client at 36 weeks' gestation has partial placenta previa and has been on bedrest at home for the previous 4 weeks. The client has started to have occasional contractions and is beginning to experience increasing vaginal bleeding. What intervention does the nurse anticipate?

1. tocolytic, observation, and supportive care
2. immediate induction and vaginal birth
3. transfusions and eventual vaginal birth
4. cesarean delivery

102. If the nurse is providing education to a male client who is HIV positive, which of the following information should the nurse include? *Select all that apply.*

1. need to use condoms for every sexual encounter
2. need to tell sexual or needle-sharing partners about HIV status
3. signs and symptoms indicating increased viral load and infections
4. importance of maintaining a healthy lifestyle
5. availability of support groups

103. If a group includes only members selected on a specific basis, such as women with a history of domestic or partner abuse, how is this type of group classified?

1. homogeneous
2. closed
3. heterogeneous
4. task

104. Which of the following is the primary focus of cognitive behavioral therapy (CBT)?

1. gaining reward by repeating good behavior
2. understanding the underlying causes of behavior
3. acknowledging the effect behavior has on others
4. identifying automatic thoughts and correcting errors in thinking

105. A nurse reviewed a client's progress in smoking cessation, praising the client for being successful but suggesting the client might stop having coffee in the morning since that caused an urge to smoke. Following this session, the client appeared upset and complained that the nurse believed she was doing poorly because she wanted a cigarette with her morning coffee. Which type of cognitive distortion is the client exhibiting?

1. overgeneralization
2. mental filter
3. all-or-nothing thinking
4. magnification

106. A client has accidentally splashed a toxic (although not caustic) substance in his right eye and the nurse must flush the eye. Which of the following steps are correct? *Select all that apply.*

1. position client head down and on the left side
2. irrigate with bulb syringe tip about one-half inch above eye
3. flush for about 5 minutes
4. hold eyelid open with thumb and index finger while flushing
5. hold an emesis basin against left face to contain irrigant

107. A postoperative client whose oxygen saturation has been stable at 96% to 98% suddenly shows a drop to 80%. What initial response is <u>most</u> indicated?

1. notify physician
2. administer oxygen
3. assess client and reposition pulse oximeter
4. collect an arterial specimen for ABGs

108. A client has had 4 pregnancies. She experienced one miscarriage at 12 weeks, had one stillborn birth at 34 weeks, a healthy son at 38 weeks, and a healthy daughter at 40 weeks. How would the client's obstetric history be classified?

1. Gravida 3, Para 2
2. Gravida 4, Para 4
3. Gravida 4, Para 3
4. Gravida 4, Para 2

109. Which of the following immunizations is usually administered to neonates within hours of birth?

1. rotavirus
2. polio
3. hepatitis A
4. hepatitis B

110. Using Naegele's rule for estimating the due date for a pregnancy, if a client's last menstrual cycle started on September 6 and ended September 10, when is the client's approximate due date?

1. June 6
2. June 13
3. June 10
4. June 17

111. In many cultures, pregnancy is viewed as a natural rather than a medical condition. How does this affect prenatal care?

1. pregnant women often seek prenatal care later and less frequently
2. these views have little effect on prenatal care
3. pregnant women believe prenatal care is harmful to the fetus
4. these views often result in increased rates of fetal mortality

112. A fundamentalist Muslim woman and her spouse come to the emergency department when the pregnant woman develops premature contractions and slight vaginal bleeding; however, the only physician available is a male. Which of the following initial responses is <u>most</u> appropriate?

1. ask the woman's permission for treatment by a male physician
2. ask the woman's husband's permission for treatment by a male physician
3. delay examination by a physician until a female physician can be located
4. proceed with examination by the male physician

113. Which cephalic presentation is most common during delivery of a neonate?

1. vertex
2. face
3. military
4. brow

114. Two Mexican immigrant families live closely together and share goods, services, and childcare. To which of the following family structures does this model correspond?

1. kinship network
2. binuclear
3. nuclear
4. extended

115. A 65-year-old client who recently retired from many years of working full-time for a company has become increasingly unmotivated and states he feels as though he has no purpose. Which of the following recommendations are <u>most</u> appropriate? *Select all that apply.*

1. volunteer or get a part-time job
2. participate in community activities
3. join a senior citizen's group
4. be thankful he can afford to retire
5. ask to have retirement reversed

116. The first-time mother of a 6-month old infant is concerned that the child's physical development is delayed because the child cannot crawl. Which of the following is the most appropriate response?

1. "Most infants can crawl by 9 months."
2. "Most infants can crawl by 6 months."
3. "Don't worry, infants vary widely in abilities."
4. "Look at all your child can do!"

117. A 14-year-old client has been diagnosed with celiac disease after a long history of diarrhea, anemia, and weight loss. What type of diet does the nurse anticipate the client will require?

1. high protein
2. dairy free
3. low carbohydrate
4. gluten free

118. A 68-year-old client states he decided not to take the herpes zoster (shingles) immunization because his friend had the immunization and still developed shingles. Which of the following information should the nurse include when discussing this issue with the client? *Select all that apply.*

1. shingles rarely occurs after immunization
2. the immunization decreases the severity of infection
3. the immunization decreases the likelihood of postherpetic syndrome
4. the immunization cuts the chance of developing shingles in half
5. the client should never take advice from friends

119. A nulliparous client has been admitted after 12 hours of mild contractions at home. On examination, the client is found to be fully effaced and dilated to 3 cm. Contractions are every 5 minutes and last approximately 60 seconds. The client asks the nurse approximately how long it should take to get to 10 cm dilation. Which of the following is the <u>most</u> appropriate response?

1. approximately 3 hours
2. approximately 4 hours
3. approximately 5 hours
4. approximately 7 hours

120. The nurse is serving on the performance improvement committee, which has agreed to some changes in procedures on the basis of evidence-based research. If the committee wants to convince staff members to comply with the changes, which of the following actions should the committee carry out first?

1. identify and gain support of key staff
2. explain the consequences of failure to comply
3. determine a reward system for compliance
4. clearly outline expectations in written format

Answer Key and Explanations for Test #2

1. 4: The period of maximal respiratory depression after subcutaneous injection of morphine sulfate is approximately 90 minutes while it is 30 minutes for intramuscular and 7 minutes for intravenous. The respiratory center sensitivity should return to normal within 3 hours, but minute volume may remain impaired for up to 5 hours, so clients should be monitored carefully for indications of respiratory depression. IV morphine peaks at approximately 20 minutes while IM peaks at 30 to 60 minutes and SQ at 50 to 90 minutes.

2. 3: Two hours of activity are necessary in each 24-hour period to prevent disuse syndrome with muscle atrophy and joint contractures, but periods of exercise should be spaced and not done all at one time. Exercises may include ambulation, active and passive range-of-motion exercises, isometric exercises, and resistive isometric exercises. Clients should be encouraged to do as much independently as possible, and children may engage in active play activities.

3.

Minor injury	Immediate care	Delayed care	Unsalvageable
1. ii Sprain, cuts	2. i Arterial bleed	3. iv Fx femur	4. iii Crush injuries

1. ii: Minor injuries can safely be attended to later. The injured are generally alert and responsive and ambulatory ("walking wounded").
2. i: People with life-threatening injuries must be tended to immediately, so they have first priority.
3. iv: People with moderate to serious injuries that are not immediately life threatening can receive delayed care and are second priority.
4. iii: Those who are unsalvageable, meaning their injuries are incompatible with life, have the lowest priority.

4. 2: As an advocate for the client, the nurse has a responsibility to inform the physician that the client's Advance Directive specifically states he is not to receive intravenous fluids. Many times, physicians order treatments without referring to the Advance Directive, so the nurse should always be aware of client's preferences and should communicate them. If the physician insists on the treatment, then the nurse should contact a supervisor to determine if there is an organizational policy regarding the issue.

5. 1 and 2: Anti-embolic compression stockings must be applied properly, or they can have a constrictive effect. The stocking must be without wrinkles and the top must not be turned down as this makes a constrictive band that can impair venous circulation. The stockings should be removed and reapplied at least every 8 hours so that the skin can be examined and wrinkles removed. The client correctly holds onto the toe and turns the stocking inside out before applying, and putting a small amount of baby powder or talcum powder on the skin may make application easier.

6. 2: Chest discomfort and hiccupping are often indications that the atrial lead of a pacemaker has become dislodged and is stimulating the phrenic nerve, resulting in persistent hiccupping. If phrenic nerve stimulation is caused by output, then reprogramming may alleviate the problem, but if leads are displaced, then they must be replaced, and this is a medical emergency. In some cases, a lead may be too close to the diaphragm, resulting in repeated stimulation, especially if the patient is very thin.

7. 1: Neurological changes associated with aging include short-term memory loss, but dementia does not normally occur unless there is an underlying disorder. Peripheral nerve cells may begin to degenerate, causing muscles of the arms and legs to atrophy. The threshold for sensory input may increase and vibratory sensation may decrease. Autonomic changes cause reduced perspiration so that core temperature is higher before sweating is induced. Post-operative delirium is more likely to occur in older adults than younger.

8. 3: *Staphylococcus aureus* is a common skin bacterium, and some strains, such as methicillin-resistant *Staphylococcus aureus* (MRSA), are especially virulent. Skin infections with pustular lesions may develop and spread quickly. Common manifestations of MRSA infections include impetigo, cellulitis, boils, abscesses, and rashes. Because the infection may spread systemically to internal organs, the infection must be aggressively treated with antibiotics.

9. 1: While ideally printed materials should be available in a number of languages, if none are available in the language needed, then the nurse should contact a medical translator. Telephone translation services are available if speakers cannot be found locally. Children should not be asked to translate for adults as they may not completely understand and may not translate correctly. The nurse should not depend on diagrams and pantomime if medications or specific treatments are involved, and non-English speakers may not have personal access to people who can adequately translate.

10. 100%: Bioavailability refers to the amount of a drug that is absorbed unchanged into the systemic circulation. Morphine is poorly absorbed through the oral route because of the way it is metabolized in the intestines and liver, but medications that are administered intravenously immediately enter the systemic circulation and the bioavailability is 100%. Intramuscular and transdermal administration of medications also have high bioavailability, so when switching a client from oral medications to another form, the dosage may need to be adjusted.

11. 3: If the umbilical cord becomes soiled with urine or feces, it should be washed with mild soap and water, rinsed, and dried. Wiping with alcohol is no longer recommended as it may increase irritation of the surrounding skin. The cord should not be covered with clothing and should be protected by folding the top of the diaper under the cord instead of covering the cord with the diaper. The baby should not be immersed in water until the cord falls off in 10 to 14 days.

12. 1.7 mL: The calculation is as follows:

Required dose X amount of solution/mg of medication.

$$85 \times 2/100$$
$$85 \times 0.02 = 1.7 \text{ mL.}$$

Using an algebraic formula

$$\begin{aligned} 100/2 &= 85/x \\ 100\,x &= 170 \\ 100x/100 &= 170/100 \\ x &= 1.7 \text{ mL} \end{aligned}$$

13.

1. ii: Place a small pillow between client's knees.
2. iv: Cross client's arms across chest in preparation for turn.
3. i: Grasping draw sheet at shoulder and lower hips, roll patient on count of three.

4. iii: (Opposite nurse) Place pillows along length of client's back to provide support and maintain the person in the side-lying position. After the client is positioned, the nurse should check body alignment and client's comfort level to determine if more pillows or rolled bath blankets are needed for support.

14. 30 g: To convert pounds to kilograms, divide pounds by 2.2 (132/2.2 = 60). Then, multiply the kilograms of weight by the per-kilogram dose (60 X 0.5 = 30 g). When converting kilograms to pounds, multiply kilograms by 2.2. Mannitol is an osmotic diuretic that is used to increase excretion of sodium and water in order to reduce ICP and brain mass, especially after traumatic brain injury. Mannitol may also be used to shrink the cells of the blood-brain barrier to facilitate other medications breaching this barrier.

15. 2: Lead V4. The 12-lead ECG gives a picture of electrical activity from 12 perspectives through placement of 10 body leads:

4 limb leads, one for each arm and leg

Precordial leads:

V1: right sternal border at 4th intercostal space
V2: left sternal border at 4th intercostal space
V3: midway between V2 and V4
V4: left midclavicular line at 5th intercostal space
V5: horizontal to V4 at left anterior axillary line
V6: horizontal to V5 at left midaxillary line

16. 4: The elbow range of motion should include the following:

Flexion: Bend elbow until the hand is level with the shoulder.
Extension: Straighten elbow until arm is almost vertical (150 degrees) without forcing.

Range-of-motion exercises for the elbow can be incorporated into activities of daily living. Eating, bathing, shaving, combing the hair, and brushing the teeth all involve both flexion and extension of the elbow.

17. 2: When conducting measurements for crutches with a client in standing position, the tips of the crutches should be placed approximately 4 to 6 inches to the side and 4 to 6 inches in front of the client's feet. The crutch pads should be 1.5 to 2 inches below the axilla and the client cautioned not to bear weight under the axilla but to hold the crutches against the lateral chest wall to prevent nerve damage. The client's elbows should be slightly flexed (15 to 30 degrees) when grasping the handgrip.

18. 4: Because the client is confused, the nurse should place the ring in a secured container, according to organizational policy, which may vary widely. The ring should not be given to a friend or family member without consent and should not be replaced on the client's finger as the client may remove it again. The nurse should document when the ring was found, where it was found, and where it was placed for safekeeping. If witnesses are required, their names should be documented as well.

19. February 2014: Depending on the formula one uses, the exact date may vary. Starting with the first day of the last menstrual period on May 1, 2013, and using Naegele's formula, subtract 3 months and add 6 days. This would place the delivery date at February 7, 2014. Another formula adds 9 months and 7 days, placing the delivery date at February 8. Still other formulas place the date at February 5. Generally, gestation is considered to be 280 days in duration.

20. 0.02: A microgram (μg) is one-millionth of a gram (g). There are 1000 milligrams in a gram and 1000 micrograms in a milligram. In order to convert micrograms to milligrams, divide the micrograms by 1000 (20/1000 = 0.02 mg). To convert milligrams to micrograms, multiply the milligrams by 1000 (0.02mg X 1000 = 20 micrograms). Other conversions:

mg to cg = mg/10; cg to mg = cg X 10
g to cg = g X 100; cg to g = cg/100
mg to g = mg/1000; g to mg = g X 1000

21. 4: The nurse should not attempt a procedure for which the nurse has not been trained and is not familiar. Chest physiotherapy may result in injury to a child if done incorrectly. The nurse should tell the physician that he has not been trained to do chest physiotherapy on children but will attempt to locate another staff person knowledgeable about the procedure. Nurses should not rely on parents or other family members to explain procedures.

22. 1, 2, and 3: Increased estrogen production during pregnancy promotes hyperplasia of vaginal mucosa and increased production of mucus. This can create a warm, moist environment that promotes *Candida* monilial infection. The client should be advised to bathe daily and wear cotton panties but to avoid wearing nylon panties or pantyhose, panty liners, and tight clothing as these can increase the temperature and prevent airflow. The client should also be advised not to douche. Topical treatments that can be used include miconazole, butoconazole, clotrimazole, tioconazole, nystatin, or terconazole.

23. 3: After withdrawing the correct dosage of heparin into a syringe, approximately 0.2 to 0.3 mL of air should be drawn into the syringe. This air helps to clear the remaining drug from the syringe and to "lock" the medication into the tissue. After the air is drawn into the syringe, the cap should be replaced carefully and the syringe pointed needle down so that the air bubble rises to the top of the syringe. Heparin injection sites should be rotated with usual sites in the upper and lower abdomen and anterior thighs.

24. 3: Lochia rubra (days 1 to 3 or 4): Dark red discharge with small clots (smaller than nickel size). Larger clots may indicate hemorrhage or bleeding from vaginal lacerations. **Lochia serosa** (days 4 to 10): Pinkish to brownish discharge, gradually lightening as the number of red blood cells decreases. **Lochia alba** (persists an additional 2 to 85 days with average of 24 days): Yellowish discharge. Lochia alba ceases when the cervix closes. This decreases the chance of uterine infection.

25. 1, 2, and 4: The Z-track injection technique is especially indicated for IM drugs that are irritating to the tissues, such as iron, haloperidol, hydroxyzine, and interferon. Procedure:

1. Fill syringe, including approximately 0.3 mL of air to provide an air lock.
2. Choose site (avoid deltoid). Don gloves and cleanse skin in a circular pattern.
3. Place 3 fingers or ulnar surface of nondominant hand on skin and pull skin laterally.
4. Inject at 90 degrees over 3 to 5 seconds in the spot that fingers or hand was initially placed.
5. Hold needle in place for 10 seconds.
6. Withdraw needle and release tissue.

26. 4: Extended kin network: Two nuclear families live closely together and share goods, services, and childcare. This model is common in Hispanic families. **Nuclear:** Husband-wife-children model in which the mother usually stays home and cares for the children while the husband is the wage earner (7% of American families). **Dual career/dual earner:** Both parents work (66% of two-parent families) although one may work more than the other. **Extended:** Multigenerational or shared households with friends or family who share childcare responsibilities.

27. 3 and 4: Sublingual and buccal medications should not be administered if the mucous membranes in the mouth are red and irritated or if the client is dehydrated, because these conditions may interfere with absorption of the medication. While severe confusion may pose a problem, as long as the client is cognizant enough to cooperate with administration, dementia alone is not a contraindication. Being edentulous is not a contraindication because sublingual wafers absorb readily and do not have to be held in place for extended periods.

28. 1, 2, 4, and 5: Production of milk sometimes outstrips demand in the first 2–3 days because the baby ingests small amounts, so the breasts often become engorged. Nursing frequently (every 2–3 hours) and gently massaging the breast toward the nipple while nursing can help reduce engorgement. If the areola is hard, some milk should be manually expressed to soften the areola before the infant latches on. Breast pumps and heat (except in a shower) may increase engorgement. Cold compresses, acetaminophen, or ibuprofen may provide relief. Engorgement usually recedes within 24 to 48 hours.

29. 4: While all solid medications, such as pills, tablets, and capsules, should be delivered to the client in a disposable paper medicine cup, all individually wrapped doses should be opened in the presence of the client after verifying the client's identification with two identifiers. Prior to administration, the client should be assessed for level of consciousness, nausea and vomiting, and difficulty swallowing. Calibrated medicine cups are used for liquid preparations of 5 mL or more, but smaller amounts should be measured in a syringe for accuracy.

30. 1: While knowledge of childcare is helpful to a new mother, it does not necessarily promote attachment between a newborn and mother. Important factors include frequent contact, starting as soon after birth as possible; breastfeeding, ideally starting within 60 minutes of birth; and utilizing rooming-in so that the baby stays with the mother rather than in a nursery, allowing the mother to respond readily to the infant's needs. New mothers should be reassured that bonding may take time and that it is normal if the mother does not feel an immediate attachment.

31. 1 and 4: Schedule I drugs, such as cocaine and LSD, have high potential for abuse and no accepted medical use. Schedule II drugs pose potential for abuse and addiction and include most commonly used narcotics (codeine, hydrocodone). Schedule III drugs, such as anabolic steroids and intermediate-acting barbiturates, have lesser potential for abuse. Schedule IV drugs, including benzodiazepines, may lead to limited physical or psychological dependence. Schedule V drugs, including cough suppressants, have low potential for abuse. Schedule VI drugs include those with low potential for abuse and addiction, such as OTC drugs like ibuprofen and diphenhydramine (Benadryl®).

32. 4: African-Americans have the greatest risk of developing diabetes mellitus type 2, although risks are also high for Mexican Americans, Native Americans and Hawaiians, and some Asian Americans, all of whom also have high rates of hypertension and obesity. Risk is also increased if a family member has the disease. Diabetes mellitus type 2 is the most prevalent type, accounting for 90% to 95% of cases of diabetes, and is closely associated with obesity.

33. 2: Nocturnal myoclonus is a toxic effect of opioid analgesics. Toxicity may occur because they have metabolites that are neuroexcitatory. The medication dosage should be reduced by at least half and a benzodiazepine administered. The drug may also be changed to an equianalgesic, but opioids should not be discontinued as the client may experience withdrawal and inadequate pain control. Naloxone is not an effective solution for toxicity, and flumazenil is a benzodiazepine antagonist.

34. 1, 3, and 4: Most people who are sexually active remain so, so even though the adolescent may be adamant that she is not going to have sex again until she is married, the nurse should advise her that ALL people need to know about safe sex and that she can share what she has learned with her friends. Many people believe that a condom is not necessary for oral sex, but they are mistaken. "I'm confused about different birth control methods" is a clear indication that information is needed.

35. 1: Naloxone (Narcan®) is an opioid antagonist and should be administered if clients exhibit signs of acute respiratory and/or circulatory depression, although it must be used cautiously with opioid addiction as clients may experience withdrawal symptoms. For an opioid overdose in an adult client, the usual initial dose is 0.4 to 2 mg intravenously, repeated at 2- to 3-minute intervals. If the client does not have adequate response after administration of 10 mg, then other causes for the symptoms should be explored.

36. 3: The maximum adult dosage of acetaminophen in 24 hours is 4 g. A single dose of 20 to 25 g can result in hepatic necrosis and liver failure with 25 g often resulting in death. The toxic reaction of acetaminophen is potentiated by alcohol. Clients often exhibit mild symptoms of nausea, vomiting, and abdominal pain in the first two days after overdose but by the second or third day, signs of liver injury become evident with elevations of transaminase, lactic hydrogenase, and bilirubin and prolonged prothrombin time. Oral N-acetylcysteine is administered to prevent or reduce liver damage.

37. 2: A complete initial assessment, ongoing assessments, frequent evaluations of lithium levels, and client education are all essential. Plasma levels of lithium must be frequently monitored for lithium toxicity, which can lead to death. The normal therapeutic range of lithium is 0.6 to 1.4 mEq/L for adults. About 1 client in 25 develops goiter from lithium-induced hypothyroidism, so clients must be evaluated for thyroid disease prior to beginning therapy and on a regular basis afterward. Clients should avoid NSAIDs and dehydration.

38. 1: Children younger than 8 years should not receive tetracycline because it can result in discoloration and inadequate calcification of permanent teeth if taken during the process of tooth calcification. Because this process is usually completed by the time the child is 8, the medication may be used in older children. The pediatric dose is 20 to 50 mg/kg orally in 4 equal doses over 24 hours. Discoloration and inadequate calcification of permanent teeth may also result from fetal exposure to tetracycline.

39. 3: The nurse should report the observations to the infection control nurse. The nurse should avoid making assumptions about cause and effect until an investigation is concluded. While increased rates of infection may indicate surgeon negligence, they can also indicate that the physician simply has more clients on the unit than other physicians, that an operating room is contaminated, that surgical procedures are not followed by all surgical staff, or that the physician has clients who are immunocompromised or more susceptible to infection because of condition.

40. 1: Bulk laxatives, such as Metamucil® and Citrucel®, are usually the safest for most people because their action most closely mimics human physiology. The polysaccharides or cellulose derivatives contained in the laxatives combine with fluids in the intestine to form gels, which stimulate peristalsis and evacuation. Clients must be advised to drink adequate liquids because bulk laxatives may induce constipation if clients are dehydrated. Clients should be encouraged to increase bulk naturally in the diet through eating bran, fruits, and vegetables.

41.

1. ii: Palpate the ulnar and radial pulses and apply pressure to both arteries.
2. i: Ask the client to open and close the hand until the skin blanches.
3. iv: Release the ulnar artery while maintaining pressure on the radial artery.
4. iii: Observe the hand for color. The hand should regain natural color within 5 seconds if circulation is adequate.

The modified Allen test is conducted to ensure that the ulnar artery provides adequate circulation, including collateral circulation, so that the radial artery can be used to obtain an arterial blood sample. The patient extends the wrist over a rolled towel and makes a fist.

42. 60 percent: Each hemoglobin molecule has four iron-containing heme sites to which oxygen can bind. As oxygen binds to the heme, the hemoglobin becomes saturated. The SO2 level is the percentage of total heme sites in the blood saturated with oxygen. At 80 to 90 PO2, hemoglobin is fully saturated so increased PO2 can't increase saturation. The critical point for PO2 is 60% because below this point there is a marked decrease in saturation. PO2 of 60 usually corresponds to SO2 of 91%, which is referred to as the "ICU" point.

43. 1: Simply not adding extra salt to food is insufficient because many foods, especially processed foods, are very high in sodium. Clients need to follow dietary guidelines and learn to read labels. DASH nutrient goals (based on a 2100 calorie diet) limit Na to 1500 to 2300 mg, total fat 27%, protein 18%, and carbohydrates 55%.

- Grains (whole grains preferred): 6 to 8 daily
- Vegetables and fruits: 4 to 5 each daily
- Milk products (non- or low-fat): 2 to 3 daily
- Lean meat, poultry, fish: ≤6 ounces daily
- Nuts, seeds, legumes: 4 to 5 weekly
- Fats and oils: 2 to 3 daily
- Sweet/added sugar: ≤5 weekly

44. 4: Once the platelet count drops below 50,000, the blood's ability to clot is impaired. If a client is scheduled for an invasive procedure, the risk of bleeding increases at this level; otherwise, risk is not generally significant until the platelet count drops to below 20,000. At this level, clients usually begin to develop signs of bleeding, such as petechial, nosebleeds, bleeding gums, and increased menstrual flow and require administration of platelets. For milder thrombocytopenia, observation and steroids are indicated with immunosuppressive therapy and splenectomy used for more severe disease.

45. 2600: The absolute neutrophil count (ANC) is calculated indirectly based on the total white blood cell count and percentages of neutrophils and bands:

ANC = Total WBC X (% neutrophils + % bands/100)
ANC = 5200 X (45 + 5/100) = 5200 X 0.50 = 2600 mm^3

A normal ANC for adults is 1800 to 7700, so this is within normal range. The risk of infection increases markedly when the ANC falls to 1000, and risk is severe at 500.

46. 4: Passwords are used to protect client's records from unauthorized access, so anyone who is authorized should be able to access the records with his/her own password. Therefore, the nurse should not allow anyone else to use his/her password. Passwords can also be used to track an individual nurse's activity in the electronic health record, so the nurse may be putting his/her own career in jeopardy by allowing someone else to use the password.

47. 1: The nurse should communicate the client's financial concerns to the social worker: "I can't afford to hire anyone to help me when I am discharged." The social worker will have knowledge about resources and qualifications for applying for assistance, such as Medicaid. The social worker can assess the client's income and support system to help determine the best plan for the client. Concerns about necessary equipment and managing self-care, such as showering safely, should be communicated to physical and occupational therapists.

48. 2: Clients who are alert and responsive have the right to refuse any treatment, so the most appropriate action is for the nurse to notify the physician and ensure that orders are in place for comfort measures, such as adequate analgesia. The nurse should not insist that the client accept treatments against her wishes, as this may be construed as coercion, and should not ask family members to intervene. Most religions view refusing life-prolonging treatments as different from active suicide, but it is inappropriate to use religious beliefs to make clients feel guilty.

49. 180: The formula for calculating total cholesterol is LDL + HDL + (triglycerides/5).

100 + 50 + (150/5) = 100 + 50 +30 = 180

An alternate formula is LDL + HDL + (Triglycerides X 0.20).

100 + 50 + (150 X 0.20) = 100 + 50 +30 = 180

The optimal total cholesterol level is below 200. Optimal LDL is below 100. Optimal HDL is ≥60. Normal triglyceride level is below 150.

50.

1. iii: Inspection
2. iv: Auscultation
3. i: Percussion
4. ii: Palpation

While the usual order of examination techniques is to begin with examination and then progress to palpation, percussion, and finally auscultation, because stimulating the abdomen may increase bowel sounds and contractions, the nurse should examine the abdomen differently from least invasive to most, beginning with inspection. This is followed by auscultation to assess normal bowel sounds, then percussion to assess for gas, fluid, and consolidated masses, and finally to palpation.

51.

1. ii: Aorta
2. iv: Renal
3. iii: Iliac
4. i: Femoral:

Auscultation should be done gently to avoid stimulating bowel contractions over the sites indicated on the diagram. For hypertensive patients, the renal arteries should be assessed bilaterally as bruits may be heard, suggesting arterial occlusion. Systolic bruits are fairly common and often benign, but bruits that have both systolic and diastolic components indicate turbulent blood flow. Aortic, iliac, and femoral bruits may be heard with peripheral arterial insufficiency.

52. 2: The client should always urinate prior to a pelvic exam. When positioning the client for the exam, the client's head should be elevated slightly as this helps relax abdominal muscles. The client should be advised to keep her arms at her side or folded across her chest and not over her head as this position may cause the abdominal muscles to tense. The nurse should explain the steps to the procedure and ensure that the speculum is warmed prior to the examination.

53.

1. iii: Apply tourniquet
2. i: Palpate vein
3. ii: Cleanse skin
4. iv: Perform venipuncture

The nurse should carefully examine the veins for potential puncture sites prior to performing the venipuncture. The nurse may apply a tourniquet or heat and hold the arm in dependent position. Once a vein has been selected, the tourniquet can be released while the nurse prepares materials. Then the tourniquet is applied, the vein palpated, and the skin cleansed, with venipuncture last. The nurse should avoid palpating the vein after the skin is cleansed unless wearing sterile gloves.

54. 4: A nasal cannula at 3L/min delivers an FiO2 of approximately 28–32%. The flow rate for nasal cannulas ranges from 0.5 L/min (21–24% FiO2) to 6 L/min (40–44% FiO2), but should not be administered at a higher flow rate because the FiO2 will not increase, and it can result in drying of the mucous membranes. Face masks, non-rebreathing masks, partial re-breathing masks, and Venturi masks can be used if a higher FiO2 is needed.

55.

1. i: Client sits upright or stands
2. iv: Client takes a deep breath
3. ii: Client places the meter in the mouth and seals lips
4. iii: Client expels air through the meter as forcefully as possible

The client should repeat this procedure 2 to 5 times, noting the highest number achieved. Following treatment, the client's PEFR should be within 20% of personal best, and if results are <80% of personal best, treatment may be inadequate for client's condition.

56. 3: Headaches occur in about one-fifth of clients following lumbar puncture, but the headaches are usually relieved by the client's lying flat and drinking ample fluids. If headaches are severe and persistent, then this usually indicates a hole in the dura mater, and an epidural blood patch may be applied with an autologous blood specimen. The blood is injected in a small amount at the site of the lumbar puncture to create a blood clot that serves as a patch.

57. 4: The optimal position for a thoracentesis is an upright position with the client sitting and leaning over an over-bed tray table with the shoulders and upper arms supported by a pillow as this position expands the intercostal space, making insertion easier. If the client is unable to tolerate a sitting position, then the client should be positioned in the side-lying position on the unaffected side so that the thoracentesis insertion site is easily accessed.

58. 4: Severe vomiting can result in metabolic alkalosis because of loss of chloride in the emesis. In a compensating measure for chloride loss, bicarbonate increases. Metabolic alkalosis may also result from gastric suctioning, diuresis, hypokalemia, and excessive mineralocorticoid or sodium bicarbonate intake. Other laboratory findings include increased pH, normal PCO_2 if compensated but increased if noncompensated. Symptoms include dizziness, confusion, anxiety, muscle cramping, tingling, seizures, tetany, tachycardia, arrhythmias, nausea, vomiting, anorexia, and compensatory hypoventilation.

59. 1 and 3: Excess fluid is removed quickly from the body during hemodialysis. This can sometimes result in fluid deficit, especially if the client has run a fever or had inadequate fluid intake. Because heparin is administered during the treatment to prevent clots from forming, the client is at increased risk of bleeding. The presence of fluid volume excess, metabolic acidosis, and pulmonary edema should be evaluated prior to hemodialysis since clients are unable to excrete adequate fluids or waste products because of impaired kidney function.

60. 3: The large accumulation of fluid that can occur with ascites makes palpating the bladder difficult, so the bladder must be emptied prior to a paracentesis in order to prevent inadvertent puncture of the bladder when the needle or trocar is inserted. Clients should be positioned in upright or high Fowler's position because this helps to keep the intestines toward the back of the peritoneal cavity, preventing intestinal laceration. Usually only 4 to 5 L of fluid are removed at one time. If larger volumes are removed, the client is at risk of hypotension.

61. 1, 2, and 4: Clients with a tracheostomy are at increased risk of fecal impaction because they cannot perform the Valsalva maneuver to bear down, so they need to be educated about bowel care and advised to use stool softeners routinely and laxatives and suppositories as needed. Additionally, they need to understand the importance of pulmonary hygiene to prevent atelectasis and infection and should be confident in all aspects of tracheostomy care, including information about what to do if the tracheostomy tube falls out.

62. 1: Because of his weakness and tremors, the client will probably have difficulty preparing meals, so referral to a home meal delivery program (such as Meals on Wheels) is probably the best referral since arrangements have already been made for personal care and housekeeping. Home meal delivery programs usually provide meals 5 to 7 days a week at low cost ($2 to $4 is common). The meals are often delivered midday with a hot entrée, and many programs also provide a sandwich or other light meal for evening as well as breakfast foods (such as cereal) for the next day.

63. 1 and 3: During a life review, clients reflect on their lives, their successes and failures, and their relationships. Some clients may begin to organize old photographs or look through photo albums. Others may want to reminisce and talk about their lives and families. Some talk about their children and parenting skills. They may talk about things they regret or choices they have made. People often try to validate that their lives had purpose through their life reviews.

64. 1 and 5: The mother is using nonstandard treatments with mayonnaise and olive oil. While some anecdotal reports suggest this is helpful, according to the CDC there is no evidence to support these treatments. The mother should use OTC or prescription shampoos intended to treat lice. While linens and clothes used by the child should be washed and dried in a hot air cycle for at least 5 minutes to prevent spread, treating pets, such as cats and dogs, does no good as they do not spread head lice.

65. 9%: According to the rule of nines, body surface area (BSA) is sectioned into areas that are primarily multiples of 9:

- Head: 9%
- Anterior trunk: 18% (9% chest and 9% abdomen)
- Posterior trunk: 18% (9% upper back and 9% lower back and buttocks)
- Legs: 18% each (9% anterior and 9% posterior)
- Arms: 9% each (4.5% anterior and 4.5% posterior)
- Genitals: 1%

The percentage of BSA that is burned is important when calculating potential fluid loss and the need for fluid and electrolyte replacement.

66. 4: A positive Homan's sign—pain on palpation of the calf with dorsiflexion of the ankle—is indicative of deep vein thrombosis (DVT) although this sign occurs in only about 10%, so the absence does not preclude DVT. DVT is associated with inactivity, such as prolonged bedrest or sitting for long periods while flying, and is a complication of surgery. Clients may have pain and tenderness, erythema, elevated temperature, and unilateral edema although some exhibit no overt symptoms.

67. 2: Increasing intracranial pressure is indicated by increasing BP with widening pulse pressure, decreasing pulse, and increasing temperature. The client's initial BP was 138/72 with a pulse pressure of 66 but is now 160/64 with a pulse pressure of 96. The initial pulse was 83 and has decreased to 70. Baseline temperature was 97.5°F/36.4°C and is now increased to 99.4°F/37.4°C. Restlessness and headache are early indications of increasing intracranial pressure. Clients may also have an alteration in consciousness, change in pupillary reactions, and increasing dyspnea.

68. 4: If an implantable cardioverter-defibrillator fires one time and is not associated with other cardiac symptoms, this is not a medical emergency, and the patient should be advised to lie down to rest until he feels recovered from the stress of the firing and to telephone the physician to report the event. Multiple firings are a medical emergency, and the client or family member should call 9-1-1 as the firings may indicate recurrent ventricular fibrillation/ventricular tachycardia or a fractured lead. A single firing associated with symptoms (chest pain, dizziness, syncope, and shortness of breath) is also a medical emergency.

69. 3: The irregular rhythm is an atrial fibrillation, which is characterized by a rapid, very irregular pulse with an atrial rate of 300 to 600 and ventricular rate of 120 to 200. Because the beats are rapid and ineffectual, the atria do not empty adequately, so blood begins to pool, increasing risk of thrombus formation and emboli. Because stroke volume decreases, cardiac output decreases, leading to myocardial ischemia and palpitations.

70. 1, 3, and 4: Because clients are at risk for bleeding, they should use soft toothbrushes. Swimming is a good choice for exercise because the water exerts even pressure. Clients should always wear a Medical Alert bracelet or necklace indicating they are taking the anticoagulant. Stools should not be black as this is a sign of bleeding. While green leafy vegetables are high in vitamin K, they can be eaten in normal amounts and do not need to be restricted.

71. 1: The nurse should hold the infusion and notify the MD that the catheter tip is incorrectly placed, as it should be in the superior vena cava rather than the right atrium. Infusing the solutions directly into the right atrium may result in tissue damage. While the catheter needs to be withdrawn a few inches and another X-ray taken to ensure correct placement, this procedure should only be done by a physician or a specially trained nurse.

72. 750 mg: The simplest solution to the problem is to convert 1 g to 1000 mg and then, since the infusion was set for 60 minutes and three-fourths of the time elapsed, simply multiply 1000 X 0.75 = 750 mg. If using an algebraic formula:

$$\begin{aligned} 1000/60 &= x/45 \\ 60x &= 45{,}000 \\ 6\,x &= 4500 \\ 6x/6 &= 4500/6 \\ x &= 750 \text{ mg} \end{aligned}$$

73. 2, 4, and 5: Pills may be crushed and diluted in 10 to 15 mL of water to be added to the NG tube feeding. Liquid forms of medications are easiest to add. Soft-gel capsules can be opened at one end and drained, but some dosage is usually lost, so dissolving the capsule in warm water first (and removing the remains of the gel capsule) is a better solution. Extended-release capsules should be opened but NOT crushed before adding to the tube. Enteric-coated tablets should not be crushed or administered per NG tube, and sublingual wafers are not absorbed through the GI tract.

74. 95%: The oximeter uses light waves to determine oxygen saturation (SPO2) and utilizes an external oximeter attached to a finger or earlobe. If a client has marked vasoconstriction, the earlobe may provide more accurate readings than the finger. Oxygen saturation should be maintained >95% although some patients with chronic respiratory disorders, such as COPD, may have lower SPO2. Oximetry is often used postoperatively to assess peripheral circulation and when patients are on mechanical ventilation.

75. 1, 3, and 4: Restraints are used to restrict movement, activity, and access. Guidelines for restraints not part of routine care (surgical restraints, arm boards) include:

- A written policy must be in place.
- An assessment must be completed prior to application of restraints.
- An alternative method should be tried before applying a restraint.
- Restraints cannot be applied without a written order.
- The least restrictive effective restraint should be used.
- The nurse must remove the restraint, assess, and document findings at least every 2 hours.

76. 3: While security measures may vary somewhat, generally infants should only be removed from the mother's room in a crib and never carried in someone's arms. Mothers should be informed to never leave their infants unattended, even for a few minutes to use the bathroom. If no family member is present, the mother should call her nurse. The mother should not assume hospital attire or ID alone are sufficient identification and should remain wary of any strangers asking questions about the infant.

77. 3 mL: A simple algebraic formula provides the answer:

Mg in suspension/mL = Desired dose/x (mL needed)

$$\begin{aligned} 200/5 &= 120/x \\ 200x &= 600 \\ 200x/200 &= 600/200 \\ x &= 3 \text{ mL dose} \end{aligned}$$

78. 2: Fifteen mg/dL is within normal limits (range is 8–21 for ages 14 to adult; 5–17 for newborns; 7–17 for children to 13 years; 10–31 for adults >90 years. Urea (nonprotein nitrogen compound) is an end product of protein metabolism. BUN is usually evaluated with creatinine. The normal ratio of BUN/creatinine is 15:1 to 24:1. A BUN >100 mg/dL is a critical value. Signs of an elevated BUN include restlessness, confusion, acidemia, nausea and vomiting, and coma.

79. 4: While there is not total agreement about the results of HbA1c tests, generally levels of ≥6.5% are considered diagnostic of diabetes mellitus. Values of 5.7 to 6.4% are considered pre-diabetic by most authorities. Lower values are within normal limits. Because hemoglobin retains excess blood glucose and red blood cells live about 120 days, the HbA1c test shows the average blood glucose levels over a 3-month period. HbA1c is used to diagnose diabetes and monitor long-term diabetic therapy.

80.

1. iv: Gently retract the lower eyelid against the orbital ridge with the thumb.
2. i: Gently retract the upper lid.
3. ii: Exert slight pressure below the eyelid and slip the index finger under the prosthesis.
4. iii: Break suction and slide the prosthesis out of the eye.

Once the prosthesis is removed, clean the prosthesis with soap and water and rinse well with running water to remove all soap and residue. Dry and polish the prosthesis. Retract eyelids, wash socket with clean washcloth or gauze pad moistened with warm water or NS. Wash eyelid margins with mild soap and water and dry.

81. 2: If a nurse accidentally punctures a finger with a needle after withdrawing blood from a client, the nurse should immediately wash the puncture area with soap and water, being careful not to apply pressure but to allow the injury to bleed freely to facilitate washing out any virus or bacteria that may have been injected into the wound. Then, the incident should be reported to a supervisor, an incident/injury report filed, and follow-up assessment carried out.

82. 1 minute: Leaving a tourniquet in place for longer than a minute may cause the blood to concentrate below the tourniquet, and this can increase values for some tests, such as packed cell volume. The tourniquet should be applied to locate an appropriate vein and then released while the nurse puts on gloves, cleanses the site, and assembles equipment. The tourniquet is then reapplied immediately before the draw.

83. 2, 3, 4, and 6: The following factors increase the risk of developing deep vein thrombosis (DVT):

- Being overweight
- Smoking
- Having surgery
- Taking oral contraceptives
- Undergoing prolonged sitting or bedrest during which the calf muscles do not contract to help circulate the blood
- Older than 60 years
- Having some medical conditions, such as blood-clotting disorder, cancer, heart failure, pregnancy, or inflammatory bowel disease
- Immobility

84. 1, 2, and 4: If a client with COPD asks the nurse why the client is having the arterial blood gas (ABG) test, the nurse should explain to the client that ABGs measure the levels of carbon dioxide, oxygen, and acidity (pH level) in the blood, help to evaluate the effectiveness of treatment, and help to determine the need for supplemental oxygen. ABGs are also carried out to help diagnose and monitor certain disorders, such as metabolic disorders and kidney disease.

85. 1: If the nurse is doing a digital removal of stool for a client with a large fecal impaction resulting from opioid use, the client feels faint, and assessment of vital signs shows a marked decrease in pulse, the bradycardia has likely resulted from stimulation of the vagus nerve. Oil retention enemas should be given prior to attempting digital removal of stool, as the procedure can be very painful for the client and cause rectal bleeding.

86. 1, 2, 4, and 5: If a 15-year-old client is admitted to the emergency department 5 hours after taking a large overdose of acetaminophen and the serum level of the drug is still 180 mcg/mL, then the client should receive the 72-hour N-acetylcysteine (NAC) protocol and supportive care in an attempt to minimize hepatic damage. Hepatic function must be monitored carefully. It is too late for GI contamination with activated charcoal. The Rumack-Matthew nomogram is used to determine the need for treatment. The client should also receive a psychiatric consultation.

87. 2: If the nurse has inserted a nasogastric tube and aspirated gastric contents to check the pH with color-coded pH paper and the aspirate is dark brown with a pH of slightly less than 5 according to the color chart, this pH usually indicates intestinal aspirate rather than gastric aspirate. Gastric aspirate may vary in color from cloudy to green to tan to brown with pH less than 4, while intestinal aspirate may be yellow or brown but the pH is usually greater than 4. Respiratory secretions may look like saliva and have a pH greater than 5.5.

88. 1, 2, and 3: Because the dosage of ECT used now is less than in the earlier days of treatment, the memory loss associated with ECT is less severe, but still may occur. Confusion for a short time after the treatment as well as headache and muscle soreness are common. Clients receive medication prior to the treatment to reduce the severity of seizures induced by ECT. ECT should not result in urinary incontinence or hallucinations.

89. 4: If a male client has been diagnosed with Huntington disease and his spouse asks the nurse if their 3-year-old son should be tested to determine if he inherited the genetic disorder, the most appropriate response is: "Most authorities recommend letting your child decide when he is older and can make an informed decision about testing." Since there is no treatment that can alter the course of the disease, there are ethical concerns regarding testing children.

90. 1, 2, 3, and 4: If following femoral catheterization for PCI the client has increasing pain in the catheterization site and the nurse notes visible edema and induration, indications of a hematoma, the nurse should anticipate applying pressure to the site to control the bleeding, marking the margins of the edematous, indurated area to determine if bleeding continues, monitoring hemoglobin and hematocrit to determine if blood transfusions are needed, and maintaining bedrest.

91. 25%: If both parents are carriers of the defective gene for a disease with an autosomal recessive inheritance, each child has a 25% chance of inheriting the gene from both parents and developing the disorder. Each child has a 50% chance of inheriting the gene from only one parent and becoming a carrier:

	N	R
N	NN	NR Carrier
R	NR Carrier	RR Disease

N = normal gene; **R** = recessive mutated gene

92. 1 and 2: If a client has been diagnosed with immune thrombocytic purpura, signs and symptoms that indicate increased thrombocytopenia are frequent nosebleeds, petechiae, and increased bruising. Clients may also experience very heavy menstruation and may have blood in the stool or urine. Because platelets are essential for clotting of the blood, the platelet count must be monitored for those with ITP, although excessive bleeding is not usually a major concern until the platelet count drops below 50,000 per microliter of blood. Vision changes, numbness, and tingling are associated with thrombocytosis.

93. 2, 3, and 4: If a client seen in the emergency department for influenza asks for an antibiotic prescription, the nurse should provide the following guidelines to help the client decrease the risk of developing an antibiotic-resistant infection:

- Do not stop taking antibiotics until the entire prescription is gone.
- Do not take antibiotics for viral infections (such as influenza and the common cold) because they do no good.
- Do not take preventive antibiotics to avoid infections.
- Follow prescription directions when taking antibiotics.

94. 3: If a client who received an IV antibiotic mistakenly believed she was receiving opioid analgesia and reported a few minutes later that the medication had relieved her pain, the most likely reason for the client's response is the placebo effect. The belief that a medication is for pain control can trigger the release of endorphins that, in turn, result in a reduced perception of pain. This does not mean that the pain the client was feeling was imaginary or exaggerated.

95. 1, 3, and 4: If a client has suffered a traumatic brain injury and is being treated in the ICU, the nurse should expect to elevate the head of the bed and keep the client's head in neutral alignment. The nurse will likely administer oxygen to maintain the PaO_2 at >90 mm Hg (85 mm Hg is hypoxic) and will administer sedation to prevent or reduce agitation. Additionally, cerebral perfusion pressure should be maintained at >70 mm Hg and body temperature maintained within normal limits.

96. 3: While there are different methods of doing a "kick count," which actually counts movements rather than kicks, the usual standard is that the fetus should have at least 10 movements within a 2-hour period. However, clients may perceive movement differently, and a fetus in a rest cycle may be less active, so one finding of decreased activity is usually not a concern. Fetal activity may be depressed if the mother takes certain drugs, such as methadone or heroin, or uses alcohol or tobacco.

97. 1, 4, and 5: Intrinsic factors that increase risk of falls in older adults include sensory impairment (decrease vision and hearing) and chronic illness that interferes with strength and/or mobility. Other intrinsic factors include medications that may cause weakness or dizziness. Extrinsic factors include environmental concerns, such as steep and unlit stairs, throw rugs, and loose carpets. While falling is not a normal experience of aging, falls are most common in people older than 65 years. Falls occurring in hospitals often occur with transfers or ineffective equipment.

98. 2: The wound shows evidence of erythema and edema and phagocytosis begins during the inflammation stage of injury repair. Stages:

1. Hemostasis: During first few minutes. Platelets seal off the vessels and secrete substances that cause vasoconstriction. Thrombin stimulates the clotting mechanism, forming a fibrin mesh.
2. Inflammation: Over days 1-4. Inflammatory response and phagocytosis occurs.
3. Proliferation: Over days 5-20. Fibroblasts produce collagen to and granulation tissue starts to form. Epithelization contracts wound.
4. Maturation: After day 21 to 2 years. Collagen tightens to reduce scarring. The tissue gains tensile strength.

99. 1, 2, and 4: If a client with heart failure has a left ventricular fraction of 38%, this is classified as heart failure (<40% EF). Normal EF is 50 to 70%. Risk of dysrhythmias occurs if the EF falls to below 35%. While the client should avoid strenuous exercise and should take frequent rest periods, maintaining a routine of regular exercise, such as walking, is important to maintain adequate cardiac output. The client should stop smoking and limit alcohol intake to 1 to 2 drinks daily.

100. 3: The type of behavior modification that is most likely to benefit a client who has a severe phobia regarding spiders is desensitization. With desensitization, the client is increasingly exposed to the thing the person fears. Clients usually begin by constructing an anxiety hierarchy that indicates the least disturbing and most disturbing aspects of the phobic item and then practicing relaxation techniques before beginning desensitization, which may begin with briefly talking about the feared item and looking at a photo of it.

101. 4: If a pregnant client at 36 weeks' gestation has partial placenta previa and has been on bedrest at home for the previous 4 weeks starts to have contractions and increasing vaginal bleeding, the nurse should anticipate a cesarean delivery because of the danger of hemorrhage from partial or complete placenta previa. Fetal lungs are usually mature after 34 weeks. With partial placenta previa, part of the placenta is implanted over the internal cervical os.

102. 1, 2, 3, 4, and 5: If the nurse is providing education to a male client who is HIV positive, the nurse should include information about the need to use condoms for every sexual encounter and the need to tell sexual or needle-sharing partners about the client's HIV status. The client should understand the signs and symptoms that may indicate an increased viral load or infection and should also understand the importance of maintaining a healthy lifestyle (eat well, avoid smoking and drinking, exercise routinely). The client should be apprised of the availability of support groups

103. 1: If a group includes only members selected on a specific basis, such as women with a history of domestic or partner abuse, this group is classified as homogeneous. A heterogenous group comprises individuals with different diagnoses, ages, and genders. A closed group is one that does not admit new members once the group has formed. A task group is one that meets in order to achieve a particular goal or complete an assignment.

104. 4: The primary focus of cognitive behavioral therapy (CBT) is identifying automatic thoughts and correcting errors in thinking. Basically, Beck theorized that clients have cognitive biases that affect their perceptions of the world, so clients need to alter the way they think about people, things, and events because cognitive distortions can lead to false assumptions. Clients are helped to identify negative thinking and to substitute these thoughts for more rational ones.

105. 2: If the nurse reviewed a client's progress in smoking cessation and praised her but suggested she stop having coffee in the morning because that caused an urge to smoke and the client became upset and complained the nurse believed she was doing poorly because she wanted a cigarette with her morning coffee, this type of cognitive distortion is a mental filter. With a mental filter, the person tends to focus only on a negative detail and overlook anything positive that has been said.

106. 2 and 4: If a client has accidentally splashed a toxic (although not caustic) substance in the right eye, the steps to flushing the eye include:

- Placing the client with head elevated to 20 degrees and on right side.
- Hold emesis basis against face on right.
- Fill bulb syringe with NS irrigant.
- Hold the right eyelid open with the thumb and index finger.
- Hold tip of syringe about one-half inch above eye and direct flow of irrigant toward the lower conjunctival sac, from inner to outer canthus.
- Flush for about 1 minute.

107. 3: If a postoperative client whose oxygen saturation has been stable at 96% to 98% suddenly drops to 80%, the initial response should be to quickly assess the client's condition and reposition the pulse oximeter. In most cases, a sudden change results from incorrect position of the pulse oximeter. Oxygen saturation should be maintained above 95%, although clients with COPD may have a lower oxygen saturation level. Pulse oximeters provide information only about oxygen, not carbon dioxide, and cannot recognize carbon monoxide.

108. 3: The obstetric history of a client who has had 4 pregnancies with one miscarriage at 12 weeks, a stillborn birth at 34 weeks, a healthy son at 38 weeks, and a healthy daughter at 40 weeks would be classified as gravida 4, para 3. Gravida refers to the number of pregnancies, regardless of the duration or outcome. Para refers to the number of births after 20 weeks, regardless of whether they are live births or not. This client had 4 total pregnancies (gravida 4) and 3 births after 20 weeks (gravida 3).

109. 4: The immunization that is usually administered to neonates within hours of birth is hepatitis B, which is followed by a second dose at 6 to 18 months. A number of other immunizations are recommended during the first year at 2 months, 4 months, and 6 months: rotavirus (to prevent infectious diarrhea), DTaP (diphtheria, tetanus, and pertussis), Hib (*Haemophilus influenzae*), and CV (pneumococcal). IPV (polio) is administered in 2 doses (2 months and 4 months). Additional immunizations begin at about 1 year.

110. 2: Naegele's rule for estimating the due date of a pregnancy is:

- Date of onset of last menstrual period (LMP) + 9 months + 7 days = estimated due date
- September 6 + 9 months = June 6 + 7 days = June 13

Naegele's rule does not account for differences in menstrual cycles or number of days in the months (using an average of 28 days), but this method accounts for approximately 280 days, the normal duration of pregnancy. Most physicians use a combination of Naegele's rule and ultrasound during the first trimester to estimate a due date.

111. 1: If pregnancy is viewed as a natural rather than a medical condition, then pregnant women often seek prenatal care later and less frequently than typical American women. However, the women from other cultures usually follow cultural traditions related to pregnancy, such as restrictions on types of food or activities. They may also seek the advice of older family members or shamans, so lack of prenatal care does not mean that the pregnancy has not been considered or is necessarily at risk.

112. 2: Because Muslim societies are patriarchal and decisions are made by the male in fundamentalist households, the woman's husband should be first asked for permission for the client to be treated by a male physician. If he agrees, then the woman's permission should be sought. If neither agrees, then the examination will need to be delayed until a female physician can be located, but the client and her husband should be advised that this delay may pose a risk to the fetus and/or the mother. If they agree to care by a male physician, then the client's body should be covered as much as possible and a female in attendance.

113. 1: The cephalic presentation that is most common during delivery of a neonate is the vertex presentation. With the presentation, the fetal head is fully flexed and the diameter is the smallest, facilitating passage through the birth canal. In most cases, the fetal attitude (relationship of body parts to each other) is flexion and the lie (relationship of fetal long axis to mother's) is longitudinal. Complications may arise if the presentation, lie, and/or attitude are different.

114. 1: If two Mexican immigrant families lives closely together and share goods, services, and childcare, this family structure is a kinship network. The families may be related or may be close friends. This family structure is quite common in Mexican-American communities. In an extended family, multiple generations live together as one family. The nuclear family comprises 2 parents and their children. A binuclear family occurs when 2 nuclear families share custody of children, who typically live part of the week with one family and part of the week with the other.

115. 1, 2, and 3: The transition from full-time employment to retirement can be difficult for people, especially those who identify closely with their positions and whose lives have revolved around work. It may take time to become used to a different pace of life, but often taking on a more active role in community activities, taking classes, joining a senior citizen's center, volunteering, or taking part-time employment can help the person repurpose his life. The client should be encouraged to explore various interests. Clients who become depressed may need to seek professional support.

116. 1: First-time mothers, especially, often have little experience with children and are unsure of what to expect, so if the mother is concerned that her child cannot crawl at 6 months, then she needs factual information about when to expect the child to crawl: "Most infants can crawl by 9 months." The nurse should also assure the mother that infants may vary in their development. A 6-month old child should be able to sit in tripod position and roll in both directions, but crawling generally follows this, and the child's gross motor skills improve over the next 3 months.

117. 4: If a 14-year-old client has been diagnosed with celiac disease after a long history of diarrhea, anemia, and weight loss, the client will require a gluten-free diet. Celiac disease is an autoimmune disorder in which products containing gluten (grains, such as wheat, rye, barley) trigger damage to the intestinal mucosa. Some clients exhibit an itching vesicular rash (dermatitis herpetiformis) on the buttocks, scalp, face, elbows, and knees. Because the damaged intestinal mucosa cannot adequately absorb nutrients, anemia, osteoporosis, muscle wasting, weight loss, and malnutrition are common.

118. 2, 3, and 4: If a 68-year-old client states that he decided not to take the herpes zoster (shingles) immunization because his friend had the immunization and still developed the infection, the nurse should explain that the immunization cuts the chance of developing shingles in half. Additionally, if the person develops shingles after the immunization, the severity of the infection is usually lessoned and the likelihood of developing postherpetic syndrome, which can result in severe and long-standing pain, is decreased.

119. 4: Because the client is nulliparous, the average rate of dilation is 1 cm per hour, so the approximate time to full dilation of 10 cm is approximately 7 hours. The woman has been progressing at the average rate. The latent phase of stage 1 usually lasts from 10 to 14 hours, and the client was in this phase for 12 hours and has now progressed to the active phase. However, the nurse should stress to the client that there are individual variations with some progressing much more quickly and others more slowly.

120. 1: If the performance improvement committee has agreed to some changes in procedures on the basis of evidence-based research and wants to convince staff members to comply with the changes, the best action to carry out first is to identify and gain support of key staff. In all organizations, there are staff members who are influential for various reasons, and they are usually easy to identify. Once these key staff members (key informants) are on board, they can often influence others to comply.

NCLEX Practice Test #3

1. A client is at risk of falls. Which of the following are important home modifications to discuss with the client? *Select all that apply.*

1. install an alarm system
2. remove wall to wall carpeting
3. remove throw rugs
4. install handrails/safety bars
5. improve lighting

2. A 64-year-old female client has recently had surgery for colon cancer and has a colostomy. The client has been resistive to educational efforts and refuses to look at the colostomy. Which of the following is the most appropriate intervention?

1. remain supportive and encourage client to express feelings
2. remind the client that she will have to soon assume self-care
3. insist that the client assist in care of the colostomy
4. ask a family member to assume responsibility for colostomy care

3. At which of the following ages would a child first be expected to be able to draw a circle and other rudimentary forms, to jump, kick a ball, and throw a ball overhand?

1. 1 to 2 years
2. 2 to 3 years
3. 3 to 4 years
4. 4 to 5 years

4.

A	B	C	D	E	F
	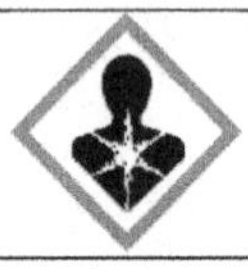		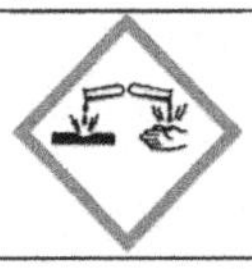		

Match the symbol above to the appropriate description.

1. Poison ____
2. Biohazard ____
3. Corrosive ____
4. Health hazard ____
5. Flame ____
6. Irritant ____

5. The nurse plans to obtain a blood sample from a venipuncture in the left median cubital vein. Which of the following are contraindications to using this vein? *Select all that apply.*

1. post left mastectomy
2. venous fibrosis felt on palpation
3. client is left-handed
4. presence of left vascular shunt for dialysis
5. median cubital vein is difficult to visualize

6. Infants and young children should be placed in rear-facing car seats until they reach a weight of at least

1. 22 lb
2. 28 lb
3. 30 lb
4. 35 lb

7. A client who had a thyroidectomy complains of numbness and tingling in the hands and feet and muscle cramps of the lower legs. The client appears slightly confused and irritable. The nurse suspects which of the following complications?

1. hypercalcemia
2. hypocalcemia
3. hyperkalemia
4. hypokalemia

8. A pregnant client is undergoing a non-stress test. During the test, the nurse instructs the client to

1. report any cramping or pain
2. report sensations of fetal movement
3. deep breathe and relax
4. try to hold completely still

9. A client is to receive 1000 mL of IV fluid in 6 hours with a drop factor of 15 gtt/mL. How many gtt/min should the nurse administer? ***Record your answer by rounding to the nearest whole number.***

Answer: _________gtt/min

10. A woman who was badly beaten by a domestic partner has come to the emergency department but is extremely fearful, stating, "My boyfriend is going to come here and shoot me, I know he will!" The most appropriate initial response is

1. contact security and place the client in a room out of sight
2. reassure the client that she is safe
3. tell the client to call the police
4. ask the client why she thinks her partner will shoot her

11. A client who was a heavy smoker and developed lung cancer constantly warns others about the dangers of smoking and refuses to allow anyone to smoke in his presence. Which type of defense mechanism does this represent?

1. sublimation
2. repression
3. conversion
4. reaction formation

12. The nurse is reviewing an adult female client's CBC. Which of the following values are outside of normal parameters? *Select all that apply.*

1. WBC: 3.0 10^3/mL
2. RBC: 4.37 10^6/uL
3. Hemoglobin 13.7 g/dL
4. Hematocrit 41.4%
5. Platelets 110 10^3/uL

13. When obtaining a blood sample from a central line using the push-pull method, after flushing the catheter with 5 to 10 mL of NS, the next step is to do which of the following?

1. aspirate a blood sample into the same syringe
2. change syringes and aspirate blood sample into new syringe
3. aspirate 6 mL of blood and reinfuse the blood one time and then aspirate blood sample in same syringe
4. aspirate 6 mL of blood and reinfuse the blood 3 times and then aspirate blood sample in new syringe

14. If a child weighs 35.2 pounds and requires 1000 mL plus 50 mL fluid for each kilogram over 10 kg as maintenance fluid every 24 hours, what is the child's required volume of fluid? *Record your answer using a whole number.*

Answer: __________mL

15. If a 6-year-old client is having a generalized seizure, the nurse should

1. place the client in supine position
2. place the client in side-lying position
3. avoid touching or moving the client
4. place a padded tongue blade between the client's teeth

16. For a newborn with suspected meconium plug syndrome, the test/procedure that will likely be used to confirm the diagnosis is

1. contrast enema
2. abdominal x-ray
3. ultrasound
4. MRI

17. Which of the following is an appropriate intervention for a newborn that experienced intrauterine drug exposure and has frequent high-pitched crying?

1. leaving child free of any constraints
2. swaddling in extended position
3. swaddling in flexed position
4. increasing exposure to ambient light

18. Which of the following is an example of an isotonic IV solution?

1. 0.45% Sodium chloride (NaCl)
2. 2.5% dextrose in water (DW)
3. 10% dextrose in water (D10W)
4. 5% DW (D5W)

19. A client with schizophrenia tells the nurse that he hates all of the doctors and nurses and wishes they would all die. Which of the following is the most therapeutic response?

1. "Things would be better for you if we were all dead?"
2. "It's important that you don't make threats."
3. "Do you have feelings about killing people?"
4. "I'm sure you don't mean that you want everyone to die."

20. A client involved in a motor vehicle accident is hospitalized with injuries after attempting to help a passenger who died at the scene. The passenger was a close friend of the client. Which of the following is likely the <u>most</u> effective approach?

1. avoid talking about the accident
2. tell the client how lucky he was to survive
3. tell the client how sorry you are about his friend's death
4. encourage the client to express his feelings

21. A physician has ordered levothyroxine 125 mcg for a client but the available medication has the dosage in mg rather than mcg. What is the correct mg dosage? *Record your answer using a whole number or a number up to three decimal points as appropriate.*

Answer: ________mg

22. When reviewing a client's medications, the nurse notes that the client is taking oral contraceptives, St. John's wort, fexofenadine, echinacea, and omeprazole. Which of the following medications/herbal preparations is of most concern?

1. Echinacea
2. St. John's wort
3. oral contraceptives
4. omeprazole

23. For a client receiving warfarin, which of the following is the critical value for the INR?

1. 2
2. >2
3. 3
4. >3

24. If a disinfectant must be mixed with water to make a 1:2 solution (one part disinfectant to 2 parts water) and a total of 2 L is needed, how many mL of disinfectant should be used to make the solution? *Record your answer by rounding to the nearest whole number.*

Answer: ________mL

25. A client with osteoarthritis of the right knee has been advised to use a cane for support. The best method to determine the correct length of the cane is to

1. measure from the wrist to the floor
2. try different sizes of cans
3. calculate based on height
4. measure from the fingertips to the floor

26. A client is to have a bladder scan to determine the volume of residual urine. The scan should be carried out within how many minutes of urination?

1. 3
2. 5
3. 10
4. 20

27. When carrying out range of motion exercises on a client's arm after an injury to the elbow, which of the following movements of the elbow should the nurse assist the client to carry out? *Select all that apply.*

1. flexion
2. extension
3. rotation
4. Abduction
5. adduction

28. An unconscious client has been brought to the emergency department after an overdose of heroin. Which reversal agent is indicated?

1. flumazenil
2. fomepizole
3. N-acetylcysteine
4. naloxone

29. Which of the following ethnic groups is most at risk for the development of hypertension?

1. African Americans
2. Caucasians
3. Asians
4. Hispanics

30. A client who must have chemotherapy is very frightened of the treatments and often becomes very agitated and hyperventilates when arriving for treatment. Which of the following complementary therapies may provide some relief for this anxiety?

1. St. John's wort
2. deep breathing and relaxation exercises
3. magnet therapy
4. acupuncture

31. A client is on a low sodium diet and the nurse is reviewing the client's food diary. Which of the following foods should the client be advised may be high in sodium? *Select all that apply.*

1. canned kidney beans
2. pickles
3. eggs
4. hot dog
5. frozen peas

32. A client has a nasogastric feeding tube in place, and the nurse aspirates fluid for pH testing prior to administering an intermittent tube feeding. What pH reading generally indicates stomach placement of the tube?

1. 2 or less
2. 5 or less
3. 5 or more
4. 6 or more

33. If an IV is to be administered through gravity flow, the IV bag should be hung at least how many feet above the client's heart?

1. 1
2. 2
3. 3
4. 4

34. The nurse is changing a postoperative client's dressing but the client shouts that the nurse is incompetent and doesn't know how to change a dressing. The best response is

1. "I've changed many dressings before, so I know what I'm doing."
2. "I can see that you are really upset. What can I do to help?"
3. "I'll get another nurse to change the dressing for you."
4. "I'm sorry, but there is no one else available to change the dressing."

35. While the nurse is having lunch in the hospital cafeteria, a coworker from another unit asks for information about the prognosis of one of the nurse's clients, who is the coworker's neighbor. The best response is

1. "He is progressing well after surgery."
2. "I'm sorry, I can't talk about clients."
3. "You know you shouldn't ask about clients."
4. "His wife will be in later and you can ask her."

36. Which of the following documentations is documented correctly?

1. MS 2 mg IM q 4 h prn
2. 83.0 mg ASA QD
3. 14 u insulin aspart SQ 10 min ac
4. Tetracycline 500 mg PO BID

37. The nurse is getting ready to transfer a client to the operating room for surgery. During the report, the nurse who cared for the client during the night stated that the client had signed the consent form. As the nurse readies the client for transfer, the nurse should

1. advise the transport team that the consent form was signed
2. verify in the record that the consent form was signed
3. ask the client if the client had signed the consent form
4. ask the transport team to verify that the consent was signed

38. The staff nurse is concerned that a physician is neglecting a client. The best course of action is to

1. confront the physician
2. discuss concerns with an immediate supervisor
3. report the physician to the chief of medicine
4. advise the client to speak up for her rights

39. A medication is supplied in a 10 mL vial that contains 60 mg. The client is to receive 35 mg in a piggyback IV. How many mL of the medication should the nurse add to the IV? *Record your answer by rounding to the nearest whole number.*

Answer: ________mL

40. If a client has tested positive for pregnancy and states that the first day of her last menstrual period was April 3, what is the client's expected delivery date?

1. December 30
2. January 3
3. January 10
4. January 14

41. A newborn is diagnosed with fetal alcohol syndrome. Which of the following are common signs and symptoms? *Select all that apply.*

1. micrognathia
2. intellectual disability
3. autistic behaviors
4. long face with prominent ears
5. hyperextensible joints

42. Which of the following is the normal range for the fetal heart rate at 32 weeks gestation?

1. 120 to 160
2. 130 to 140
3. 160 to 180
4. 180 to 200

43. A client is to receive 3/5 of a bottle of a 10-ounce bottle of magnesium citrate. How many mL should the nurse administer? *Record your answer using a whole number.*

Answer: ________mL

44. The nurse has four clients that need attention. In which order should the nurse attend to the clients' needs?

A. Client A is receiving a NS infusion per IV pump with a piggyback antibiotic
B. Client B has returned to the unit from the recovery room after removal of an ovarian cyst and is requesting pain medication
C. Client C is hospitalized with complaints of weakness and dizziness and complains of sudden onset of severe headache
D. Client D is two days postoperative and is scheduled for a routine dressing change

1. First: ____.
2. Second: ____.
3. Third: ____.
4. Fourth: ____.

45. The nurse is alone in a room with a client who has slid down in the bed and needs to be repositioned. The best course of action is for the nurse to

1. stand at the head of the bed and grasp the client under the arms and pull toward the head of the bed
2. suggest the client bend the knees and push the body up toward the head of the bed
3. call for assistance and reposition the client with the draw sheet
4. obtain a Hoyer lift to reposition the client

46. The nurse is going to irrigate the ear of a 15-year-old client with impacted cerumen. When irrigating, the nurse should

1. pull the pinna up and back
2. pull the pinna down and back
3. pull the pinna down and forward
4. avoid repositioning the pinna

47. The nurse asks a newly-hired unlicensed assistive personnel to carry out a task usually done by UAPs, but the UAP states he is uncertain how to carry out the procedure. Which of the following is the best response?

1. ask a different UAP to carry out the task
2. explain to the UAP how to carry out the task
3. assist and supervise the UAP in carrying out the task
4. do the task without assistance

48. A 58-year-old male client who weighs 114 kg and has limited mobility needs to transfer from his bed to a stretcher in order to go to imaging for an MRI. Which of the following is best method to transfer the client from bed to stretcher?

1. transfer board
2. 3-person lift
3. stand-assist device
4. Hoyer lift

49. Under which of the following circumstances may a designee exercise authority to make decisions about a client under a Medical Power of Attorney?

1. any time the client is in need of medical care
2. when the client is seriously ill
3. only when the client indicates the designee may assume authority
4. only when the client is unable to make decisions

50. Which of the following individuals has the legal right to make personal healthcare decisions? *Select all that apply.*

1. a 22-year-old with a history of mental illness
2. a 17-year-old living with friends because her parents are drug addicts
3. a 15-year-old who is legally married
4. a 90-year-old with deafness living in an assisted living facility
5. a 16-year-old homeless youth

51. A 16-year-old client is scheduled for a chemotherapy treatment for leukemia. The client is adamant about refusing to take the treatment and is combative when the nurse approaches although the client's parents insist that the treatment be administered. Which of the following is the best response?

1. withhold treatment as the client has a right to refuse treatment
2. withhold treatment at present and notify the physician
3. administer the treatment, utilizing restraints if necessary
4. explain to the client that the client has no legal rights

52. The nurse is monitoring the end-tidal carbon dioxide ($EtCO_2$) waveform through capnography. Label the following waveforms according to what the waveform indicates:

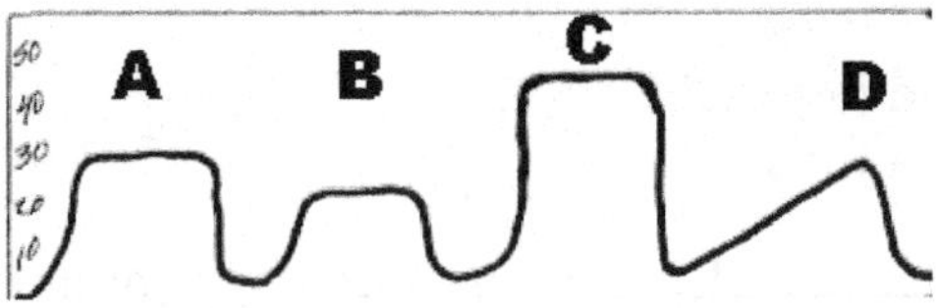

1. obstruction: ____
2. normal: ____
3. hyperventilation: ____
4. hypoventilation: ____

53. Following a stroke, a client has difficulty swallowing and chokes frequently. A referral to which of the following therapists is indicated to assess swallowing and provide treatment?

1. Physical therapist
2. Occupational therapist
3. Speech therapist
4. Respiratory therapist

54. Which of the following diseases must be reported to the CDC? *Select all that apply.*

1. Viral meningitis
2. Rubeola (measles)
3. Gonorrhea
4. Rubella (German measles)
5. Tuberculosis

55. A physician directs a nurse to carry out a procedure that is outside of the nurse's scope of practice. The nurse should

1. carry out the procedure since it is directed by a physician
2. ask a supervisor for advice about doing the procedure
3. refuse, advising the physician that the procedure is outside of the nurse's scope of practice
4. ask the physician to supervise while the nurse is doing the procedure

56. A client has been diagnosed with cancer and asks the nurse's advice about whether to have surgery or radiation. The nurse is aware that surgery offers the best chance of recovery. Which of the following is the most appropriate response?

1. provide the client with resources and information about the cancer and treatment options
2. advise the client to follow the advice of the physician
3. tell the client that the best course of action is to have surgery
4. remind the client that the client must make the decision

57. A client will soon be discharged from the hospital but is concerned because the client's insurance will not cover the cost of an expensive drug that the physician has prescribed. Which of the following is the <u>best</u> response?

1. suggest that the client ask the physician to substitute a different drug
2. provide the client information about patient assistance programs
3. encourage the client to express feelings of concern
4. suggest the client consider a Go-Fund-Me page to ask for assistance

58. The nurse is concerned that a client received the wrong medication and had a severe adverse reaction. The client recovered, and an incident report was filed but the client was not advised of the error. What is the <u>most</u> appropriate response?

1. inform the client of the medication error
2. express concerns to a supervisor
3. report the issue to the ethics committee
4. ask the physician why the client was not informed

59. A client is receiving an intravenous infusion. Which of the following are indications of catheter embolus? *Select all that apply.*

1. Hypotension
2. Hypertension
3. Edema and coolness of skin about insertion site
4. Pain at insertion site and along the vein
5. Moist productive cough and crackles in lung bases

60. A client receiving an intravenous infusion has indications of fluid overload with dyspnea, orthopnea, hypertension, and moist cough. The nurse immediately notifies the physician. Which of the following interventions are also indicated? *Select all that apply.*

1. Maintain patent catheter at very slow flowrate
2. Discontinue the infusion
3. Elevate the head of the bed
4. Administer intermittent positive pressure breathing therapy
5. Administer oxygen

61. The nurse, serving as team leader, has delegated a task to a fellow RN. After delegating, the delegating nurse's responsibility is to

1. leave the task and outcomes to the fellow RN to monitor
2. ask the fellow RN if the task was completed
3. assume the task was completed and document accordingly
4. follow up to ensure the task was completed and outcomes appropriate

62. Which of the following are important risk factors for lung cancer? *Select all that apply.*

1. smoking
2. vitamin B supplement
3. family history of lung cancer
4. high protein diet
5. radon exposure

63. An adolescent was struck by a car and brought to the emergency room unconscious. Because he was not carrying an ID, the nurse has been unable to locate a parent or family member to provide consent. The client has a ruptured spleen and the physician states the client needs immediate life-saving surgery. The nurse should

1. contact administration for a consent waiver
2. hold client transfer until a family member is found
3. sign the consent form since no one else is available to do so
4. transfer the client to surgery without a consent form signed

64. While the nurse is accessing a client's electronic medical record, a coworker (not assigned to the client) leans over the nurse and begins to read the client's record. The nurse should

1. allow the coworker to read the record
2. ask the coworker to stop reading
3. immediately block view or close-out the screen
4. threaten to report the nurse to a supervisor

65. The nurse notes that a transfer procedure is time consuming because of redundant steps and has developed a streamlined procedure. The nurse should

1. personally use the streamlined procedure
2. tell the other staff members to use the streamlined procedure
3. propose the new procedure to the performance improvement committee
4. print up instructions for the new procedure and let others decide whether to use it

66. A client states that she is severely allergic to avocados, kiwi fruit, and bananas. The nurse should suspect that the client may also be allergic to

1. latex
2. antibiotics
3. lanolin
4. plastic

67. When assessing a client for risk of falls, the nurse should be aware that the primary risk factors include which of the following? *Select all that apply.*

1. polypharmacy
2. male gender
3. history of falls
4. cigarette smoking
5. hypertension

68. A train disaster has occurred and the hospital is expecting a large surge of incoming clients. Which of the following current clients should be considered for rapid discharge in order to reduce the census and free up hospital beds? *Select all that apply.*

1. client scheduled for elective reduction mammoplasty
2. stable client three-days postoperative after vaginal hysterectomy
3. stable client one-day postoperative after craniotomy for removal of meningioma
4. client with status asthmaticus who still exhibits mild-to-moderate wheezing
5. client postoperative colon resection with 35,000 WBC count

69. The nurse notes that the electrical cord of a portable ECG machine is slightly cracked. Which of the following responses is <u>most</u> appropriate?

1. take no action as this poses no risk
2. apply electrical or other tape about the cracked area
3. use the equipment but notify repair services later
4. remove the equipment from use, label, and notify repair services

70. The nurse is assisting with triage at the site of an accident. Rank order the following injured individuals from most critical to least critical.

A. Individual with a slowly oozing wound on the right forearm
B. Individual with a fractured left wrist
C. Individual with an obstructed airway
D. Individual with head injury, conscious but somnolent and combative

1. Most critical: ____.
2. Next: ____.
3. Next: ____.
4. Least critical: ____

71. A 20-year-old university student complains of aching joints, chronic fatigue, fever (>100 °F/37.8 °C), and a butterfly rash across the cheeks and bridge of the nose. Which of the following disorders do these signs and symptoms suggest?

1. rheumatoid arthritis
2. systemic lupus erythematosus
3. scleroderma
4. multiple sclerosis

72. A client has been recently diagnosed with Parkinson's disease, and the nurse is educating the client and family about the condition. Which of the following symptoms are typical of Parkinson's disease and should be included in the discussion? *Select all that apply.*

1. peripheral numbness
2. rigidity
3. tremors
4. spasticity
5. bowel dysfunction

73. A client is scheduled for insertion of a central venous catheter in an upper central vein (not the femoral vein). Which of the following positions is usually utilized for clients during the insertion procedure?

1. upright
2. semi-Fowler's
3. supine, flat
4. Trendelenburg

74. An infant with hyperbilirubinemia is to have conventional phototherapy with a regular blue fluorescent light (non-Halogen) and to wear eye shields during treatment. Which of the following is true regarding the use of eye shields? *Select all that apply.*

1. apply eye shields tightly
2. perform eye care before applying eye shields
3. ensure the eyes are closed when applying shields
4. perform eye care at least every 4 hours
5. turn child's face away from the phototherapy lights when removing eye shields

75. The nurse is caring for a client with osteoporosis. Which of the following signs and symptoms would the nurse expect to find? *Select all that apply.*

1. Heberden's nodules on distal interphalangeal joints of fingers
2. ulnar deviation of the fingers
3. boutonniere deformity of proximal fingers
4. pain that may intensify with changes in barometric pressure
5. morning stiffness that decreases after about 30 minutes of activity
6. Swan neck deformity of fingers

76. When utilizing nasopharyngeal suctioning for a client unable to cough up secretions, once the catheter is inserted to the proper depth, the correct suction procedure is to

1. apply intermittent suction for a maximum of 5 seconds
2. apply intermittent suction for a maximum of 15 seconds
3. apply continuous suction for a maximum of 5 seconds
4. apply continuous suction for a maximum of 15 seconds

77. A client has returned from surgery with a urostomy after removal of the bladder because of cancer. How much urine does the nurse expect that the urostomy will produce per hour?

1. ≥10 mL
2. ≥ 20 mL
3. ≥30 mL
4. ≥40 mL

78. Correctly identify the cardiac abnormalities in the exhibit below.

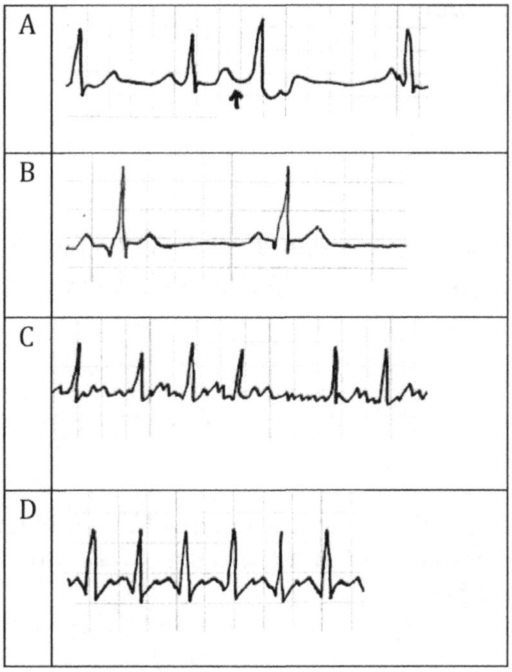

1. atrial fibrillation: ____
2. premature ventricular contractions: ____
3. ventricular tachycardia: ____
4. sinus bradycardia:____

79. A client is at 22 weeks gestation. Which of the following may be indicative of preeclampsia? *Select all that apply*.

1. negative urine dipstick for protein
2. BP 148/96
3. proteinuria: 0.4 g/24-hour urine collection
4. retinal vasodilation
5. hyperreflexia

80. A client is to be discharged with a medication labeled 25 mg per 5 mL and the client needs to take 150 mg BID but will use a tablespoon measure because the metric system is confusing to the client. How many tablespoons are equal to 150 mg of the medication? *Record your answer using a whole number*.

Answer: ________Tbsp.

81. An 80-year-old client confesses to the nurse that she has not bathed for over 2 weeks because she feels unsteady in the shower and dislikes tub baths. Which of the following is the <u>most</u> appropriate advice?

1. hire an aide to assist with bathing
2. take sponge baths
3. utilize a shower chair
4. take tub baths only

82. An older client has been admitted to the hospital after prolonged diarrhea. Which of the following are signs of dehydration? *Select all that apply.*

1. bradycardia
2. poor skin turgor
3. dry mucous membranes
4. concentrated urine
5. hypertension

83. A client has a diabetic ulcer with minimal to moderate exudate and a small amount of eschar that requires debridement. Which of the following dressing choices is <u>most</u> appropriate?

1. gauze
2. hydrogel
3. alginate
4. hydrocolloid

84. A physician has written an order for a client to receive 4 tablespoons of Milk of Magnesia at bedtime, but the nurse must convert this dosage to mL. What mL dosage should the nurse administer? *Record your answer using a whole number.*

Answer: _________mL

85. Which of the following are contraindications for the use of oral contraceptives for a 36-year-old client? *Select all that apply.*

1. smoking
2. benign liver tumor
3. history of deep vein thrombosis (DVT)
4. alcohol use (moderate)
5. HIV infection

86. If the mechanical ventilation waveform shows the expiratory flow is below baseline, as in the exhibit below, which of the following does this indicate?

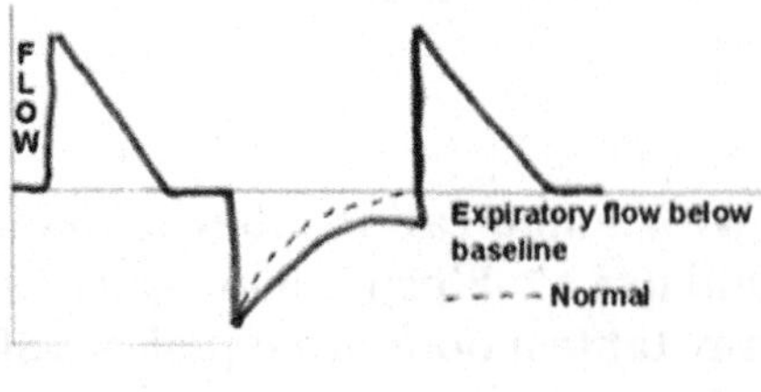

1. air trapping
2. lung overdistention
3. increased airway resistance
4. decreased airway resistance

87. A client is hospitalized after a traumatic brain injury and exhibits increasing intracranial pressure. The goal of treatment is to maintain the cerebral perfusion pressure between

1. 40 and 50 mm Hg
2. 50 and 60 mm Hg
3. 70 and 100 mm Hg
4. 100 and 110 mm Hg

88. A client's weight is 121 pounds but the client's weight in kilograms is need to calculate a drug dosage. What is the client's weight in kilograms? ***Record your answer using a whole number.***

Answer: ________kilograms

89. A client whose oxygen saturation has ranged from 96% to 98% has a sudden drop to 82% although the client's condition appears unchanged. Which of the following is the most appropriate initial response?

1. administer oxygen
2. notify the physician
3. check placement and functioning of the oximeter
4. check the client's vital signs

90. Which of the following are reciprocal attachment behaviors exhibited by a newborn? ***Select all that apply.***

1. roots and latches onto the mother's breasts
2. cries when hungry
3. engages in entrainment
4. sleeps in parent's arms
5. grasps parent's finger

91. The nurse is doing a venipuncture on a sitting client in order to obtain a blood sample, but before the blood can be withdrawn, the client complains of feeling faint and appears pale and shaky. The most appropriate response is for the nurse to

1. immediately remove the needle
2. complete the blood draw
3. keep the needle in place and ask the client to take deep breaths
4. ask for assistance to support the client while finishing the blood draw

92. If assessing arterial blood gases, the nurse must be aware that the normal range for PO_2 is

1. 35 to 45 mm Hg
2. 50 to 70 mm Hg
3. 80 to 95 mm Hg
4. 90 to 100 mm Hg

93. A client with type 2 diabetes reports that he has stayed on his low carbohydrate diet and takes metformin daily. His Hgb A1c is 8.2. Which of the following does this Hgb A1c indicate?

1. the client's diabetes is well-controlled
2. the client may need to increase intake of carbohydrates or lower the dosage of metformin
3. the client's diabetes is not well-controlled
4. the client is probably being untruthful about his diet and medication use

94. A client with anorexia nervosa states, "I was so happy when I was thinner. I need to lose weight so I can be happy again." This is an example of which of the following types of cognitive distortion?

1. overgeneralization
2. catastrophizing
3. personalization
4. emotional reasoning

95. A client has been diagnosed with schizophrenia. Which of the following signs and symptoms does the nurse expect the client may exhibit? *Select all that apply.*

1. impulsivity
2. flat affect
3. rapid mood swings
4. disordered speech
5. hallucinations

96. A client with hemolytic uremic syndrome is to receive eculizumab IV. The medication is supplied in a 300-mg single use vial with 10 mg/mL. If the client is to receive 900 mg IV one time weekly, how many mL of the drug will the nurse administer for each treatment? *Record your answer using a whole number.*

Answer: ________mL

97. A nurse is preparing to enter an isolation room to care for a client and has completed hand hygiene, prepared the supplies and equipment that will be needed, made introductions to the client, and advised the client of the procedure. When applying PPE, in which order should the nurse carry out the following steps?

A. Apply surgical mask or respirator
B. Apply clean gloves
C. Apply goggles
D. Tie gown securely at neck and waist
E. Apply gown

1. Step 1____
2. Step 2____
3. Step 3____
4. Step 4____
5. Step 5____

98. The nurse is attempting to irrigate an NG feeding tube with 30 mL of water but is unable to instill the solution. Which of the following is the next appropriate step?

1. remove the NG tube and insert another tube
2. position the client on the left side and attempt irrigation again
3. try again, applying more pressure
4. gently pull the NG tube out about 5 cm and then reinsert before attempting irrigation again

99. When an NG feeding tube is placed initially, which of the following is the <u>most</u> appropriate method of ensuring correct placement?

1. check the color of aspirant
2. carry out a pH measurement of aspirant
3. conduct air auscultation
4. x-ray to confirm placement

100. A diabetic client has been hospitalized for surgical debridement of a diabetic ulcer, and the physician is concerned that the client may develop hyperglycemia or hypoglycemia because of poor control of the diabetes. Which of the following symptoms should the nurse be alert for as indications of hyperglycemia? *Select all that apply.*

1. blurred vision
2. polyuria
3. cardiac dysrhythmia
4. polydipsia
5. inappropriate behavior
6. increased perspiration

101. When assessing a 75-year-old client for risk of falls, the nurse conducts the timed up and go (TUG) test. What is the normal time required for a client to complete standing, walking 3 meters, turning, returning back, and sitting down?

1. 4 to 6 seconds
2. 7 to 10 seconds
3. 11 to 14 seconds
4. 15 to 20 seconds

102. Which of the following fractures poses the greatest risk for older adults?

1. wrist
2. vertebral
3. radial/ulnar
4. hip/femur

103. A client has suffered an ischemic stroke in the right hemisphere. Which of the following should the nurse anticipate?

1. the client has left paralysis and left visual field defect
2. the client has expressive, receptive, and/or global aphasia
3. the client remains uncharacteristically positive
4. the client has difficulty with mathematics, reading, and writing

104. The nurse is caring for a client in the recovery room after the client's abdominal surgery. The client's base BP prior to surgery was 130/84. Recovery room BP record is as follows:

- 1:00 PM 126/84
- 1:15 PM 128/82
- 1:30 PM 124/80
- 1:45 PM 116/72
- 2:00 PM 110/66
- 2: 15 PM 100/62

Which of the following is the <u>most</u> appropriate response?

1. notify the surgeon of the change in BP
2. continue to monitor the client as usual
3. increase the rate of oxygen flow to the client
4. notify the surgeon if the systolic BP falls below 90

105. Which of the following statements by a newly diagnosed client with diabetes type 1 indicates the need for further education?

1. "I should check my blood sugar level before meals and at bedtime."
2. "I can eat whatever I want if I increase my insulin to cover the food."
3. "I can see that being diabetic is going to be somewhat difficult."
4. "I should keep a record of where I give the injections so I don't forget."

106. Which of the following is an absolute contraindication for the use of isotretinoin as a treatment for acne.

1. age younger than 18
2. sensitivity to vitamin D
3. pregnancy
4. hearing deficit

107. A client has a newly-applied cast on the left foot and ankle. The client complains of severe itching on the bottom of the foot. Which of the following interventions may help to relieve the itching?

1. encourage the client to do deep breathing and relaxation exercises
2. gently insert a tongue blade inside the cast and rub the area that itches
3. elevate the left leg and foot above the heart
4. blow cold air from a hair dryer into the cast toward the area that itches

108. A client receiving total parenteral nutrition (TPN) exhibits sudden onset of respiratory distress with cough and dyspnea, and oxygen saturation level falls to 88%. On examining the client, the nurse finds that the IV tubing has become disconnected so that part of the catheter system is open to the air. The immediate response before notifying the physician should be to

1. clamp the catheter and place client in left lateral Trendelenburg position
2. clamp the catheter and place the client in supine position with head of bed elevated
3. reconnect the tubing immediately and provide oxygen
4. remove the catheter and provide oxygen

109. Anticipatory guidance for a 16-year-old should include which of the following? *Select all that apply.*

1. responsibilities of marriage/family
2. financial management
3. risk-taking behaviors (drugs, drinking, reckless driving)
4. age-appropriate sports activities
5. information about abstinence/birth control

110. The nurse must insert a urinary catheter into the bladder of a client with osteoarthritis of the hips. When the nurse positions the client in dorsal recumbent position, the client complains of pain in both hips. Which of the following is the most appropriate response?

1. assure the client that the procedure will be done quickly
2. place pillows under the legs to provide some support
3. administer analgesia before completing the catheterization
4. place the client in side-lying (Sims) position

111. A client undergoing a colonoscopy is administered IV midazolam as part of moderate sedation. Which of the following is a primary concern when monitoring a patient receiving midazolam?

1. heart rate
2. respiratory status
3. level of consciousness
4. peripheral circulation

112. Which of the following foods has the greatest potential for interaction with drugs?

1. milk products
2. grapefruit
3. potatoes
4. cabbage

113. A 4-year-old client weighing 39.6 pounds is to receive an infusion of IV ceftriaxone sodium at 75 mg/kg/d in a divided dose every 12 hours. How many mg should the child receive with each infusion? *Record your answer using a whole number.*

Answer: ________mg

114. A client recovering from open heart surgery complains of pain at 9 on a 1-to-10 scale, but when the nurse returns within 5 minutes with analgesia, the client is talking with a visitor, smiling, and appears relaxed. Which of the following is the most appropriate action?

1. hold the medication until the client asks again
2. ask the client to rate the pain again
3. administer the analgesia
4. tell the client that it appears the pain has reduced

115. A client with a 3-week-old infant tells the nurse that her infant has started to sleep up to 6 hours at a time during the night. Which of the following is the most appropriate response?

1. "Newborns can get too dehydrated if they sleep more than 4 hours."
2. "You are so lucky. That gives you a chance to rest."
3. "You should never let a neonate sleep that long."
4. "That's really unusual. There may be something wrong with your infant."

116. Which of the following vaccinations are recommended for all adults 50 to 65 years and older? *Select all that apply.*

1. herpes zoster (shingles)
2. hepatitis B
3. pneumococcal polysaccharide
4. human papillomavirus
5. influenza

117. A client was recently diagnosed with pancreatic cancer and is undergoing chemotherapy. When the laboratory technician has difficulty obtaining a blood specimen because the client has very small veins, the client becomes very upset and complains that the technician is incompetent and should be fired. The <u>most</u> appropriate response is

1. "I can see how distressed you are."
2. "The technician was trying her best."
3. "You should file a complaint with human resources."
4. "You have bad veins, so obtaining a specimen is difficult."

118. The nurse observes a coworker sign out a narcotic for a client but sees the nurse take the medication into the nurse's restroom and then return to the nursing station without seeing the client and without the medication. Which of the following actions is most appropriate?

1. confront the coworker about the issue
2. report the observation to a supervisor
3. report the observation the state board of nursing
4. monitor the coworker carefully to see if this is a pattern

119. A 10-year-old client is scheduled for surgery and the hospital allows parents to be with the child during anesthesia induction. The nurse assists the child's mother to gown and explains the parent's role during induction, but the mother begins to cry when she prepares to enter to operating room. Which of the following is the <u>most</u> appropriate response?

1. "Crying will frighten your child, so you need to try to control yourself."
2. "I know how worried you are. Let's just take a minute to prepare yourself."
3. "Would you rather not be with your child during the induction?"
4. "Go ahead and cry. It will make you feel better."

120. A client's medication order is for 300 mg of a liquid medication that is available at 75 mg per mL. How many mL should the nurse administer to the client? *Record your answer using a whole number.*

Answer: ________mL.

Answer Key and Explanations for Test #3

1. 3, 4, and 5: If a client is at risk of falls, home modifications that the nurse should discuss with the client include removing throw rugs as they may slide or cause the client to trip, installing handrails on stairs and safety bars in the bathroom, and improving lighting, such as by ensuring that burned out bulbs are replaced and improving lighting as needed in hallways and stairways. Removing clutter from walkways is especially important. Clients should be advised to take care around pets and to discourage animals from jumping on the client.

2. 1: If a 64-year-old female client has recently had surgery for colon cancer and has a colostomy, but the client has been resistive to educational efforts and refuses to look at the colostomy, the most appropriate intervention is to remain supportive and encourage the client to express her feelings. Clients cope with a changed body image in different ways, and the client may need extra time to process the changes and to cope emotionally.

3. 2: At ages 2 to 3 (toddler), the child would first be expected to be able to draw a circle and other rudimentary forms, to jump, kick a ball, and throw a ball overhand. At this stage of development, the child should be able to walk up and down stairs, undress, and build a tower of at least 4 blocks. The child should be learning to dress. Most children are toilet trained between 2 and 3 years of age although some, especially girls, may be toilet trained earlier.

4.

1	Poison	F	
2	Biohazard	C	
3	Corrosive	D	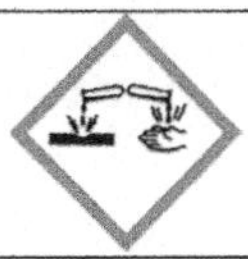
4	Health hazard	B	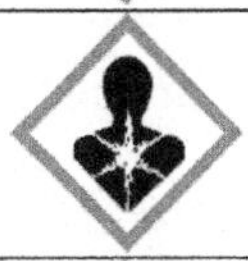
5	Flame	E	
6	Irritant	A	

5. 1, 2, and 4: If the nurse plans to obtain a blood sample from a venipuncture in the left median cubital vain, contraindications to using this vein include post left mastectomy because of impaired circulation, especially if any evidence of lymphedema is present, venous fibrosis felt on palpation, and presence of a left vascular shunt for dialysis. Venipuncture should be avoided if the site is edematous or if there is an IV in the arm as this may dilute the specimen. Other contraindications include the presence of cellulitis or hematoma.

6. 4: Infants and young children should be placed in rear-facing car seats until they reach a weight of at least 35 pounds, which is the maximum weight for most car seats. Parents should be made aware that they should position the child according to weight and not age as children's sizes may vary widely. After the rear-facing car seat, all children under age 8 or 4 feet 9 inches tall must be secured in a car seat or booster seat in the back seat of the motor vehicle because the airbag in the front poses a danger to young children.

7. 2: If a client who had a thyroidectomy complains of numbness and tingling in the hands and feet and muscle cramps in the lower legs and the client appears slightly confused and irritable, the nurse should suspect that the client has developed hypocalcemia, which may occur if the parathyroid glands were inadvertently removed or traumatized during the thyroidectomy. The client should receive calcium supplements and vitamin D. In most cases, calcium levels will stabilize within a few days.

8. 2: If a pregnant client is undergoing a non-stress test, during the test the nurse instructs the client to report sensations of movement so these reports can be compared to the record of movement. The client's report and the record should correlate 50 to 90% of the time. Monitoring with an ultrasound transducer for FHR and a tocodynamometer for fetal movement is carried out for 20 to 40 minutes or longer if the fetus is sleeping. Scoring:

- 2: Normal score with ≥2 FHR accelerations of 15 bmp above baseline for ≥15 seconds in a 20-40-minute period. (Reactive).
- 0: Abnormal score with 1-0 accelerations of FHR in 40 minutes. (Nonreactive).

9. If a client is to receive 1000 mL of IV fluid in 6 hours with a drop factor of 15 gtt/mL, the nurse should administer 42 gtt/min. The total volume (1000 mL) is first divided by the number of hours:

- 1000 / 6 = 166.66

This result is then divided by 60 because there are 60 minutes in an hour:

- 166.66 / 60 = 2.77 mL/min

This result is then multiplied by the drop factor—15.

- 2.77 × 15 = 41.55 = 42 gtt/min

10. 1: If a woman who was badly beaten by a domestic partner has come to the ED but is extremely fearful, stating, "My boyfriend is going to come here and shoot me, I know he will!" the most appropriate initial response it to contact security and place the client in a room out of sight. Ensuring the client's safety and the safety of others is of primary importance, especially if the perpetrator of the abuse is believed to have a weapon. Once the client feels safe, then the nurse can discuss notifying the police although many victims refuse to do so.

11. 4: If a client who was a heavy smoker and developed lung cancer constantly warns others about the dangers of smoking and refuses to allow anyone to smoke in his presence, the type of defense mechanism this represents is reaction formation. Reaction formation is utilized when a client is able to control unacceptable feelings (the desire to smoke) by focusing on the opposite behavior or desire (the abstinence and dangers of smoking).

12. 1 and 5: The WBC count generally ranges from 4.8 to 10.80 10^3/mL and a count below 3.5 is generally considered an indication of leukopenia, which indicates an impaired immune system. The platelet count should range from 150 to 450 10^3/uL. A count of 111 indicates thrombocytopenia although there is little risk of bleeding until the level decreases to less than 50. The normal range for hemoglobin is 12 to 16 g/dL and hematocrit, 37 to 47%.

13. 4: When obtaining a blood sample from a central line using the push-pull method, after flushing the catheter with 5 to 10 mL of NS, the next step is to aspirate 6 mL of blood and reinfuse the blood 3 times and then attach a new syringe and aspirate the blood sample. If possible, a blood sample should be obtained from a peripheral vein because obtaining a sample from the central line increases the risk of complications, such as infection or occlusion.

14. If a child weighs 35.2 pounds and requires 1000 mL plus 50 mL fluid for each kilogram over 10 kg as maintenance fluid every 24 hours, the child's required volume of fluid is 1300 mL.

The child's weight is first converted to kilograms:

- 35.2 / 2.2 = 16 kg

The fluid volume for the first 10 kg is 1000 mL and 50 mL is added for each additional kg:

- 50 × 6 = 300.
- 1000 mL + 300 mL = 1300 mL

15. 2: If a 6-year-old client is having a generalized seizure, the nurse should ease the child to the floor if standing when the seizure begins and place the client in side-lying position to prevent aspiration. The nurse should not try to restrain the child but should pad side rails if in bed or move objects out of the way if on the floor. Nothing should be placed between the teeth. The child should be monitored during the seizure and the recovery period.

16. 1: For a newborn with suspected meconium plug syndrome (AKA functional colonic obstruction), the test/procedure that will likely be used to confirm the diagnosis is contrast enema. A plain abdominal X-ray may show distended loops of bowel but cannot identify the cause. A contrast enema will show the blockage and, in many cases, may serve to relieve the obstruction as well. Meconium plug syndrome most often occurs in full-term newborns, infants of diabetic mothers, or newborns with hypermagnesemia.

17. 3: An appropriate intervention for a newborn that experienced intrauterine drug exposure and has frequent high-pitched crying is swaddling the infant in flexed position, keeping the arms close to the body. Holding the newborn close to the body and rocking the infant slowly and rhythmically may also soothe the child. The light should be kept low to decrease stimulation. Soft music or a warm bath may also help. Some newborns will calm when offered a pacifier, sometimes with sugar solution.

18. 4: 5% DW is an isotonic IV solution.

Hypotonic	Isotonic	Hypertonic
2.5% DW	5% DW	>5%DW
0.2% NaCl	0.9% NaCl	D10W
0.33% NaCl	Lactated Ringer.	3% NaCl
0.45% NaCl	Ringer's solution	5% NaCl
		5% NaCl + DW

19. 1: If a client with schizophrenia tells the nurse that he hates all of the doctors and nurses and wishes that they would all die, the most therapeutic response is to paraphrase, "Things would be better for you if we were all dead?" Paraphrasing encourages the client to confirm or refute the statement and to provide more information, and paraphrasing is not judgmental or threatening to the client. Paraphrasing should, however, be used sparingly.

20. 4: If a client involved in a motor vehicle accident is hospitalized with injuries after attempting to help a passenger (a close friend) who died at the scene, the most effective approach is to encourage the client to express his feelings, but the nurse should not force the discussion but should take time to listen. The client may be quite traumatized and may feel guilty about surviving, especially if he was at fault in the accident.

21. If a physician has ordered levothyroxine 125 mg for a client but the available medication has the dosage in mg rather than mcg, the correct dosage is 0.125 mg. The formula to convert mcg to mg is:

- mcg / 1000 = mg
- 125 / 1000 = 0.125 mg

22. 2: While the nurse should review adverse effects of all of the client's medications and herbal preparations, the herbal preparation of most concern is St. John's wort, which interacts with numerous prescription medications and should, therefore, be avoided. In fact, St. John's wort interacts negatively with oral contraceptives (decreases effectiveness), fexofenadine (increases adverse effects), and omeprazole (decreases effectiveness).

23. 4: For a client receiving warfarin, the critical value for the INR is >3. The normal value for the INR is <2, but for clients receiving warfarin, the value should be between 2 and 3 because of the increased clotting time associated with anticoagulation. However, if the value exceeds 3, the risk of bleeding increases. During initial treatment, the client should have the INR tested frequently, at least every week for the first 3 months after which the time between tests may be extended if values are stable.

24. If a disinfectant must be mixed with water to make a 1:2 solution (one part disinfectant to 2 parts water) and a total of 2 L is needed, 667 mL of disinfectant should be used to make the solution.

- 1 L equals 1000 mL, so 2L = 2000 mL.
- 1:2 equals 3 parts.
- 2000 / 3 = 666.66 = 667
- 1 part is equal to 667 mL.

25. 1: If a client with osteoarthritis of the right knee has been advised to use a cane for support, the best method to determine the correct length of the cane is to measure from the crease in the wrist to the floor while the client is standing and wearing usual shoes (because the client will most often have shoes on when using the cane). When used for support, the cane is generally held in the opposite hand, so if the deficit is on the right, the client would hold the cane in the left hand.

26. 3: If a client is to have a bladder scan to determine the volume of residual urine, the scan should be carried out within 10 minutes of urination. If a longer time period has elapsed, the client should be asked to urinate again. For the scan, the client is placed in supine position with the head slightly elevated. If the client is female and has had a hysterectomy, the "male" designation should be used rather than the "female" because the uterus is missing.

27. 1 and 2: When carrying out range of motion exercises on a client's arm after an injury to the elbow, the nurse should assist the client to carry out extension and flexion. Hinge joint, such as the elbow, knee, interphalangeal joints and ankle, can move only along one axis. Hinge joints are a type of synovial joint that join two or more bones. In a synovial joint, the bones at the joint are surrounded by a synovial capsule and synovial fluid.

28. 4: If an unconscious client has been brought to the emergency department after an overdose of heroin, the reversal agent that is indicated is naloxone (Narcan®). Naloxone is available as an injection, nasal spray, and prefilled auto-injector and is carried by many first responders. The dose for an adult overdose is 0.4 to 2 mg IV, IM, or SQ, repeated every 2 to 3 minutes as needed. The dosage from children age one month and older is 0.01 mg/Kg IV or IM for first dose and 0.1 mg/kg for second.

29. 1: The ethnic group that is most at risk for the development of hypertension is African American. The rate of hypertension among African Americans is about 46% and 45% for Native Hawaiians and other Pacific Islanders. The rate among Asians is about 40%, about 34% for Hispanics, and about 35% for Caucasians. Some African Americans may carry a gene that makes them more sensitive to sodium intake, leading to hypertension. Hypertension also correlates with obesity.

30. 2: If a client who must have chemotherapy is very frightened of the treatments and often becomes very agitated and hyperventilates when arriving for treatment, the complementary therapy that may provide some relief for this anxiety is deep breathing and relaxation exercises. St. John's wort may interfere with the action of some chemotherapeutic agents. Acupuncture may help to relieve pain and nausea. There is no evidence to support magnet therapy.

31. 1, 2, and 4: Canned vegetables and legumes, such as kidney beans, are often high in sodium as are processed meats, such as hot dogs, salami, and other luncheon meats. Pickles are especially high in sodium. Frozen vegetables, such as frozen peas, usually do not include added sodium unless they are frozen with a sauce. Clients should be cautioned that sodium is added to many products, such as cereals and bread, so they should learn to read labels to check sodium content.

32. 2: The pH of gastric fluids usually ranges from 1.5 to 5, and feedings should be withheld and placement further verified if the pH is greater than 5; however, the pH may be 5 or greater in those receiving continuous feedings. A pH of greater than 6 may occur from fluid obtained from the small intestine of those who are fasting or obtained from pleural fluid.

33. 3: If an IV is to be administered through gravity flow, the IV bag should be hung at least 3 feet above the client's heart, so the height may need to be adjusted if the client changes from flat to sitting position to ensure a steady an even flow rate. The higher the IV bag, the greater the gravitational pull. If the flow rate must be increased, then elevating the bag should speed the flow.

34. 2: If a nurse is changing a postoperative client's dressing but the client shouts that the nurse is incompetent and doesn't know how to change a dressing, the best response is, "I can see that you are really upset. What can I do to help?" Often, when a client erupts in anger, the real reason is not that at which the client is directing anger. For example, the client may have pain or may be fearful or may have received bad news. Acknowledging the client's feelings and showing a willingness to listen may encourage the client to express feelings.

35. 2: If, while the nurse is having lunch in the hospital cafeteria, a coworker from another unit asks for information about the prognosis of one of the nurse's clients, who is the coworker's neighbor, the best response is, "I'm sorry, I can't talk about clients." This keep the focus on the self rather than the coworker, so it's not accusatory, but reinforces the client's right to confidentiality. Disclosing information about the family is also a breach of confidentiality.

36. 4: Tetracycline 500 mg PO BID is documented correctly. MS should not be abbreviated as it could mean morphine sulfate or magnesium sulfate. Trailing zeros, such as in 83.0 should be avoided but leading zeros (such as 0.8) should be utilized." Unit" should be written out and not abbreviated as "u." QD and QOD and variations (q.o.d., etc.) should be avoided as they may be misread.

37. 2: When a nurse is readying a client for transfer to the operating room for surgery, the nurse should always verify that the consent form has been signed by checking the client's record and should not depend on the word of others because sometimes mistakes are made. The nurse should not depend on the transport team to verify the consent, and the client may not be a reliable reporter, especially if the client has been premedicated.

38. 2: If a nurse is concerned that a physician is neglecting a client, the best course of action is to discuss concerns with an immediate supervisor. It's important to utilize the chain of command when concerns arise about client care because immediate perceptions may be wrong, or there may be issues about which the nurse is unaware. A supervisor is in a better position to make a decision about the course of action to follow.

39. If a medication is supplied in a 10 mL vial that contains 60 mg and the client is to receive 35 mg, the client should receive 6 mL.

- 60 / 10 = 6 mg per mL
- 35 (required dose) / 6 = 5.83 mL = 6 mL.

40. 3: If a client has tested positive for pregnancy and states that the first day of her last menstrual period was April 3, then the expected delivery date is January 10. In order to calculate the expected delivery date, count back three months from the first day of the last menstrual period—to January 3—and then add 7 days (January 3 plus 7 equals January 10). The average duration of gestation is 280 days. Another way to calculate is to count 280 days from the first day of the last menstrual period. The expected delivery date is an estimate and the actual delivery date may occur before or after the expected date.

41. 1 and 2: If a newborn is diagnosed with fetal alcohol syndrome, common signs and symptoms include micrognathia and intellectual disability. Other characteristics include hypoplastic maxilla, hypoplastic philtrum (groove under the nose) and short palpebral fissures (eye slits between upper and lower lids). The newborn may have various other neurological deficits as well, including microcephaly, hearing deficits, and motor delays. The prenatal growth deficit persists after birth with slow growth. As the child ages, learning and attention disorders may become evident.

42. 1: The normal range for the fetal heart rate at 32 weeks gestation is 120 to 160 bpm. Some variability in the heart rate is normal with tachycardia considered a rate of greater than 160 for 10 minutes and bradycardia a rate of less than 120 for 10 minutes. Fetal heart tones are generally heard per fetoscope at about 20 weeks and earlier with ultrasound. The fetus should be palpated to determine position before listening for the heart beat with a fetoscope because the heart is best heard through the fetal back.

43. If a client is to receive 3/5 of a 10-ounce bottle of magnesium citrate, the nurse should administer 180 mL.

- 3/5 = 6/10 = 6 ounces.
- Each ounce equals 30 mL.
- 6 × 30 = 180 mL.

44. If a nurse has four clients that need attention, the nurse should attend to the client's needs in this order:

1. First: C. The sudden headache may indicate a stroke, ruptured aneurysm, or other severe problem, so this client needs immediate attention.
2. Second: B. Clients returning from surgery should be assessed as soon as possible and pain medication provided if needed.
3. Third: A. The IV should be assessed next to make sure it is infusing without difficulty, but the IV pump alarm should sound if there is a problem.
4. Fourth: D. A routine dressing change is not generally time-sensitive.

45. 3: If the nurse is alone in a room with a client who has slid down in the bed and needs to be repositioned. The **best** course of action is for the nurse to call for assistance of one or two other staff members and reposition the client with the draw sheet. The nurse should never try to pull the client by grasping under the arms as this may injure both the nurse and the client. Asking the client to slide up in bed may result in friction and shear, and a Hoyer lift should not be necessary for repositioning.

46. 1: If the nurse is going to irrigate the ear of a 15-year-old client with impacted cerumen, when irrigating, the nurse should pull the pinna up and back as this is the correct positioning for those 3 years and older. For those younger than 3, the pinna should be pulled down and back. These maneuvers help to straighten the ear canal and make irrigation easier. The irrigation should be done slowly to avoid excess pressure in the ear canal.

47. 3: If the nurse asks a newly-hired unlicensed assistive personnel to carry out a task usually done by UAPs, but the UAP states he is uncertain how to carry out the procedure, the best response is for the nurse to assist and supervise the UAP in carrying out the task as this provides a learning opportunity. Part of the responsibility of the nurse is to help to educate other staff members and to supervise the care provided by UAPs.

48. 1: If a 58-year-old male client who weighs 114 kg (250 lb) and has limited mobility needs to transfer from his bed to a stretcher, the best method to transfer the client from the bed to the stretcher is to use a transfer board. Three-person lifts are no longer recommended as they may result in injury to staff. Two staff members should logroll the client onto one side, and then the transfer board is positioned under the draw sheet and the client rolled back over the board. The stretcher is placed next to the bed and one staff member on each side uses the draw sheet to slide the client onto the stretcher while the third staff person holds onto the transfer board.

49. 4: A designee may exercise authority to make decisions about a client under a Medical Power of Attorney only when the client is unable to make decisions as determined by the client's physician, psychologist, or nurse practitioner. In order to make decisions, the client must be able to understand the implications of healthcare decisions, understand options and make an informed decision, and communicate wishes. If the client has a Living Will, then the designee with the Medical Power of Attorney must follow the client's wishes.

50. 1, 3, and 4: Mental illness does not interfere with a person's legal right to make personal healthcare decisions unless the client has been declared legally incompetent. If a client is legally married (at any age), that client is able to make healthcare decisions. Disability and age do not affect an individual's right to make healthcare decisions. A homeless youth has no legal right to make healthcare decisions unless legally emancipated.

51. 2: If a 16-year-old client is scheduled for a chemotherapy treatment for leukemia, but the client is adamant about refusing to take the treatment and is combative when the nurse approaches although the client's parents insist that the treatment be administered, the best response is to withhold the treatment at present and notify the physician. While a 16-year-old has no legal rights, forcing the client to take treatment that the client is refusing should be a last resort.

52. $EtCO_2$ waveforms per capnography:

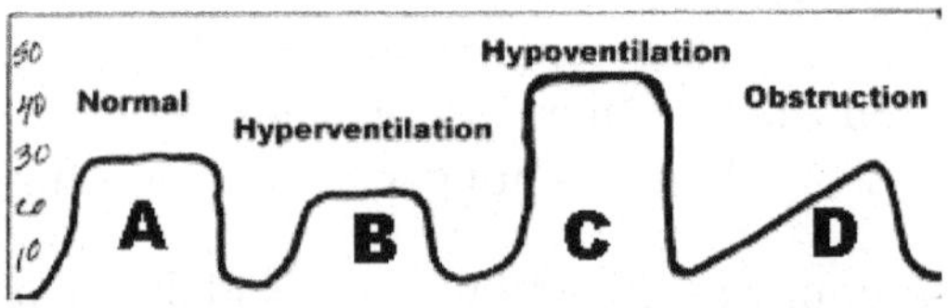

1. obstruction: D.
2. normal: A.
3. hyperventilation B.
4. hypoventilation: C.

$EtCO_2$ is the partial pressure/concentration of carbon dioxide at the end of expiration. Hyperventilation lowers the waveform and increases the number of waveforms while hypoventilation raises the waveform but decreases the number of waveforms. A "shark fin" sloped waveform indicates obstruction, such as may occur with asthma, COPD, or bronchospasm.

53. 3: If, following a stroke, a client has difficulty swallowing and chokes frequently, a referral to a speech therapist is indicated to assess swallowing and provide treatment. The speech therapist may assist the client with exercises to strengthen the muscles involved with swallowing and with techniques to compensate in order to reduce the risk of aspiration, such as through positioning and swallowing techniques as well as diet modification (such as by thickening liquids and using pureed or soft foods).

54. 3, 4, and 5: Gonorrhea, rubella (German measles) and tuberculosis all must be reported to the CDC. However, rubeola, a milder form of measles, does not have to be reported. Meningococcal meningitis must be reported but not viral meningitis. Reporting of communicable diseases is essential for public health in order for the government to compile statistics and be made aware of outbreaks that may require intervention, such as campaigns to encourage vaccination.

55. 3: If a physician directs a nurse to carry out a procedure that is outside of the nurse's scope of practice, the nurse should refuse and advise the physician that the procedure is outside of the nurse's scope of practice. The nurse is legally responsible for personal actions, and acting outside of the scope of practice could result in legal and/or civil action against the nurse if a problem arises. The scope of practice is determined by the state board of nursing and the nurse's licensure and certification.

56. 1: If a client has been diagnosed with cancer and asks the nurse's advice about whether to have surgery or radiation, and the nurse is aware that surgery offers the best chance of recovery, the most appropriate response is to provide the client with resources and information about the cancer and treatment options. The nurse should avoid advising the client about the course of action to take as this may unduly influence the client.

57. 2: If a client will soon be discharged from the hospital but is concerned because the client's insurance will not cover the cost of an expensive drug that the physician has prescribed, the best response is to provide the client information about patient assistance programs. For example, RxAssist.org provides a database search engine to help individuals find assistance programs offered by drug companies. In some cases, the physician may be able to substitute a less expensive drug, but this is not always the case.

58. 2: If the nurse is concerned that a client received the wrong medication and had a severe adverse reaction but recovered and an incident report was filed but the client was not advised of the error, the most appropriate response is to express concerns to a supervisor. The nurse should not inform the client. In fact, most clients are not advised of errors as part of risk management procedures although some organizations are now taking a different more open approach.

59. 1 and 4: Indications of catheter embolus (a piece of the catheter breaks loose and migrates in the venous system) include hypotension and pain at insertion site and along the vein. The client may also exhibit cyanosis, especially of the nail beds on the affected side. The pulse may be weak and rapid and the client may lose consciousness. Emergency response is to remove the catheter and check for breaks and apply a tourniquet distally to the site. The physician should be notified immediately.

60. 1, 3, and 5: If a client receiving an intravenous infusion has indications of fluid overload with dyspnea, orthopnea, hypertension, and moist cough, and the nurse has notified the physician, other interventions that are indicated include maintaining a patent catheter at a very slow flowrate because emergency medications may be indicated. Elevating the head of the bed may help to relieve orthopnea and oxygen may relieve dyspnea. The client must be carefully monitored and emergency interventions carried out as needed.

61. 4: If a nurse, serving as team leader, has delegated a task to a fellow RN, the responsibility for ensuring that the task was completed and outcomes appropriate remains with the delegating nurse, so simply asking if the task was completed is not sufficient. Additionally, the nurse should never assume a task was completed and document accordingly unless the completion is verified. When delegating, the nurse should always be mindful of the 5 rights of delegation: right task, right circumstance, right person, right direction, and right supervision.

62. 1, 3, and 5: Important risk factors include smoking, which is associated with about 90% of cases. Exposure to secondhand smoke is also a risk factor. Those with a family history of lung cancer have double the risk of developing the disease and should especially avoid smoking. Other risk factors include radon exposure and asbestos exposure, which leads to mesothelioma. A diet high in carbohydrates is also a risk factor. Smokers who take beta carotene supplements increase the risk of getting lung cancer.

63. 4: While consent is usually required for all procedure unless waived by the individual, in an emergency situation when the client's life is at risk and no one is available to sign the consent form, the procedure (in this case for the ruptured spleen) can be carried out. The nurse should immediately transfer the client to the operating room for surgery. In descending order, those who can provide consent if the client is unable to do so include the spouse, adult children, parent, siblings, other relatives, and friends.

64. 3: If, while the nurse is accessing a client's electronic medical record, a coworker (not assigned to the client) leans over the nurse and begins to read the client's record, the nurse should immediately block the view or close-out the screen to prevent the coworker from reading as this is a breach of confidentiality. Only those who are authorized to access a client's record may legally do so. If a nurse allows others to view the record, this nurse is also at fault.

65. 3: If the nurse notes that a transfer procedure is time consuming because of redundant steps and has develop a streamlined procedure, the nurse should propose the new procedure to the performance improvement committee so that the procedure can be reviewed and a decision made about implementation. Once procedures have been established, questioning them and revising those that are inefficient are important steps, but these should not be carried out unilaterally.

66. 1: If a client states that she is severely allergic to avocados, kiwi fruit, and bananas, the nurse should suspect that the client may also be allergic to latex (latex-fruit syndrome) because of cross-reactivity associated with IgE antibodies and antigens in latex and fruits/vegetables. Some fruits and vegetables contain proteins that are similar to those in latex. Other fruits and vegetables that may be involved include peaches, papayas, and nightshades (potatoes, tomatoes, bell peppers, and eggplants).

67. 1 and 3: When assessing a client for risk of falls, the nurse should be aware that the primary risk factors include polypharmacy, especially if the client takes 5 or more medications, and a history of falls. Other risk factors include older age, muscle weakness, female gender, gait abnormalities, and postural hypotension. Those who drink alcohol also put themselves of increased risk. All clients should be assessed for a risk of falls even though risk factors may not be evident.

68. 1 and 2: If a train disaster has occurred and the hospital is expecting a large surge of incoming clients, the clients that should be considered for rapid discharge in order to reduce the census and free up beds include clients scheduled for elective procedures, such as a reduction mammoplasty, because delaying surgery does not present a risk to the client. A stable client who is three-days postoperative after vaginal hysterectomy may also be considered for discharge because the average length of stay is generally 2 to 3 days. The clients with the craniotomy, status asthmaticus, and elevated WBC count may need more observation and treatment before discharge.

69. 4: If the nurse notes that the electrical cord of a portable ECG machine is slightly cracked, the nurse should immediately remove the equipment from use, label it, and notify repair services. Because of the risk of a spark, no damaged electrical equipment should be used, and the nurse should not attempt repairs. Before using electrical equipment, the nurse should always check for fraying cords or other problems. Any electrical equipment that a client brings to a facility should be inspected by the appropriate personnel and labeled for safety before use is permitted.

70. If the nurse is assisting with triage at the site of an accident, injured individuals would be ranked from most critical to least critical in the following order:

1. Most critical: C. Individual with obstructed airway because this condition is incompatible with life and requires immediate intervention.
2. Next: D. Individual with head injury, conscious but somnolent and combative because these signs may indicate increasing intracranial pressure.

3. Next: A. Individual with slowly oozing wound on the right forearm because bleeding should be stopped as soon as possible. The nurse might instruct the individual to apply pressure to the wound even while attending to other individual.
4. Least critical: B. Individual with a fractured left wrist is least critical because the individual can likely wait 35 or 40 minutes without increased risk.

71. 2: If a 20-year-old university student complains of aching joints, chronic fatigue, fever (>100 °F/37.8 °C), and a butterfly rash across the cheeks and bridge of the nose, these signs and symptoms suggest a diagnosis of systemic lupus erythematosus, which is an autoimmune disorder that results in the body attacking its own tissues, such as in the joints and organs. The severity of the condition may vary. Antibody tests should be carried out as well as tissue biopsies because symptoms of SLE are often nonspecific.

72. 2 and 3: If a client has been recently diagnosed with Parkinson's disease and the nurse is educating the client and family about the condition, the symptoms that the nurse should include in the discussion are rigidity and tremors. Clients are also likely to have a propulsive shuffling gait as they tend to walk quickly with the head bent forward. Some clients develop dementia and auditory and visual hallucinations are common. Over time clients develop micrographia and dysphonia.

73. 4: Clients undergoing insertion (or removal) of a central venous catheter into an upper central vein are generally placed in the Trendelenburg position unless there are contraindications, such as increased intracranial pressure, because the Trendelenburg position increases the central venous pressure. The Trendelenburg position causes the vein to dilate, making the target vein easier to identify, and decreases the risk of air embolism. Clients should also be well hydrated because hypovolemia may make insertion more difficult.

74. 3 and 4: If an infant with hyperbilirubinemia is to have conventional phototherapy with a regular blue fluorescent light (non-Halogen) and to wear eye shields during treatment, the nurse should take care to avoid applying the eye shields too tightly as the pressure may damage the child's eyes. The eyes should be closed when the shields are applied in order to protect the corneas. Routine eye care to check the eyes should be carried out every 4 hours, but the phototherapy lights must be turned off prior to removing the eye shields.

75. 1, 4, and 5: If a client has osteoporosis, the nurse would expect that the client may exhibit Heberden's nodules on distal interphalangeal joints of the fingers and Bouchard's nodules on proximal interphalangeal joints. Stiffness of the affected joints is common in the morning and usually decreases within 30 minutes of activity. Pain tends to worsen over time, and the client may find that the pain intensifies with changes in barometric pressure (such as when the weather is cold and damp).

76. 2: When utilizing nasopharyngeal suctioning for a client unable to cough up secretions, once the catheter is inserted to the proper depth, the correct suction procedure is to apply intermittent suction for a maximum of 15 seconds. The catheter should be slowly withdrawn while suctioning and rotated back and forth. The depth of insertion for adults is about 16 cm; for older children, 8 to 12 cm; and for infants and children, 4 to 7.5 cm.

77. 3: If a client has returned from surgery with a urostomy after removal of the bladder because of cancer, the nurse should expect that the urostomy will produce ≥30 mL/hr as this is the normal urinary output, and kidney function should remain unchanged. If the urinary output falls, the client's intake may need to be increased. If the urine is cloudy or has a foul odor, then urinary culture and sensitivities should be done to determine if an infection has occurred.

78.

1	C	Atrial fibrillation	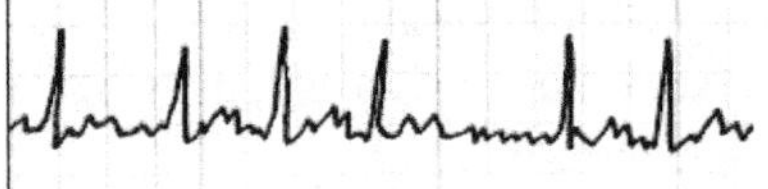
2	A	Premature ventricular contractions	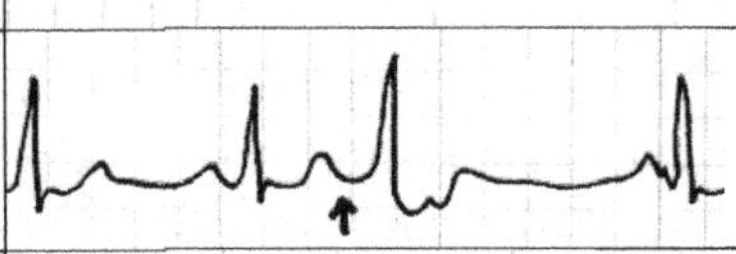
3	D	Ventricular tachycardia	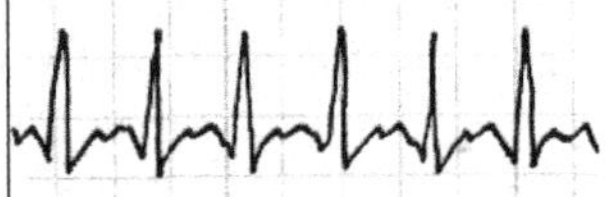
4	B	Sinus bradycardia	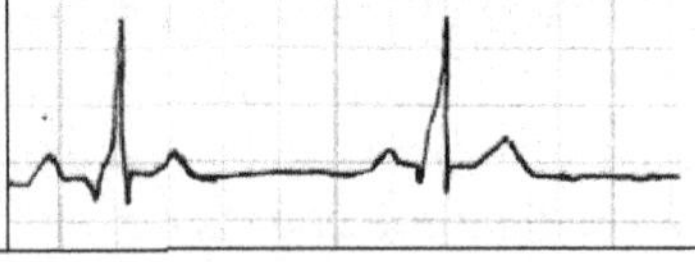

79. 2, 3, and 5: If a client is at 22 weeks gestation, one of the first indications is hypertension (>140/90) along with proteinuria of ≥0.3 g/24-hour urine collection or ≥1+ with urine dipstick (although proteinuria is no longer a required diagnostic for preeclampsia, as some patients present as preeclamptic without proteinuria). Other indications include hyperreflexia and generalized vasoconstriction, usually identified through examination of retina. The platelet count may drop, resulting in impaired coagulation. The client may experience severe headache and confusion because pf impaired cerebral circulation. If not promptly treated, preeclampsia may progress to life-threatening eclampsia with seizures.

80. If a client is to be discharged with a medication labeled 25 mg per 5 mL and the client needs to take 150 mg BID but will use a tablespoon measure because the metric system is confusing to the client, the client needs to take 2 tablespoons to equal 150 mg:

- 25 / 5 × 150 / x
- 25x = 750
- 25x / 25 = x; 750 / 25 = 30 mL
- x = 30 mL
- 30 mL / 15 (mL in a Tbsp) = 2 Tbsp.

81. 3: If an 80-year-old client confesses to the nurse that she has not bathed for over 2 weeks because she feels unsteady in the shower and dislikes tub baths, the most appropriate advice is to utilize a shower chair. Showers are generally safer than tub baths for those who are older and/or unsteady because getting in and out of the tub can be difficult if the client is weak, and there is increased risk of slipping and falling. Safety bars in the shower should also be recommended so that the client has a secure place to hold onto when sitting on or rising from the shower chair.

82. 2, 3, and 4: If an older client has been admitted to the hospital after prolonged diarrhea, signs of dehydration may include poor skin turgor, dry mucous membranes (usually evident in the mouth), and concentrated urine. Other indications may include tachycardia, fever, dizziness, confusion, and postural hypotension. For fluid replacement, the client may need not only water but also electrolytes. Dehydration may result from any condition that involves loss of body fluids, such as diarrhea, as well as from inadequate fluid intake or exposure to heat.

83. 4: If a client has a diabetic ulcer with minimal to moderate exudate and a small amount of eschar that requires debridement, the most appropriate dressing choice is a hydrocolloid (such as DuoDERM®, Exuderm®, and Replicare®). Hydrocolloids form a gelatinous mass that keeps the wound hydrated and provides an environment in which autolytic debridement can occur. Hydrocolloids can be used with wounds that have minimal to moderate exudate.

84. If a physician has written an order for a client to receive 4 tablespoons of Milk of Magnesia at bedtime, the nurse should administer 60 mL:

- 1 tablespoon is equal to 15 mL.
- 15 × 4 = 60 mL.

85. 1, 2, and 3: Contraindications for the use of oral contraceptives include smoking and a history of deep vein thrombosis (DVT). Women over age 35 who smoke are especially at risk of stroke and should use a different form of birth control. Other contraindications include coronary artery disease, breast cancer (estrogen dependent), liver tumor (benign or malignant), and known or suspected pregnancy. Those with undiagnosed vaginal bleeding should also avoid oral contraceptives.

86. 1: If the mechanical ventilation waveform shows the expiratory flow is below baseline, as in the exhibit, this is an indication of air trapping. Air trapping (auto-PEEP) occurs if the air that is inhaled is not completely exhaled because some of it is trapped in the lungs. This most often occurs with clients with COPD or asthma because of decreased elasticity of the lungs. Air trapping can lead to barotrauma, hypotension, and cardiovascular collapse.

87. 3: If a client is hospitalized after a traumatic brain injury and exhibits increasing intracranial pressure, the goal of treatment is to maintain the cerebral perfusion pressure between 70 and 100 mm Hg in order to ensure that blood flow to the brain is adequate. The CPP is calculated by subtracting the ICP from the mean arterial pressure (MAP). If the CPP calls below 50 mm Hg, irreversible neurologic damage occurs. If the ICP and the MAP are equal, then circulation to the brain stops.

88. If a client weighs 121 pounds but the client's weight must be calculated in kilograms, the weight in pounds must be divided by 2.2 because there are 2.2 kilograms in each pound.

- 121 / 2.2 = 55 kg.

89. 3: If a client whose oxygen saturation level has ranged from 96% to 98% has a sudden drop to 82% although the client's condition appears unchanged, the initial response should be to check the placement and functioning of the oximeter as it can become easily dislodged. If the oximeter is functioning properly, the client should begin to show signs of hypoxia and should receive oxygen and a respiratory assessment and the physician notified.

90. 1, 3, and 5: Reciprocal attachment behaviors exhibited by a newborn are those behaviors that facilitate attachment between the parent and the newborn and include rooting and latching onto the mother's breasts, engaging in entrainment (moving synchronously with the rhythm and tone of the mother's voice) and grasping parent's finger. The parent perceives these interactions as positive and rewarding. For example, when the infant grasps the parent's finger, this is a reflexive action, but the parent often perceives it as a sign of love.

91. 1: If the nurse is doing a venipuncture on a sitting client in order to obtain a blood sample, but before the blood can be withdrawn, the client complains of feeling faint and appears pale and shaky, the most appropriate response is for the nurse to immediately remove the needle. This is likely a vasovagal reaction, and, if the client faints and falls forward, it could dislodge the needle and cause trauma to the vein. The nurse should support the client and assist the client to lower the head and take deep breaths until the reaction passes.

92. 3: If assessing arterial blood gases, the nurse must be aware that the normal range for PO_2 is 80 to 95 mm Hg. The PO_2 measures the pressure of free oxygen dissolved in the plasma, not oxygen carried by hemoglobin. Some medications (theophylline, urokinase) increase the PO_2 while others (althesin, barbiturates, meperidine, isoproterenol, and granulocyte-macrophage stimulating factor decrease the PO_2. The PO_2 for cord blood is lower, ranging from 8 to 24 mm Hg.

93. 3: If a client with type 2 diabetes reports that he has stayed on his low carbohydrate diet and takes metformin daily but his Hgb A1c is 8.2, this suggests that the client's diabetes is not well-controlled. Whether or not this is because the client is being untruthful about his diet and medication cannot be determined without further inquiry. Diabetic patients are generally advised to keep the Hgb A1c below 7 (normal value for non-diabetics should be below 5.7).

94. 1: A client with anorexia nervosa states, "I was so happy when I was thinner. I need to lose weight so I can be happy again." This is an example of **overgeneralization** because the client is assuming that the earlier event (being thin and happy) will remain true in another situation (the present). **Catastrophizing** is imagining the worst: "When people look at me, all they think about is how fat I am." **Personalization** is focusing everything on the self: "Everybody is watching me eat." **Emotional reasoning** is connecting emotional feelings to reality: "I feel invincible when I am thin."

95. 2, 4, and 5: If a client has been diagnosed with schizophrenia, the client may exhibit a flat affect, disordered speech, hallucinations, and delusions. The client may also exhibit unusual behavior and may become socially isolated, showing little interest in activities. Acts of violence toward self (cutting) are more common than violence toward others although that may occur. Impulsivity and rapid mood swings are more common with bipolar disorder.

96. If a client with hemolytic uremic syndrome is to receive eculizumab IV and the medication is supplied in a 300-mg single use vial with 10 mg/mL, if the client is to receive 900 mg IV one time weekly, the nurse must administer 90 mL of the drug for each treatment.

- 300 / 10 = 30 doses = 30 mL because each dose 10 mg dose is 1 ml.
- 300 mg is in each vial, so three 30 mL vials are needed.
- 30 × 3 = 90 mL total.

97. If a nurse is preparing to enter an isolation room to care for a client and has completed hand hygiene, prepared the supplies and equipment that will be needed, made introductions to the client, and advised the client of the procedure, when applying PPE, the nurse should carry out the following steps.

- Step 1: E. Apply the gown.
- Step 2: D. Tie the gown securely at the neck and waist.
- Step 3. A. Apply surgical mask or respirator.
- Step 4: C. Apply goggles or appropriate side shields if wearing glasses.
- Step 5: B. Apply clean gloves.

98. 2: If the nurse is attempting to irrigate an NG feeding tube with 30 mL of water but is unable to instill the solution, the next appropriate step is to position the client on the left side and attempt the irrigation again. The tip of the NG tube is sometimes lying against the abdominal wall, so changing position will often dislodge the NG tube. Excessive force should be avoided because it may damage the tissue.

99. 4: When an NG feeding tube is placed initially, the most appropriate method of ensuring correct placement is an x-ray to confirm placement. Subsequently, the nurse should check the measurement of the exposed tube to ensure it's the same as originally documented and may use a combination of other methods, such as checking the color of aspirant (should be cloudy and green, tan, brown, or off-white) and check the pH of gastric aspirate (should be 1 to 5). Air auscultation (injecting air and listening over epigastric area for sound of air) is not reliable.

100. 1, 2, and 4: Hyperglycemia is characterized by blurred vision, polyuria, and polydipsia. The client may complain of headache and trouble concentrating and may become increasingly weak and fatigued. Left untreated, hyperglycemia may cause organ damage and retinal damage leading to blindness. Hypoglycemia, on the other hand, is characterized by shakiness, cardiac dysrhythmia, irritability, anxiety, confusion, and inappropriate behavior (the client may appear intoxicated) and increased perspiration.

101. 2: When assessing a client with the timed up and go (TUG) test, the normal time required for a client to complete standing, walking 3 meters, turning, returning back and sitting down is 7 to 10 seconds. If the client requires 14 seconds or longer, this indicates increased risk for falls. The nurse may also assess gait speed in 5 meters. If the client walks at a rate slower than 0.6 meters/second, this is predictive of mobility limitations.

102. 4: The fracture that poses the greatest risk to older adults is the hip/femur fracture, most often involving the femoral neck and the intertrochanteric region. During initial treatment, mortality rates are 10% with over 25% dying over the following year. Hip fractures often occur because of weakness in the bones resulting from osteoporosis and, in fact, the fracture may be spontaneous, causing the client to fall rather than the result of a fall.

103. 1: If a client has suffered an ischemic stroke in the right hemisphere, the nurse should anticipate that the client has left paralysis and left visual field defect. Language skills usually remain intact although the client may have some short-term memory loss and difficulty following directions. Clients may also act impulsively and have poor judgement. The client's fine motor skills may be impaired, resulting in difficulty dressing and carrying out tasks that involve the use of tools.

104. 1: If the nurse is caring for a client in the recovery room after the client's abdominal surgery and the BP is initially stable but then falls 5 or more mm Hg every 15 minutes, the nurse should notify the surgeon as this may be an indication of bleeding and/or the development of shock. Generally, the surgeon should be notified if the systolic BP falls below 90, but the nurse should not wait since a clear pattern of decreasing blood pressure is evident.

105. 2: The statement by a newly diagnosed client with diabetes mellitus type 1 that indicates the need for further education is, "I can eat whatever I want if I increase my insulin to cover the food." While diabetic regimens are somewhat less restrictive than previously, clients must understand the need for an appropriate well-balanced diet with routinely scheduled mealtimes so that insulin requirements can be calibrated and glucose levels stabilized.

106. 3: Pregnancy is an absolute contraindication for use of isotretinoin as a treatment for acne because it can cause severe birth defects. Females taking the drug must have 2 negative pregnancy tests before beginning treatment, must utilize two forms of birth control, and must have monthly pregnancy tests before each course of treatment. If pregnancy should occur during treatment, the drug must be discontinued immediately, and the client is usually advised to terminate the pregnancy.

107. 4: If a client with a newly-applied cast on the left foot and ankle complains of severe itching at the bottom of the foot, the intervention that may help to relieve itching is to blow cold air from a hair dryer into the cast toward the area that itches. The nurse should never insert anything inside the cast, and elevating the cast may relieve swelling and discomfort but is not likely to relieve itching.

108. 1: If a client receiving total parenteral nutrition (TPN) exhibits sudden onset of respiratory distress with cough and dyspnea, and oxygen saturation level falls to 88%; and, on examining the client, the nurse finds that the IV tubing has become disconnected so that part of the catheter system is open to the air, the immediate response before notifying the physician should be to clamp the catheter and place the client in left lateral Trendelenburg position to prevent the air from entering the right side of the heart and the pulmonary arteries. These signs and symptoms are indicative of air embolism. The client may be provided oxygen as necessary.

109. 3 and 5: Anticipatory guidance for a 16-year-old should include a discussion of relationships and risk-taking behaviors (such as drinking, drugs, reckless driving, vaping, and smoking) and information about abstinence and birth control. The client at this age should be taught about breast and testicular self-examinations and may benefit from discussion about their future life and academic plans although they may not have specific plans or may be unsure of how to reach goals they do have.

110. 4: If the nurse must insert a urinary catheter into the bladder of a client with osteoarthritis of the hips; but, when the nurse positions the client in dorsal recumbent position, the client complains of pain in both hips, the most appropriate response is to change the client's position to the left side-lying (Sims) position. This position also allows adequate visualization of the perineum. The upper leg should be flexed at the knee and supported by a pillow.

111. 2: If a client undergoing a colonoscopy is administered IV midazolam as part of moderate sedation, monitoring the client's respiratory status is a primary concern because midazolam can cause a client to go into respiratory depression and arrest. Resuscitation equipment, oxygen and drugs should be available, and the client must be monitored by a qualified professional (other than the physician doing the procedure) during the procedure.

112. 2: The food that has the greatest potential for interaction with drugs is grapefruit (both the fruit and the juice) because it contains furanocoumarins, which block the action of CYP3A4 enzymes that metabolize drugs. This can result in increased levels of the drug in the system. Grapefruit interacts with statins, calcium channel blockers, loratadine, and multiple other drugs. Some other fruits, including oranges, apples, pomelos, and pomegranates, may also interact with drugs.

113. If a 4-year-old client weighing 39.6 pounds is to receive an infusion of IV ceftriaxone sodium at 75 mg/kg/d in a divided dose every 12 hours, the child should receive 675 mg with each infusion.

First, 39.6 pounds is converted to kg:

- 39.6 / 2.2 = 18.

Since the child is to receive 75 mg per kg per day, the total daily dose is:

- 75 × 18 = 1350 mg

The total dose is given in divided doses every 12 hours. There are two 12-hour periods in a day:

- 1350 / 2 = 675 mg

114. 3: If a client recovering from open heart surgery complains of pain at 9 on a 1-to-10 scale, but when the nurse returns within 5 minutes with analgesia, the client is talking with a visitor, smiling, and appears relaxed, the nurse should administer the analgesia as requested. The outward appearance of a client does not always mirror what the client is feeling, especially if the client doesn't want to worry visitors. If the client's pain has actually subsided, the client will likely tell the nurse.

115. 1: If a client with a 3-week-old infant tells the nurse that her infant has started to sleep up to 6 hours at a time during the night, the most appropriate response is, "Newborns can get too dehydrated if they sleep more than 4 hours." Additionally, infants who are dehydrated may become lethargic, so the nurse should review the child's feeding schedule and carefully assess the infant to determine if the infant's weight gain is as expected.

116. 1, 3, and 5: The vaccinations that are recommended for all adults to 50 to 65 years and older include herpes zoster (shingles), which is recommended at age 50 or older; pneumococcal polysaccharide, which is recommended at age 65 or older, and influenza, which is recommended annually for all individuals who are 6 months or older. Some clients may require additional vaccinations, such as hepatitis B, depending on their individual health histories and risk factors.

117. 1: If a client recently diagnosed with pancreatic cancer and undergoing chemotherapy becomes upset and complains that a technician is incompetent and should be fired because the technician had difficulty obtaining a blood specimen, the most appropriate response is one that focuses on the client's feelings rather than the situation: "I can see how distressed you are." Anger is a common response to the grief and stress associated with being diagnosed with cancer, so the client should be encouraged to express feelings.

118. 2: If the nurse observes a coworker sign out narcotic for a client but sees the nurse take the medication into the nurse's restroom and then return to the nursing station without seeing the client and without the mediation, the nurse should immediately report the observation to a supervisor. The nurse should not confront the coworker directly as this may result in a verbal conflict and provide warning that the coworker will be investigated.

119. 2: If a 10-year-old client is scheduled for surgery and the hospital allows parents to be with the child during anesthesia induction, but the mother begins to cry when she prepares to enter to operating room, the most appropriate response is one that recognizes the client's emotions but allows her time to stop crying as that may frighten the child even more: "I know how worried you are. Let's just take a minute to prepare yourself."

120. If a client's medication order is for 300 mg of a liquid medication that is available at 75 mg per mL, the nurse should administer 4 mL of medication.

- 300 / 75 = 4 mL OR
- 75/1 × 300/x
- 75 × x = 75x; and 1 × 300 = 300
- 75x / 75 = x; 300 /75 = 4
- X = 4 mL

Image Credits

LICENSED UNDER CC BY 2.5 (CREATIVECOMMONS.ORG/LICENSES/BY/2.5/DEED.EN)

Bell's Palsy: "Bell's palsy diagram" by Patrick J. Lynch, medical illustrator (https://commons.wikimedia.org/wiki/File:Bells_palsy_diagram.svg)

LICENSED UNDER CC BY 3.0 (CREATIVECOMMONS.ORG/LICENSES/BY/3.0/DEED.EN)

Colostomy: "Colostomy Types" by Wikimedia user BruceBlaus (https://commons.wikimedia.org/wiki/File:Blausen_0247_Colostomy.png)

PICC Catheter: "Peripherally-inserted Central Catheter (PICC)" by Blausen Medical Communications, Inc. (https://commons.wikimedia.org/wiki/File:Blausen_0193_Catheter_PICC.png)

Heart: "Blood Flow Through the Heart" by Wikimedia user BruceBlaus (https://commons.wikimedia.org/wiki/File:Blausen_0452_Heart_BloodFlow.png)

Scoliosis: "Scoliosis" by Wikimedia user BruceBlaus (https://commons.wikimedia.org/wiki/File:Blausen_0785_Scoliosis_01.png)

Lobes of the Brain: "Brain Lobes" by Wikimedia user BruceBlaus (https://commons.wikimedia.org/wiki/File:Blausen_0111_BrainLobes.png)

LICENSED UNDER CC BY-SA 4.0 (CREATIVECOMMONS.ORG/LICENSES/BY-SA/4.0/DEED.EN)

Venous Access Port: "Illustration depicting a catheter in a venous access port" by Wikimedia user BruceBlaus (https://commons.wikimedia.org/wiki/File:Venous_Access_Port_Catheter.png)

Tunneled CVAD: "Central Venous Access Device (Tunneled) by Wikimedia user BruceBlaus (https://commons.wikimedia.org/wiki/File:Central_Venous_Access_Device_(Tunneled).png)

Nasogastric Intubation: "An illustration depicting nasogastric intubation" by Wikimedia user BruceBlaus (https://commons.wikimedia.org/wiki/File:Nasogastric_Intubation.png)

How to Overcome Test Anxiety

Just the thought of taking a test is enough to make most people a little nervous. A test is an important event that can have a long-term impact on your future, so it's important to take it seriously and it's natural to feel anxious about performing well. But just because anxiety is normal, that doesn't mean that it's helpful in test taking, or that you should simply accept it as part of your life. Anxiety can have a variety of effects. These effects can be mild, like making you feel slightly nervous, or severe, like blocking your ability to focus or remember even a simple detail.

If you experience test anxiety—whether severe or mild—it's important to know how to beat it. To discover this, first you need to understand what causes test anxiety.

Causes of Test Anxiety

While we often think of anxiety as an uncontrollable emotional state, it can actually be caused by simple, practical things. One of the most common causes of test anxiety is that a person does not feel adequately prepared for their test. This feeling can be the result of many different issues such as poor study habits or lack of organization, but the most common culprit is time management. Starting to study too late, failing to organize your study time to cover all of the material, or being distracted while you study will mean that you're not well prepared for the test. This may lead to cramming the night before, which will cause you to be physically and mentally exhausted for the test. Poor time management also contributes to feelings of stress, fear, and hopelessness as you realize you are not well prepared but don't know what to do about it.

Other times, test anxiety is not related to your preparation for the test but comes from unresolved fear. This may be a past failure on a test, or poor performance on tests in general. It may come from comparing yourself to others who seem to be performing better or from the stress of living up to expectations. Anxiety may be driven by fears of the future—how failure on this test would affect your educational and career goals. These fears are often completely irrational, but they can still negatively impact your test performance.

Review Video: 3 Reasons You Have Test Anxiety
Visit mometrix.com/academy and enter code: 428468

Elements of Test Anxiety

As mentioned earlier, test anxiety is considered to be an emotional state, but it has physical and mental components as well. Sometimes you may not even realize that you are suffering from test anxiety until you notice the physical symptoms. These can include trembling hands, rapid heartbeat, sweating, nausea, and tense muscles. Extreme anxiety may lead to fainting or vomiting. Obviously, any of these symptoms can have a negative impact on testing. It is important to recognize them as soon as they begin to occur so that you can address the problem before it damages your performance.

Review Video: 3 Ways to Tell You Have Test Anxiety
Visit mometrix.com/academy and enter code: 927847

The mental components of test anxiety include trouble focusing and inability to remember learned information. During a test, your mind is on high alert, which can help you recall information and stay focused for an extended period of time. However, anxiety interferes with your mind's natural processes, causing you to blank out, even on the questions you know well. The strain of testing during anxiety makes it difficult to stay focused, especially on a test that may take several hours. Extreme anxiety can take a huge mental toll, making it difficult not only to recall test information but even to understand the test questions or pull your thoughts together.

Review Video: How Test Anxiety Affects Memory
Visit mometrix.com/academy and enter code: 609003

Effects of Test Anxiety

Test anxiety is like a disease—if left untreated, it will get progressively worse. Anxiety leads to poor performance, and this reinforces the feelings of fear and failure, which in turn lead to poor performances on subsequent tests. It can grow from a mild nervousness to a crippling condition. If allowed to progress, test anxiety can have a big impact on your schooling, and consequently on your future.

Test anxiety can spread to other parts of your life. Anxiety on tests can become anxiety in any stressful situation, and blanking on a test can turn into panicking in a job situation. But fortunately, you don't have to let anxiety rule your testing and determine your grades. There are a number of relatively simple steps you can take to move past anxiety and function normally on a test and in the rest of life.

Review Video: How Test Anxiety Impacts Your Grades
Visit mometrix.com/academy and enter code: 939819

Physical Steps for Beating Test Anxiety

While test anxiety is a serious problem, the good news is that it can be overcome. It doesn't have to control your ability to think and remember information. While it may take time, you can begin taking steps today to beat anxiety.

Just as your first hint that you may be struggling with anxiety comes from the physical symptoms, the first step to treating it is also physical. Rest is crucial for having a clear, strong mind. If you are tired, it is much easier to give in to anxiety. But if you establish good sleep habits, your body and mind will be ready to perform optimally, without the strain of exhaustion. Additionally, sleeping well helps you to retain information better, so you're more likely to recall the answers when you see the test questions.

Getting good sleep means more than going to bed on time. It's important to allow your brain time to relax. Take study breaks from time to time so it doesn't get overworked, and don't study right before bed. Take time to rest your mind before trying to rest your body, or you may find it difficult to fall asleep.

Review Video: The Importance of Sleep for Your Brain
Visit mometrix.com/academy and enter code: 319338

Along with sleep, other aspects of physical health are important in preparing for a test. Good nutrition is vital for good brain function. Sugary foods and drinks may give a burst of energy but this burst is followed by a crash, both physically and emotionally. Instead, fuel your body with protein and vitamin-rich foods.

Also, drink plenty of water. Dehydration can lead to headaches and exhaustion, especially if your brain is already under stress from the rigors of the test. Particularly if your test is a long one, drink water during the breaks. And if possible, take an energy-boosting snack to eat between sections.

Review Video: How Diet Can Affect your Mood
Visit mometrix.com/academy and enter code: 624317

Along with sleep and diet, a third important part of physical health is exercise. Maintaining a steady workout schedule is helpful, but even taking 5-minute study breaks to walk can help get your blood pumping faster and clear your head. Exercise also releases endorphins, which contribute to a positive feeling and can help combat test anxiety.

When you nurture your physical health, you are also contributing to your mental health. If your body is healthy, your mind is much more likely to be healthy as well. So take time to rest, nourish your body with healthy food and water, and get moving as much as possible. Taking these physical steps will make you stronger and more able to take the mental steps necessary to overcome test anxiety.

Review Video: How to Stay Healthy and Prevent Test Anxiety
Visit mometrix.com/academy and enter code: 877894

Mental Steps for Beating Test Anxiety

Working on the mental side of test anxiety can be more challenging, but as with the physical side, there are clear steps you can take to overcome it. As mentioned earlier, test anxiety often stems from lack of preparation, so the obvious solution is to prepare for the test. Effective studying may be the most important weapon you have for beating test anxiety, but you can and should employ several other mental tools to combat fear.

First, boost your confidence by reminding yourself of past success—tests or projects that you aced. If you're putting as much effort into preparing for this test as you did for those, there's no reason you should expect to fail here. Work hard to prepare; then trust your preparation.

Second, surround yourself with encouraging people. It can be helpful to find a study group, but be sure that the people you're around will encourage a positive attitude. If you spend time with others who are anxious or cynical, this will only contribute to your own anxiety. Look for others who are motivated to study hard from a desire to succeed, not from a fear of failure.

Third, reward yourself. A test is physically and mentally tiring, even without anxiety, and it can be helpful to have something to look forward to. Plan an activity following the test, regardless of the outcome, such as going to a movie or getting ice cream.

When you are taking the test, if you find yourself beginning to feel anxious, remind yourself that you know the material. Visualize successfully completing the test. Then take a few deep, relaxing breaths and return to it. Work through the questions carefully but with confidence, knowing that you are capable of succeeding.

Developing a healthy mental approach to test taking will also aid in other areas of life. Test anxiety affects more than just the actual test—it can be damaging to your mental health and even contribute to depression. It's important to beat test anxiety before it becomes a problem for more than testing.

Review Video: Test Anxiety and Depression
Visit mometrix.com/academy and enter code: 904704

Study Strategy

Being prepared for the test is necessary to combat anxiety, but what does being prepared look like? You may study for hours on end and still not feel prepared. What you need is a strategy for test prep. The next few pages outline our recommended steps to help you plan out and conquer the challenge of preparation.

Step 1: Scope Out the Test

Learn everything you can about the format (multiple choice, essay, etc.) and what will be on the test. Gather any study materials, course outlines, or sample exams that may be available. Not only will this help you to prepare, but knowing what to expect can help to alleviate test anxiety.

Step 2: Map Out the Material

Look through the textbook or study guide and make note of how many chapters or sections it has. Then divide these over the time you have. For example, if a book has 15 chapters and you have five days to study, you need to cover three chapters each day. Even better, if you have the time, leave an extra day at the end for overall review after you have gone through the material in depth.

If time is limited, you may need to prioritize the material. Look through it and make note of which sections you think you already have a good grasp on, and which need review. While you are studying, skim quickly through the familiar sections and take more time on the challenging parts. Write out your plan so you don't get lost as you go. Having a written plan also helps you feel more in control of the study, so anxiety is less likely to arise from feeling overwhelmed at the amount to cover.

Step 3: Gather Your Tools

Decide what study method works best for you. Do you prefer to highlight in the book as you study and then go back over the highlighted portions? Or do you type out notes of the important information? Or is it helpful to make flashcards that you can carry with you? Assemble the pens, index cards, highlighters, post-it notes, and any other materials you may need so you won't be distracted by getting up to find things while you study.

If you're having a hard time retaining the information or organizing your notes, experiment with different methods. For example, try color-coding by subject with colored pens, highlighters, or post-it notes. If you learn better by hearing, try recording yourself reading your notes so you can listen while in the car, working out, or simply sitting at your desk. Ask a friend to quiz you from your flashcards, or try teaching someone the material to solidify it in your mind.

Step 4: Create Your Environment

It's important to avoid distractions while you study. This includes both the obvious distractions like visitors and the subtle distractions like an uncomfortable chair (or a too-comfortable couch that makes you want to fall asleep). Set up the best study environment possible: good lighting and a comfortable work area. If background music helps you focus, you may want to turn it on, but otherwise keep the room quiet. If you are using a computer to take notes, be sure you don't have any other windows open, especially applications like social media, games, or anything else that could distract you. Silence your phone and turn off notifications. Be sure to keep water close by so you stay hydrated while you study (but avoid unhealthy drinks and snacks).

Also, take into account the best time of day to study. Are you freshest first thing in the morning? Try to set aside some time then to work through the material. Is your mind clearer in the afternoon or evening? Schedule your study session then. Another method is to study at the same time of day that you will take the test, so that your brain gets used to working on the material at that time and will be ready to focus at test time.

STEP 5: STUDY!

Once you have done all the study preparation, it's time to settle into the actual studying. Sit down, take a few moments to settle your mind so you can focus, and begin to follow your study plan. Don't give in to distractions or let yourself procrastinate. This is your time to prepare so you'll be ready to fearlessly approach the test. Make the most of the time and stay focused.

Of course, you don't want to burn out. If you study too long you may find that you're not retaining the information very well. Take regular study breaks. For example, taking five minutes out of every hour to walk briskly, breathing deeply and swinging your arms, can help your mind stay fresh.

As you get to the end of each chapter or section, it's a good idea to do a quick review. Remind yourself of what you learned and work on any difficult parts. When you feel that you've mastered the material, move on to the next part. At the end of your study session, briefly skim through your notes again.

But while review is helpful, cramming last minute is NOT. If at all possible, work ahead so that you won't need to fit all your study into the last day. Cramming overloads your brain with more information than it can process and retain, and your tired mind may struggle to recall even previously learned information when it is overwhelmed with last-minute study. Also, the urgent nature of cramming and the stress placed on your brain contribute to anxiety. You'll be more likely to go to the test feeling unprepared and having trouble thinking clearly.

So don't cram, and don't stay up late before the test, even just to review your notes at a leisurely pace. Your brain needs rest more than it needs to go over the information again. In fact, plan to finish your studies by noon or early afternoon the day before the test. Give your brain the rest of the day to relax or focus on other things, and get a good night's sleep. Then you will be fresh for the test and better able to recall what you've studied.

STEP 6: TAKE A PRACTICE TEST

Many courses offer sample tests, either online or in the study materials. This is an excellent resource to check whether you have mastered the material, as well as to prepare for the test format and environment.

Check the test format ahead of time: the number of questions, the type (multiple choice, free response, etc.), and the time limit. Then create a plan for working through them. For example, if you have 30 minutes to take a 60-question test, your limit is 30 seconds per question. Spend less time on the questions you know well so that you can take more time on the difficult ones.

If you have time to take several practice tests, take the first one open book, with no time limit. Work through the questions at your own pace and make sure you fully understand them. Gradually work up to taking a test under test conditions: sit at a desk with all study materials put away and set a timer. Pace yourself to make sure you finish the test with time to spare and go back to check your answers if you have time.

After each test, check your answers. On the questions you missed, be sure you understand why you missed them. Did you misread the question (tests can use tricky wording)? Did you forget the information? Or was it something you hadn't learned? Go back and study any shaky areas that the practice tests reveal.

Taking these tests not only helps with your grade, but also aids in combating test anxiety. If you're already used to the test conditions, you're less likely to worry about it, and working through tests until you're scoring well gives you a confidence boost. Go through the practice tests until you feel comfortable, and then you can go into the test knowing that you're ready for it.

Test Tips

On test day, you should be confident, knowing that you've prepared well and are ready to answer the questions. But aside from preparation, there are several test day strategies you can employ to maximize your performance.

First, as stated before, get a good night's sleep the night before the test (and for several nights before that, if possible). Go into the test with a fresh, alert mind rather than staying up late to study.

Try not to change too much about your normal routine on the day of the test. It's important to eat a nutritious breakfast, but if you normally don't eat breakfast at all, consider eating just a protein bar. If you're a coffee drinker, go ahead and have your normal coffee. Just make sure you time it so that the caffeine doesn't wear off right in the middle of your test. Avoid sugary beverages, and drink enough water to stay hydrated but not so much that you need a restroom break 10 minutes into the test. If your test isn't first thing in the morning, consider going for a walk or doing a light workout before the test to get your blood flowing.

Allow yourself enough time to get ready, and leave for the test with plenty of time to spare so you won't have the anxiety of scrambling to arrive in time. Another reason to be early is to select a good seat. It's helpful to sit away from doors and windows, which can be distracting. Find a good seat, get out your supplies, and settle your mind before the test begins.

When the test begins, start by going over the instructions carefully, even if you already know what to expect. Make sure you avoid any careless mistakes by following the directions.

Then begin working through the questions, pacing yourself as you've practiced. If you're not sure on an answer, don't spend too much time on it, and don't let it shake your confidence. Either skip it and come back later, or eliminate as many wrong answers as possible and guess among the remaining ones. Don't dwell on these questions as you continue—put them out of your mind and focus on what lies ahead.

Be sure to read all of the answer choices, even if you're sure the first one is the right answer. Sometimes you'll find a better one if you keep reading. But don't second-guess yourself if you do immediately know the answer. Your gut instinct is usually right. Don't let test anxiety rob you of the information you know.

If you have time at the end of the test (and if the test format allows), go back and review your answers. Be cautious about changing any, since your first instinct tends to be correct, but make sure you didn't misread any of the questions or accidentally mark the wrong answer choice. Look over any you skipped and make an educated guess.

At the end, leave the test feeling confident. You've done your best, so don't waste time worrying about your performance or wishing you could change anything. Instead, celebrate the successful completion of this test. And finally, use this test to learn how to deal with anxiety even better next time.

Review Video: 5 Tips to Beat Test Anxiety
Visit mometrix.com/academy and enter code: 570656

Important Qualification

Not all anxiety is created equal. If your test anxiety is causing major issues in your life beyond the classroom or testing center, or if you are experiencing troubling physical symptoms related to your anxiety, it may be a sign of a serious physiological or psychological condition. If this sounds like your situation, we strongly encourage you to seek professional help.

Tell Us Your Story

We at Mometrix would like to extend our heartfelt thanks to you for letting us be a part of your journey. It is an honor to serve people from all walks of life, people like you, who are committed to building the best future they can for themselves.

We know that each person's situation is unique. But we also know that, whether you are a young student or a mother of four, you care about working to make your own life and the lives of those around you better.

That's why we want to hear your story.

We want to know why you're taking this test. We want to know about the trials you've gone through to get here. And we want to know about the successes you've experienced after taking and passing your test.

In addition to your story, which can be an inspiration both to us and to others, we value your feedback. We want to know both what you loved about our book and what you think we can improve on.

SCAN HERE

The team at Mometrix would be absolutely thrilled to hear from you! So please, send us an email at tellusyourstory@mometrix.com or visit us at mometrix.com/tellusyourstory.php and let's stay in touch.

Additional Bonus Material

Due to our efforts to try to keep this book to a manageable length, we've created a link that will give you access to all of your additional bonus material.

Please visit https://www.mometrix.com/bonus948/nclexpn to access the information.